Psychological Bases of Sport Injuries

Third Edition

David Pargman, Ph.D.

Professor Emeritus
Florida State University

Editor

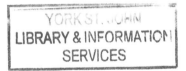
Fitness Information Technology
A Division of the International Center for Performance Excellence
262 Coliseum, WVU-PE PO Box 6116
Morgantown, WV 26506-6116

Library of Congress Card Catalog Number: 2006939829

ISBN: 978-1-885693-75-4

Cover Design: Jamie Merlavage
Cover Photo: iStockphoto
Production Editor: Valerie Gittings
Typesetter: Jamie Merlavage
Proofreader: Danielle Costello
Printed by: Sheridan Books

12 11 10   2 3 4 5

Fitness Information Technology
A Division of the International Center for Performance Excellence
West Virginia University
262 Coliseum, WVU-PE
PO BOX 6116
Morgantown, WV 26506-6116
800.477.4348 (toll free)
304.293.6888 (phone)
304.293.6658 (fax)
Email: icpe@mail.wvu.edu
Website: www.fitinfotech.com

To the memory of Michael L. Steuerman—humanitarian, athlete, coach, and dear friend, whose passing occurred during the preparation of this book

Contents

SECTION 1: Preventing Athletic Injury

SECTION 2: Rehabilitating the Injured Athlete

About the Editor

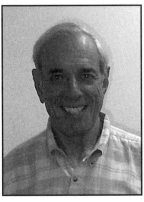

David Pargman is emeritus professor of educational psychology at Florida State University, where he served as program leader for educational psychology and coordinator for graduate studies in sport and exercise psychology. Prior to his 31 years of service at Florida State University, he taught at Boston University and the City College of New York. Dr. Pargman received the master's degree from Teachers College, Columbia University, and a Ph.D. from New York University.

Dr. Pargman is author or co-author of six other books that deal respectively with stress and performance, fitness and wellness, and sport psychology. He has been major professor to more than 40 Ph.D. graduates and is a fellow of the American College of Sports Medicine, the Association for the Advancement of Applied Sport Psychology, and the Research Consortium of the American Alliance of Health, Physical Education, Recreation and Dance. He is also a Certified Sport Psychology Consultant for the Association for the Advancement of Applied Sport Psychology and is listed in the United States Olympic Committee Sport Psychology Registry.

Dr. Pargman has served as visiting professor at the University of Akron, Ohio, USA; Srinakharinwirot University, Bangkok, Thailand; University of San Marcos, Lima Peru; University of the Andes, Merida, Venezuela; Lund University, Lund, Sweden; and the University of Zulia, Maricaibo, Venezuela. He is currently on the Editorial Board of the Journal of Studia Kinanthropologia (Czech Republic) and the Board of Directors of the Multidisciplinary Institute of Neuropsychological Development (Cambridge, Massachusetts, USA).

Dr. Pargman was a member of his college track and cross-country team and has since competed in hundreds of road races.

Foreword

The importance of psychological factors in sport injury first became clear to me as a team physician for a high school football team. In a hard-fought, low scoring game, the opposing team suddenly scored two quick touchdowns. The discouragement and dejection on the home team was obvious. Over the next few series of plays, two of the defensive linemen were hurt. When the team went on offense, a parent in the stands screamed at his son (the star running back), "Where the hell are your guts?" On the next series, he carried the ball three times in succession, and on the final time, he cut too sharply and twisted his knee. I was struck by the coincidence of three injuries right after their depressed mood. Or was it a coincidence? As I observed more games and other sports, I became aware of the frequent connection between injury, psychological factors, and game circumstances.

Considering the frequency and significance of psychological factors in sport injury, it is somewhat surprising that there are so few books offering comprehensive coverage of this complex subject. Since its initial publication in 1993, "Psychological Bases of Sport Injury" has been a major reference source for practitioners and graduate students in sport psychology, providing a thorough examination of the psychological aspects of prevention, treatment, and rehabilitation of sport injury. This new Third Edition contains many interesting new chapters, as well as updating existing ones. An intriguing new one on sensory-neural pathways gives practitioners some understanding of the neuroanatomy involved in the sensation of pain.

One of the strengths of this edition is the emphasis on the prevention. In his introduction, David Pargman highlights the importance of one's ability to process information as a factor in the frequency of sport injury. Several of the new chapters address additional factors in decreasing the occurrence of injury in sport. For example, the need for specificity in stress management interventions, the importance of coping skills, identifying target populations who are prone to injury, and counseling approaches to predict injuries.

Psychological factors are both antecedents and consequences of athletic injury, and frequently, psychological recovery from injury takes longer than physical recovery.

It is, therefore, gratifying to see several chapters on psychological rehabilitation and recovery. The complicated nature of the recovery process and return to competition is well illustrated in the discussions of the influence of personality factors; the interaction and collaboration of the practitioner and the patient; the importance of coach support, the value of modeling, imagery, and group approaches to help the athlete; and the use of counseling and other psychological strategies. There are also important discussions of opposite outcomes, such as permanent injury and suicide. To illustrate some of the principles involved in applied practice, chapters on specific cases are included, as well as a discussion of ethical and legal issues.

This third edition will continue to be a valuable resource for sport psychologists, sports medicine professionals, coaches, and athletes who seek more knowledge and understanding about the complexity of tasks facing injured athletes. The contributors are experienced applied practitioners and research scientists from diverse backgrounds who clarify the psychological factors involved in prevention, treatment, and rehabilitation of athletic injury.

Burt Giges, M.D.
Clinical Professor, Department of Psychology, Springfield College, MA
President-Elect, Association for the Advancement of Applied Sport Psychology

Preface

This, the third edition of *Psychological Bases of Sport Injuries,* retains the same focus employed by its two previous editions, namely an emphasis upon psychological issues related to sport injury. Implicit in this focus is that from both causal and rehabilitative perspectives an exclusively medical, organic, or biomechanical approach to sport injury is clearly incomplete and insufficient. Injured athletes are advantaged when their treatment incorporates methods predicated upon psychological models. Those who construct and administer programs of rehabilitation are therefore obliged to appreciate the value of psychological strategies as they assist all kinds of athletes—professional, collegiate, and secondary school, as well as those who participate on a purely recreational basis.

An outstanding array of authors contributed to this volume. Some were prior contributors to the first and second editions and have graciously complied with my request to revisit and refurbish their material. Therefore, nine authors are, so to speak, old timers who have provided new references, ideas, and recommendations. Eleven are new contributors whose fine work I had encountered in the research literature, in conference presentations, or through my professional grapevine. I extended invitations to them to join the third edition and they acceded. Authors hail from Sweden, Canada, Australia, Korea, New Zealand, and the United States. Thus, this edition reflects diverse educational and cultural experiences on behalf of authors as well as the athletes they write about.

Among the chapters not included in the two previous editions are three case study reports: one by Renee Newcomber Appaneal and Megan Granquest, another by Barbara Meyer and Kyle Ebersole, and a third by Mark Andersen. Each delineates in fascinating manner the authors' personal encounters with injured athletes and methods employed while addressing rehabilitation.

Another new chapter is one by Wendy Sternberg that provides a highly detailed overview of the perceptual-cognitive experience known as pain. The pain phenomenon is invariably associated with sport injury, and professionals seeking to administer to injured athletes require an understanding of its dimensions.

In the book's opening chapter, Tony Morris and Young-Eun Noh make a case for dance being an athletic endeavor and accordingly address various psychological issues related to dance injury—particularly injury prevention. Two other new and valuable chapters provide insight into the prevention of sport injury that should be of considerable assistance to coaches and trainers. One is written by Ralph Maddison and Harry Prapavessis, and the other by Urban Johnson.

Leslie Podlog and Robert Eklund make a fine contribution to this edition with their elaboration upon important considerations related to return to full athletic participation following injury. That is, after the healing has taken place.

In her chapter, Teresa Bianco discusses issues that coaches in particular should be apprised of as they fulfill their essential role in assisting the injured athlete rehabilitate and return to action.

Trent Petrie's chapter is devoted to a particular kind of rehabilitative strategy and its advantages, namely group counseling. He identifies cautions and guidelines associated with two different methods.

Frances Flint has written two chapters in this volume. One is a refurbished piece that was included in both the first and second editions. The other is new and emphasizes the importance of matching psychological strategies of rehabilitating athletes to type of injury as well as individual athlete needs and attributes.

As was the case with this book's two previous editions, counselors, therapists, coaches, athlete trainers, and students preparing to work in some way with injured athletes should profit from its contents. Outstanding and experienced authors comprehensively address diverse topics related to the psychology of injury. It was my great pleasure to organize and preside over the preparation of this project.

David Pargman
Tallahassee, Florida

Acknowledgments

I wish to express heartfelt gratitude to all the authors who contributed their excellent chapters. They have generously detailed their personal experiences with injured and disabled athletes and have forwarded their ideas, criticisms, and recommendations, and in so doing have provided basic ingredients for a fine volume. Obviously, without their willingness to extend themselves, this book would not have materialized. I also wish to thank my assistant, Kimberlee Bethany Bonura for the assistance she rendered in a multitude of ways. Her commitment to this project and the effort she invested in seeing it to completion are much appreciated. —D.P.

Sport Injury: An Introduction and Overview of Related Psychological Issues

Sport demands rigorous, physically challenging, and, often, risky gross motor activity. As a result, injury is a likely consequence of active involvement. Some sports require inordinately high torques and pressures upon the skeletal system that are effectuated explosively and dramatically in uncomfortable or even hostile environments. Severely inclement weather, for example, may, in and of itself, present formidable physical barriers to the athlete (ice, heavy rain, snow- or mud-covered terrain, etc.). In addition, emotions such as anger, fear, and exuberance, which are often present prior to or during competitive efforts, may compound the experience's risk and danger. Athletes at elite levels may be particularly vulnerable to injury because some of the above climatic or topological circumstances, although risky and dangerous, do not necessarily cause competitions to be cancelled. For instance, soccer and football games go on despite inclement weather.

Sport participants of low skill level may be particularly susceptible to injury because their movements are often imprecise and mechanically deficient. Be that as it may, active involvement in sport is accompanied by a heightened probability of physical trauma. And almost always when injury strikes, the athlete suffers disadvantage—sometimes of a long-lasting or even permanent kind. Although some good can accrue from sport injury (Udry, 1999), the experience is essentially negative. The consequences of injury to an individual athlete may also seriously impinge upon the welfare of an entire team or athletic program. When a starter goes down, his or her absence may be sorely felt by all participants and result in reconfiguration of offensive or defensive strategy.

Ironically, despite significant amounts of technological improvement in the design of athletic equipment and facilities, the incidence of sport injury has actually increased during the past 15–20 years (Orchard & Powell, 2003). Dramatic increases in muscular strength and explosive power of athletes (Sokolove, 2004) due to new training procedures now place greater loads and more stress upon the long bones and joints of competitors. Yet, the skeletal framework itself remains unchanged, thus raising its susceptibility to trauma (Pargman, 2006). Other factors contributing to recent increases in sport injury (at least in North American society) include the following:

1. More people are involved in sport and sport/recreational activities because of encouragement by health professionals who view exercise (sport is undeniably a form of exercise) as an important contributor to mental and physical well-being. Regular physical activity is considered by most physicians as a strategy for body weight regulation and an impediment to the development of certain illnesses.

2. Shockingly high salaries and lucrative product endorsement opportunities offered to professional athletes in many sports stimulate risk-taking behavior. In order to avoid being replaced by younger aspiring athletes waiting in the wings, elite athletes may be inspired to put themselves in harm's way and throw caution to the wind. This may also be true of high school competitors eager to be offered college or university athletic scholarships. Their inspiration to excel may encourage overtraining or other forms of imprudent and unsafe behavior.

3. Artificial playing surfaces that permit athletes to move faster than on natural turf might also account for an increase in the probability of many kinds of injuries.

   In a nutshell, involvement in sport makes injury a reality.

The term *sport injury*

Diversity in definitions of the term *sport injury* is apparent in the literature and probably accounts for some disagreement in reported research findings. Authors and researchers frequently diverge in their interpretations, usually differing with regard to the number of days of practice or competition missed due to physical trauma incurred on or in the playing field or other performance facility. Some scholars emphasize "major negative life changes events" in their definition (Gould, Udry, Bridges & Beck, 1997), while others incorporate the need for rehabilitation as a result of physical damage as the essential ingredient. The National Injury Registration Systems (Lysens, Weerdt, & Nieuwboer, 1991) identifies but a one-day limit upon participation in order for an athlete to be considered injured. Petscher (2005) considered a three-day period of activity cessation as a requirement. And Pargman (2006) entirely avoids dependence upon a chronological criterion and defines sport injury as: "Debilitation resulting in the inability to function as competently as before the occurrence of physical trauma during sport participation." Although athletes may abide by pragmatic and subjective criteria such as pain or impaired movement, researchers (for obvious reasons) tend to favor objective and quantifiable guidelines such as days absent from practice and/or competition.

Injury causality

Sport injury is often attributable to environmental factors such as icy or slippery playing surfaces (Orchard & Powell, 2003), equipment failure, or intrapersonal factors such as inadequate preparation or not having mastered skills necessary to compete at a particular level (Engebretsen & Bahr, 2003). Along these lines is the fact that the physical fitness level of athletes has been shown to be positively correlated with frequency of injury (Arnason, Sigurdsson, Gudmundsson, Holme, Engebretsen, & Bahr, 2004). In addition, a teammate's failure to properly execute a defined responsibility (fulfilling a blocking assignment in American football) may cause injury to another. An imprudent or incorrect coaching decision may also be a causal factor.

It may be argued that within-athlete psychological factors are also causally related to sport injury. In the 1960s when sport psychology was establishing an identity as a research-oriented sub-discipline, a good deal of scientific inquiry was directed toward personality traits, and ultimately, attempts were made to link them with sport injury. However, such linkages have not been clearly established to date. But other psychological factors such as self-concept and locus of control have been shown to be associated with success in sport injury rehabilitation (Grove & Bianco, 1999), as well as severity and incidence of injury (Pargman & Lunt, 1989). Some personality traits such as neuroticism have been associated with type of preferred coping responses in reaction to distress. Injury is certainly stressful, and those scoring high in neuroticism tend to evince high levels of maladaptive behavior (Costa & McRae, 1989; Kardum & Hudek-Knezevic, 1996). Such correlations carry implications for sport injury rehabilitation. Grove, Stewart, & Gordon (1990) were able to establish a connection between explanatory style, dispositional optimism, and hardiness, and various psychological processes, in athlete recovery from reconstruction surgery.

Other psychological factors may also have some connection to sport injury, to wit, self-abusive behavior manifest in training overuse. Whether the abuse is due to naiveté or an exceedingly strong motivation to succeed, some athletes undertake entirely inappropriate workloads and thereby injure themselves. Psychological abuse on the part of others may also contribute to injury. Improper training assignments by coaches and strength-training consultants may also be responsible for trauma.

Yet another psychological framework may be helpful in clarifying sport injury. Pargman has speculated that information-processing style and efficiency vary among athletes, as they do with all persons. When these styles are inconsistent with cognitive demands of a particular sport task, injury may be the unfortunate consequence. Athletes whose cognitive style is mismatched with information-processing requirements inherent in their particular sport may not be able to efficiently satisfy momentary cognitive challenges. Error in behavior is a probable consequence that may accordingly account for injury. Information processing involves receipt of environmental stimuli by the brain, their interpretation and passage through the working memory, storage in long-term memory, and eventually, some sort of action. Athletes who process or construct knowledge accurately and efficiently are likely to execute necessary behaviors with a relatively low probability of injury.

Along these lines is *field dependence/independence*, an example of cognitive style conceptualized by Witkin, Dyk, Patterson, Goodenough, and Karp (1962) and subsequently elaborated upon by many others over the years. Witkin and his colleagues maintained that some individuals are efficient in extracting a good deal of information from the visual field in order to resolve mental challenges, whereas others do so with less facility. Witkin hypothesized a continuum anchored at each end by the former and latter tendencies that he labeled field dependent and field independent, respectively. Pargman was able to relate score on a written test of field dependence/independence (employing geometric shapes in a framework of lines and forms) to incidence of injury in college football players (Pargman, 1976; Pargman, Sachs, & Deshaies, 1978). Athletes whose perceptual/cognitive style was indicative of relatively greater visual independence were among the least frequently injured. It may be that football players who are able to efficiently extract meaningful cues from their environmental visual field (higher field dependent score) are less likely to incur injury because they are better able to receive and process important visual stimuli from the environment. In other words, they are proficient in attending to and interpreting vital information and, accordingly, making judgments and decisions that better insulate them from injury. A more comprehensive discussion of the applicability of Witkin's theoretical field dependent/independence construct (eventually these terms were subsumed under the more general heading of *psychological differentiation*) may be found in Pargman (1993).

When information processing is efficacious, correct skill execution is likely. Since decision making in sport is a function of cognitive capability, and poor choices may be precipitators of athletic injury, it is critical that the coaching and teaching of sport skills be done with insight into developmental factors that influence the information processing abilities of athlete learners. Athletes of different ages and different developmental stages process information differently and cognitive styles are idiosyncratic in that all athletes do not accommodate new information or store and retrieve it in like manner. A more comprehensive treatment of this notion is to be found in Pargman (2006, a) and Pargman (2006, b).

The Stress/Injury Model

Another approach to clarifying injury in sport has been promulgated by Andersen and Williams (1998). Their model, referred to as the *Stress/Injury Model,* suggests an interplay among cognitive, physiological, attentional, behavioral, interpersonal, social, and stress history variables. All of these impinge upon the psychological state of athletes and influence their behavior. Accordingly, athletes who cope with these forces in a non-stressful manner are likely to avoid athletic injury. When coping responses are weak or inadequate, stress stimuli accumulate and eventually take their toll; the consequences include increased susceptibility to fatigue, illness, or injury (Smith, Smoll, & Ptacek, 1990).

In the stress/injury model, emphasis is placed upon cognitive appraisal or what the athlete thinks about during competition or practice. Athletes whose thoughts dwell on stress or potential or past injury, for example, are ripe for trauma. Furthermore, increased levels of sport-related anxiety encourage appraisal of environmental stimuli as stressful. Another element of the model is the athlete's personality, which Andersen and Williams hypothesized influences the way in which he or she appraises and responds to stressors. For instance, those with high levels of trait anxiety and/or neuroticism would process many environmental stimuli as potentially problematic (stressful), in contrast to those with comparatively low scores. And once again, an abundance of such perceptions provide for an increased susceptibility to injury. However, this hypothesized inclusion of a personality dimension of the model, as attractive as it may appear, is in need of empirical support, which as yet has not been definitively provided.

Return to competition

Many injured athletes are eager to resume competitive activities after sustaining trauma, and an available body of literature addresses a number of psychological variables that appertain to reentry.

Personal adjustment to physical incapacitation must precede rehabilitative efforts, and attitudes and affect are foundational to the athlete's successful return to practice or competition. Feelings of loss, decreased self-esteem, frustration, and anger are responses that challenge the athlete's quest for recovery and reinstatement within the community of competitors (Tracy, 2000). Those who participate at elite levels are likely to experience higher intensities of such negative reactions than recreational athletes (Meyers, Sterling, Calvo, Marely, & Duhon, 1991). It is therefore necessary for counselors, athletic trainers, and psychologists who preside over rehabilitative programs to determine the importance of sport in their clients' lives. Athletes who reveal sport to be essential components of their mental well-being will encounter a relatively burdensome rehabilitative experience. Along these lines is the timeliness of the injury; that is, at what point in the competitive season did the injury occur, or at what stage in the athlete's development as a competitor did it occur (Gayman & Crossman, 2003)?

Two additional factors that influence emotional and cognitive responses to injury are medical assessment of long-range incapacitation and overall prognosis (Albut, McShane, Gordin, & Dobson, 1988). Discouraging news from physicians and athletic trainers may engender negative cognitions and emotional reactions. Good news is potentially inspirational and may serve to inhibit anxious and depressive responses. The athlete's rehabilitative efforts and acceptance of incapacitation are also contingent upon his or her personal evaluation of rehabilitative success to date. Recovering athletes who conclude that they are progressing and improving in their quest for pre-injury function are thereby assisted in their efforts. Those who are unable to "see the light at the end of the tunnel" are motivationally handicapped.

Because the time frame immediately following injury usually reveals the greatest mood disturbances (Leddy, Lambert, & Ogles, 1994), intervention and psychological evaluation of the athlete should commence as near as possible to the disabling event. Brewer, Linder, and Phelps (1995), Gould et al. (1997), and Udry (1997) have recommended that injured athletes be led to an internal locus of control as early as possible, thus placing responsibility for rehabilitation on their own regulatory efforts.

Support from others—social support

Among the most influential forces acting upon rehabilitation from sport injury is *social support*. When attempting to cope with injury-related stress and anxiety, athletes may deplete their supply of psychological skills and conclude that continuation with rehabilitative efforts is in vain and that they "will never come back." Hobfall and Stokes (1988) suggest that at this point the resource pool available to injured athletes may be extended by turning to others in their environment. Hardy, Burke, and Crace (1999) have identified four elements that comprise the social support process: (a) the support provider, (b) the support recipient, (c) the transaction between the provider and the recipient, and (d) the outcomes of the transaction.

Support may take many forms and have numerous sources, and athletes themselves must assume at least partial responsibility for identifying them. Teammates, coaches, parents, family members and friends, trainers, counselors, and sport psychologists are examples of social supporters. Support may be emotional, informational, or tangible (offer of transportation, food, or money). Supporters may also provide reality confirmation (empathy) and encouragement to find alternative ways of thinking about injury and disability (reframing). Among those who have studied and written about the power of social support in the recovery from athletic injury are Reese, Smith, and Sparkes (2003), Ievleva and Orlick (1991), and Silva and Hardy (1991).

Teammates may help the injured athlete avoid feelings of isolation by sustaining contact and relationships as well as providing assurance of heartfelt acceptance at social and recreational functions. Among the helpful interventions provided by teammates are listening support, emotional support, confirmation support (confirmation of the athlete's perspective of the situation), task appreciation support (acknowledgement of the athlete's efforts at rehabilitation), and personal knowledge sharing (sharing expertise gained through the supporter's prior experiences with similar injury and incapacitation (Richman, Rosenfeld & Hardy, 1993).

Coaches should encourage teammates to give attention to injured athletes despite feelings of awkwardness (Wiese-Bjornstal & Smith, 1999). The disabled athlete may be assigned record-keeping responsibilities or officiating tasks during scrimmages.

Parents, family members, and friends (non-athletes) are additional sources of social support. Athletes may feel more comfortable sharing feelings and perspectives about their injury with those who are not directly connected to their athletic endeavors than with teammates and coaches. In particular, parents play vital supportive roles with youth athletes. Their strong commitments and concerns for their very own offspring place them in highly influential and potentially effective supportive roles. Brewer (2003) has described the variability in responses to sport injury on behalf of children of different development stages. Therefore, in order to offer optimal levels of support to their disabled children, well-intentioned and highly motivated parental supporters should consider their children's stages of cognitive and psychosocial development.

Pain—a consequence of sport injury

Pain receptors dispersed throughout the entire body transmit information to the brain about tissue damage, on-site retention of fluid, and disruption of organic and systemic function. Such events are common sequels of sport injury. This information is then aligned with memories of previous experiences, perhaps acquired from other sources (books, etc.),and interpreted in the brain's *nociceptor system*. Pain is therefore a perceptual-cognitive phenomenon and very much a psychological entity. *Nociception* refers to the processing of sensory communications and their interpretation. Interpretation varies according to prior learning and experience. Some evidence exists that gender and the prevailing culture of the particular sport itself may also have bearing upon the ways in which athletes respond to pain (Meyers, Bourgois, & Leunes, 2001). The athlete's history with injury and relevant attitudes also influence the trauma's interpretation.

Risk-taking tendencies may also be gender specific, although this is debatable (Pike & Maguire, 2003; Theberge, 2000; Young & White, 1995). More likely it is the level of competition rather than gender that influences the extent to which pain is perceived and reacted to.

The intensity of pain is not well correlated with seriousness or severity of injury. Ironically, acute discomfort may be indicative of modest trauma, and moderate pain may reflect significant tissue damage.

Heil and Fine (1999) discuss various aspects of *pain tolerance,* a term that connotes something other than what *coping* brings to mind. Tolerance is the ability to deal with pain over time, whereas coping implies use of strategies (cognitive, chemical, etc.) designed to reduce or erase it entirely. According to Heil and Fine the degree of pain that can be tolerated is contingent upon four factors: (a) expectation that pain can and will be tolerated (it's part of being an athlete), (b) a strong goal orientation (something that must be done in order for the injured athlete to recover and eventually be successful), (c) absorption in the work in progress (being focused on athletically related endeavors such as practice and competition enables the injured athlete to dissociate from pain stimuli), and (d) the assumption of limited pain duration (being confident that the discomfort will wane and soon disappear). Tolerance connotes acceptance and adjustment to discomfort, whereas coping infers definitive strategic efforts to manage it.

Assisting the injured athlete with psychological interventions

Professionals who administer to injured athletes have at their disposal a multitude of psychological interventions. *Imagery* and *modeling* are two such examples.

Mental imagery employs symbolic representations that enable injured athletes to believe they are undergoing successful rehabilitation. Sensations are built in virtual fashion (rather than in actuality) by the athlete in the so-called mind's eye, ear, nose, hand, etc. Accordingly, the body's physiological processes are stimulated to respond authentically (Fiore, 1988; Hanley & Chinn, 1989; May & Johnson, 1973). In effect, the participant is encouraged to experience a sort of vicarious progress toward healing, which in turn, hopefully, exerts a positive influence upon his or belief in a successful recovery. The athlete initiates imagery volitionally, but prior training is necessary in order to attain an adequate level of imaging skill. Such training typically requires the leadership of an experienced teacher. For optimal results it is also advisable to implement imagery following accomplishment of a state of deep muscular relaxation such as potentially achieved by the Jacobson progressive muscular relaxation procedure (see Pargman, 2006). Imaging may also be applied to enable the injured athlete to understand and accept the long-term consequences of the disability and, as Green (1999) suggests, create a mindset and resolve for recovery. In addition, imagery may be applied to reduce or eliminate counterproductive thoughts and pain sensations. Another way of describing the benefit of imagery within the context of athletic injury is to conclude that it provides for mental and physical healing in conjunction with each other.

Modeling, or observational learning, is a powerful strategy for motivating learners with many different skills, behaviors, and attitudes (Bandura, 1986; McCullagh, Weiss, & Ross, 1989; Weiss & Klint, 1987). A learner observes the model and places in memory a symbolic representation of that which is to be acquired, which in turn serves as a guide for behavior. The most potent effects of modeling accrue from models that are similar to the learner in as many respects as possible. For instance, models of the same age, gender, and ability will enable more efficient learning than models who do not permit the learner to conclude that, "If he can do it, so can I." Frances Flint (1999) has applied observational learning to the psychological rehabilitation of injured athletes. She has done this by exposing recovering athletes to videotaped behaviors of others who have successfully recovered. The observers were thus able to imitate attitudes about effort, positive beliefs about recovery, and appropriate execution of assigned rehabilitative regimens. Because inappropriate models also abound in locker rooms, training facilities, and in all sorts of the injured athlete's immediate environments, care must be given to filtering them out. Athletic trainers, coaches, parents, physical therapists, and athletes themselves must not emulate incorrect models lest they ultimately acquire attitudes and behaviors that are counterproductive to successful rehabilitation.

Adherence to rehabilitative protocols is another problematic issue for some injured athletes as well as the therapists and social supporters invested in their optimal recovery. Some injured athletes have difficulty in conforming to prescribed rehabilitative programs. They fail to appear regularly for therapy or do not abide by prohibitions or programs prescribed by physicians, physical therapists, or athletic trainers. Their professed recognition of the importance of assigned rehabilitative programs not withstanding, some injured athletes do not follow instructions. Brewer, Avondoglio, Cornelius et al. (2000) have offered explanations that may clarify such failure to comply. Among these is the degree of and nature of the athlete's identification with sport, or the meaningfulness of the experience. Grove and Bianco (1999) identified personality factors as correlates of adherence, and other researchers such as Duda, Smart, and Tappe (1989) and Fischer, Domm, and Weust (1988) have established a link between adherence and self-motivation and social support in injured athletes. Grove and Bianco have reported that athletes recovering rapidly from injury tend to attribute their recovery to stable, internal, and controllable factors in comparison to those who recover slowly. Attributions are reasons persons provide for event outcomes in which they have been involved. Those utilizing attributions such as "It wasn't my fault—my teammate made a mistake" are designating *external attributions* as causes of an outcome (loss of a competition). In contrast is the attribution "I'm to blame—it was my fault" by which the athlete reports an *internal attribution*. A *controllable attribution* puts emphasis upon the person's perception that he or she had the ability to influence the outcome of the experience. *Stability* refers to the consistently sustained attributions that do not vary over time.

Injured athletes (Olympic skiers) who were able to identify at least one positive outcome of their injury did better in rehabilitation efforts than those who could not

(Gould et al. 1997). Injured athletes receiving various kinds of social support tend to adhere better to rehabilitative assignments in comparison to those without support (Bianco & Eklund, 2001; Udry, 1996).

Summary

Sport injury is common among those participating in this demanding and rigorous experience. Despite advances in sport facility and equipment design, the incidence of injury has steadily increased during the past two decades.

When considering various aspects of sport injury, psychological factors merit analysis and a few, such as risk-taking tendencies and self-concept, were discussed in this chapter. Some causal linkages have been hypothesized; however, more viable connections have been established between motivation for and success in rehabilitation.

Among the factors discussed as being causally related to injury in sport are stress appraisal, effectiveness of stress-coping capabilities, and history of past stressors, all of which have been incorporated into a model proposed by Andersen and Williams (1998). Certain personality and cognitive style variables were also discussed in terms of their possible connections to sport injury. Faulty information processing, whereby knowledge encoding and retrieval are weak or compromised, was also speculated to be a causal factor in sport injury.

The perceptual cognitive experience known as pain was described and addressed as an all too frequent correlate of injury. A distinction was drawn between pain tolerance and pain coping.

Next the chapter turned to selected psychological factors that relate to rehabilitation from athletic injury, notably social support, and certain personality variables such as neuroticism, dispositional optimism, and pessimism.

Mental imagery and modeling, two approaches that may be incorporated in rehabilitation regimens, were also presented. And lastly, adherence to programs of rehabilitation for injured athletes was discussed. Some athletes have difficulty in maintaining participation in much needed prescriptive regimens designed to enhance their recovery processes. Reasons for such difficulty and strategies for overcoming low levels of adherence were reviewed.

References

Albert, N. J., McShane, D., Gordin, R., & Dobson, W. (1988, September). *The emotional effects of injury on female collegiate gymnasts.* Paper presented at the Seoul Olympic Scientific Congress, Seoul, South Korea.

Andersen, M. B., & Williams, J. M. (1988). A model of stress and athletic injury: Prediction and prevention. *Journal of Sport and Exercise Psychology, 10,* 299-306.

Arnason, A., Sigurdsson, S., Gudmundsson, A., Holme, I., Engebretsen, L., & Bahr, R. (2004). Physical fitness, injuries, and team performance in soccer. *Medicine and Science in Sports and Exercise, 36,* 278-285.

Bandura, A. (1986). *Social foundations of thought and action: A social cognitive theory.* Englewood Cliffs, NJ: Prentice-Hall.

Bianco, T., & Eklund, R. C. (2001). Conceptual considerations for social support research in sport and exercise settings: The case of sport injury. *Journal of Sport and Exercise Psychology, 23,* 85-107.

Brewer, B. W. (2003). Developmental differences in psychological aspects of sport-injury rehabilitation. *Journal of Athletic Training, 38,* 152-153.

Brewer, B., Avondoglio, J. B., Cornelius, A. E., Van Raalte, J. L., Brickner, J. C., Petitpas, A. J., Kolt, G. S., Pizzari, T., Schoo, A. M. M., Emery, K., & Hatten, S. J. (2002). Construct validity and interrater agreement of the Sport Injury Rehabilitation Adherence Scale. *Journal of Sport Rehabilitation, 11*, 170-178.

Brewer, B. W., Linder, D. E., & Phelps, C. M. (1995). Situational correlates of emotional adjustment to athletic injury. *Clinical Journal of Sport Medicine, 5*, 241-245.

Costa, P. T., & McRae, R. R. (1987). Validation of the five factor model of personality across instruments and observers, *Journal of Personality and Social Psychology, 52*, 81-90.

Duda, J. L., Smart, A. E., & Tappe, M. K. (1989). Predictors of adherence in the rehabilitation of athletic injuries: An application of personal investment theory. *Journal of Sport and Psychology, 11*, 367-381.

Fiore, N. A. (1988). The inner healer: Imagery for coping with cancer and its therapy. *Journal of Mental Imagery, 12*, 79-82.

Fisher, A. C., Domm, M. A., & Wuest, D. A. (1988). Adherence to sports injury rehabilitation programs. *The Physician and Sports Medicine, 16*, 47-51.

Flint, F. (1999). Seeing helps believing: Modeling in injury rehabilitation. In D. Pargman (Ed.), *Psychological bases of sport injuries* (2nd ed., pp. 221-233). Morgantown, WV: FIT.

Gayman, A., & Crosman, J. (2003). A qualitative analysis of how the timing of the onset of sports injuries influences athlete reactions. *Journal of Sport Behavior, 26*, 255-271.

Gould, D., Udry, E., Bridges, D., & Beck, L. (1997a). Down but not out: Athlete responses to season-ending injuries. *Journal of Sport and Exercise Psychology, 19*, 224-248.

Gould, D., Udry, E., Bridges, D., & Beck, L. (1997b). Stress sources encountered when rehabilitating from season-ending ski injuries. *The Sport Psychologist, 11*, 361-378.

Green, L. B. (1999). The use of imagery in the rehabilitation of injured athletes. In D. Pargman (Ed.), *Psychological bases of sport injuries* (2nd ed., p. 238). Morgantown WV: FIT.

Grove, J. R., & Bianco, T. (1999). Psychological correlates of psychological processes during injury rehabilitation. In D. Pargman (Ed.), *Psychological bases of sport injuries* (2nd ed., pp. 89-110). Morgantown, WV: FIT.

Grove, J. R., Stewart, R., & Gordon, S. (1990). Emotional reactions of athletes to knee rehabilitation. Annual Meeting of the Australian Sports Medicine Federation, Alice Springs.

Hanley, G. L., & Chinn, D. (1989). Stress management: An integration of multidimensional arousal and imagery theories with case study. *Journal of Mental Imagery, 13*, 107-118.

Heil, J., & Fine, P. (1999). Pain in sport: A biopsychological perspective. In D. Pargman (Ed.), *Psychological bases of sport injuries* (2nd ed., pp. 13-28). Morgantown, WV: FIT.

Hobfoll, S. E., & Stokes, J. P. (1988). The process and mechanics of social support. In S. W. Duck (Ed.), *Handbook of personal relationships: Theory, research, and interventions* (pp. 497-517). New York: John Wiley and Sons.

Ievleva, L., & Orlick, T. (1991). Mental links to enhanced healing: An exploratory study. *The Sport Psychologist, 5*, 25-40.

Kardum I. & Hudek-Knezevic, J. (1996). The relationship between Eysenck's personality traits, coping styles and moods. *Personality and Individual Differences, 20*, 341-350.

Leddy, M. H., Lambert, M. J., & Ogles, B. M. (1994). Psychological consequences of athletic injury among high-level competitors. *Research Quarterly for Exercise and Sport, 65*, 347-354.

Lysens, R. L., Weerdt, W., & Nieuwboer, A. (1991). Factors associated with injury proneness. *Sports Medicine, 12*, 281-289.

May, J., & Johnson, H. (1973). Psychological activity to internally elicited arousal and inhibitory thoughts. *Journal of Abnormal Psychology, 82*, 239-245.

McCullagh, P., Weiss, M. R., & Ross, D. (1989). Modeling considerations in motor skill acquisition and performance: An integrated approach. In K. B. Pandolf (Ed.), *Exercise and sport sciences reviews* (Vol. 17, pp. 475-513). Baltimore: Williams and Wilkins.

Meyers, M. C., Bourgeois, A. E., & LeUnes, A. Pain coping response of collegiate athletes involved in high contact, high injury-potential sport. *International Journal of Sport Psychology, 32*, 29-42.

Meyers, M. C., Sterling, J. C., Calvo, R. D., Marley, R., & Duhon, T. K. (1991). Mood state of athletes undergoing orthopaedic surgery and rehabilitation: A preliminary report. *Medicine and Science in Sports and Exercise, 23*, S138.

Orchard, J. W., & Powell, J. W. (2003). Risk of knee and ankle sprains under various weather conditions in American football. *Medicine and Science in Sports and Exercise, 35*, 1118-1123.

Pargman, D. (2006). *Managing performance stress: Models and methods.* New York: Routledge.

Pargman, D. (2006). "Sport Injury: A Psychological Perspective," in *Psychology of Sport Training*, B. Blumenstein & R. Lidor (Eds.), Mayer & Mayer. In press.

Pargman, D. "Individual Differences: Cognitive and Perceptual Styles," in *Handbook on Research in Sport Psychology*, R. N. Singer, M. Murphey, L. K. Tennant (Eds.), Macmillan, 1993.

Pargman, D. (1976). Visual disembedding and injury in college football players. *Perceptual and Motor Skills, 42,* 762.

Pargman, D., & Lunt, S. D. (1989). The relationship of self-concept and locus of control to the severity of injury in freshmen collegiate football players. *Sports Training, Medicine, and Rehabilitation, 1,* 1-6.

Pargman, D., Sachs, M., & Deshaies, P. (1976). Field-dependence-independence and injury in college football players. *American Corrective Therapy Journal, 30,* 174-176.

Petscher, Y. (2004). Incidence of Sport Injury in Female Collegiate Athletes across the Four Phases of the Menstrual Cycle. Unpublished Master's Thesis, Florida State University.

Pike, E. C., & Macguire, J. A. (2003). Injury in women's sport: Classifying key elements of "risk encounters." *Sociology of Sport Journal, 20,* 232-251.

Reese, T., Smith, B., & Sparkes, A. (2003). The influence of social support on the lived experiences of spinal cord injured sportsmen. *The Sport Psychologist, 17,* 135-156.

Richman, J. M., Rosenfeld, L. B., & Hardy, C. J. (1993). The social support survey: A validation study of a clinical measure of the social support process. *Research on Social Work Practice, 3,* 288-311.

Silva, J. M., & Hardy, C. J. (1991). The sport psychologist: Psychological aspects of injury in sport. In F. O. Mueller, & A. Ryan (Eds.), *The sports medicine team and athletic injury prevention* (pp. 114-132). Philadelphia: FA Davis.

Smith, R., Smoll, F., & Ptacek, J. (1990). Conjunctive moderator variables in vulnerability and resiliency: Life stress, social support and coping skills, and adolescent sport injuries. *Journal of Personality and Social Psychology, 58,* 360-370.

Sokolove, M. (2004, Jan. 18). The lab animal. *The New York Times Magazine,* pp. 28-33, 48, 54, 58.

Theberge, N. (2000). *Higher goals: Women's ice hockey and the politics of gender.* New York: State University of New York Press.

Tracey, J. (2003). The emotional response to the injury and rehabilitation process. *Journal of Applied Sport Psychology, 15,* 279-293.

Udry, E. (1996). Social support: Exploring its role in the context of athletic injuries. *Journal of Sport Rehabilitation, 5,* 151-163.

Udry, E. (1999). The paradox of injuries: Unexpected positive consequences. In D. Pargman (Ed.), *Psychological bases of sport injuries* (pp. 79-88). Morgantown, WV: FIT.

Weiss, M. R., & Klint, K. A. (1987). "Show and tell" in the gymnasium: An investigation of developmental differences in modeling and verbal rehearsal of motor skills. *Research Quarterly for Exercise and Sport, 58,* 234-241.

Wiese-Bjornstal, D., & Smith, A. M. (1991). Counseling strategies for enhanced recovery of injured athletes within a team approach. In D. Pargman (Ed.), *Psychological bases of sport injuries* (pp. 125-155). Morgantown, WV: FIT.

Witkin, H. A., Dyk, R. B., Fattuson, H. F., Goodenough, D. R., & Karp, S. A. (1962). *Psychological differentiation: Studies of development.* New York: Wiley.

Young, K., & White, P. (1995). Sport physical danger and injury: The experience of elite women athletes. *Journal of Sport and Social Issues, 19,* 45-61.

Section One | Preventing Athletic Injury

Each of the three chapters in Section 1 deals with sport injury prevention.

In the first chapter, Tony Morris and Young-Eun Noh focus upon the dance experience, which they feel satisfies definitional criteria for sport. The reader is reminded that the number of injuries in this domain is both prodigious and problematic. The authors suggest that the Andersen and Williams psychosocial model used to clarify sport injury is also relevant to the world of dance.

In the section's second chapter, Ralph Maddison and Harry Prapavesis discuss cognitive behavioral stress management interventions intended to reduce the occurrence of sport injury.

The third chapter in this section, written by Urban Johnson, overviews important issues related to psychosocial antecedents of sport injury and provides measures to be taken to prevent injuries in competitive soccer athletes.

Chapter One

Research-based Injury Prevention Interventions in Sport and Dance

Tony Morris and Young-Eun Noh
Victoria University

As discussed in many other chapters in this book, injury is a major problem in sport at all levels and also in other physical performance activities, such as dance. Further, physical trauma alone cannot account for the extent of injury that is observed (Petrie & Perna, 2004). A number of researchers have approached injury from a psychological perspective, proposing that psychosocial stress is a significant factor influencing injury in sport (Andersen & Williams, 1988; Smith, Smoll, & Ptacek, 1990; Wiese-Bjornstahl, Smith, Shaffer, & Morrey, 1998). The model proposed by Andersen and Williams has gained popularity, acting as the framework for a range of research. Andersen and Williams proposed that three classes of variable influence the occurrence of psychological stress. These are personality variables, such as competitive trait anxiety, hardiness, and locus of control; history of stressors, including life event stress, daily hassles, and past injury history; and coping resources, such as coping behaviors, stress management, and social support. According to the model, as stress increases in performance contexts, muscles become tight and tense and attentional focus is disrupted. These changes make the performer more vulnerable to injury. Researchers have published a substantial amount of evidence supporting the influence of the key variables in this model on injury (Petrie & Perna, 2004; Williams & Andersen, 1998). History of stressors, especially life stress and daily hassles have been widely studied, whereas coping resources have received less research attention. Most coping research is supportive, but researchers have generally reported the influence of coping to be less strong than life stress and daily hassles (Petrie & Perna, 2004).

In their model, Andersen and Williams (1988) proposed that psychological interventions can be used to reduce the impact of psychosocial stress, so that athletes experience lower levels of muscle tension and less attentional distraction, hence there is less risk of injury. To date, intervention research has been limited. Nonetheless, studies in which athletes were trained in stress management have shown favorable results (e.g., Davis, 1991; Kerr & Goss, 1996). The application of general stress management programs may not be best practice in stress reduction and injury risk management, however. One reason why we argue that a generalized stress management program might not be maximally effective is because it does not target the specific sources of stress in that context. For example, young female gymnasts living away from home in a highly disciplined environment might primarily experience stress because of the absence of social support. We might expect the impact of stress inoculation training in this case to be limited. To reduce their stress substantially, what these young gymnasts need is social support, preferably from their family! Another reason we would consider general stress management programs to be less than best practice is because they might be wasteful of time, effort, and money. Whatever the level of injury-risk reduction that is achieved with such a program, it could be that as much or more could be attained with a more targeted intervention. An example here might be the application of a general stress management program when the main concern for the performers is that their coaches place a lot of stress on them and they do not know how to handle stress emanating from that highly influential source. Training in specific coping skills to manage that stressor would probably be much less time-consuming and more readily effective than a generalized stress management intervention.

In research and practice on injury-risk reduction, sport psychologists might not be aware of the specific contextual factors, so general stress management programs could be claimed to offer the best way to cover all the possibilities. We propose that researchers should devise studies to examine the relative effectiveness of different interventions, based on information gleaned from in-depth qualitative studies about stressors in that specific context. Similarly, exploration by practitioners, using discussion and observation, could form the basis for customized interventions. To support our argument for the adoption of techniques that can help researchers and practitioners to direct interventions more effectively, we describe here two studies we conducted to identify the sources of stress and show how we used the information gleaned from these studies to devise a context-specific intervention.

Given the extent of coverage of the theory and research on sport injury, we only briefly review research on the prevalence of injury, leading to a limited description of the Andersen and Williams (Williams & Andersen, 1998) model of psychosocial stress and injury. Then we provide a summary of the main research supporting the model. In the largest part of the chapter, we discuss the principle of using research or evaluation to guide intervention design and report the two studies that we conducted with dancers to identify sources of stress and ways of coping. Then we describe the intervention study in which we examined an intervention designed to address the stressors we identified. Finally, we make some recommendations for practitioners and researchers, based on our research.

Prevalence of Injury in Sport and Dance

As the number of people participating in physical activity to promote health has increased, sport and exercise can present an inevitable danger, involving accidents and injuries. Consequently, physical injury is considered to be one of the major factors for concern related to the risks of sport/exercise participation, a factor that can cause people to stop exercising or not to start at all. Despite advances in equipment, physical conditioning techniques, and coaching expertise, sport injury has not decreased (Bond, Miller, & Chrisfield, 1988; Petrie & Perna, 2004).

Uitenbroek (1996) reported that 32.5% of participants in the United Kingdom were injured as a result of engaging in sport or exercise. In the United States, an estimated 3 to 17 million sport- and recreation-related injuries are incurred among adults and children per year. A recent population survey conducted by the National Institutes of Health in the USA reported that adults who were over 25 years old had experienced 2.29 million injuries related to physical activities annually from 1997 to 1999 (Ruibal, 2005). Finch, Valuri, and Ozanne-Smith (1998) reported that, in Australia, 20% of child visits and 18% of adult visits to hospital emergency rooms were associated with sport-related injuries. Further, serious injuries can lead to long-term health problems and increased medical expenses. High school athletes participating in 12 sports sustained injuries and produced medical costs of $19 million during one year, in the state of North Carolina (Weaver et al., 1999).

Because dance is similar to sport in terms of the levels of physical and performance demands, at high levels in particular, injuries are also common in dance. Dancers undertake a number of practice sessions, rehearsals, and performances at progressively higher levels of intensity to maintain their position in the group. Because of demanding workloads, the pursuit of perfection, and the quest to perform advanced techniques, dancers often incur overuse injuries and syndromes (Hamilton, 1999; Ryan & Stephens, 1989; Teitz, 1991). Dance injuries produce substantial financial and emotional costs to individual dancers, the health system, and insurance companies.

Bowling (1989) found that dance injuries, at the elite level, were often caused by the demands of performing advanced techniques. He reported that those who had chronic injuries experienced severe pain continually, and just over two-fifths of the dancers studied had sustained at least one injury in the previous six months that had affected their dancing. Recently, Kim and Heo (2003) reported that 95% of a large sample of ballet dancers in Korea had experienced injuries during practice and performance since they had started dancing.

Garrick and Requa (1993) found that 104 professional ballet dancers incurred 309 injuries, for which insurance disbursed nearly USD $400,000 for medical costs, during a three-year period. Dancers had 2.97 injuries on average, but the data were skewed. In particular, Garrick and Requa stated it was remarkable that 23% of these dancers incurred 52% of all injuries. Similarly, Solomon, Micheli, Solomon, and Kelley (1995) reported that 137 injuries occurred among 70 professional ballet dancers. Ten percent of these dancers accounted for a total of 23% of the injuries, that is, around 4.6 injuries each. The rest of the dancers in the study by Solomon et al. averaged 1.7 injuries for two years (1993-1994). For these 137 injuries, insurance companies paid USD $249,272. Efforts to reduce the frequency of injuries in sport and dance are warranted, both to ensure the long-term health of individuals and to reduce the substantial financial and emotional costs for families and insurance companies.

Models of Psychosocial Stress and Injury in Sport and Dance

Over the past three decades, sport science researchers have made efforts to discover how to prevent sport injuries. Examination of physical and biomechanical factors has led to the conclusion that these variables alone cannot account for all the injuries that occur, so psychological factors have been examined (Andersen & Williams, 1988, 1999; Maddison & Prapavessis, 2005; Petrie, 1992, 1993a, 1993b; Smith, Ptacek, & Smoll, 1992).

Figure 1.
Stress-Injury Model

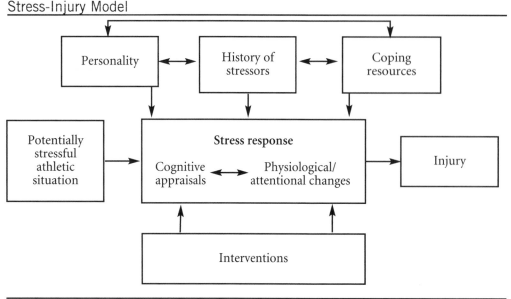

According to the stress-injury model proposed by Andersen and Williams (1988), when athletes experience stressful situations, they react with a stress response. Increases in stress are likely to be associated with

- narrowing attention,
- greater distractibility, and
- higher levels of muscle tension.

These changes increase the probability of injuries. Andersen and Williams suggested that psychosocial factors, such as

- personality,
- history of stressors, and
- coping resources

influence the stress response and, thus, the likelihood of injury occurrence.

Williams and Andersen (1998) reviewed the substantial research that tested aspects of their psychosocial model. The vast majority of this work supported the model, especially with respect to the roles of history of stressors, life event stress, and daily hassles. The involvement of coping resources, such as coping skills and social support, has been shown to moderate the effects of stress on sport injuries (Hardy, O'Connor, & Geisler, 1990; Maddison & Prapavessis, 2005; Petrie, 1993b; Smith, Smoll, & Ptacek, 1990).

In dance, many researchers have investigated the physical factors related to injuries:

- pathogenesis,
- epidemiological, mechanical, and anatomical characteristics, and
- environmental factors.

(Bronner & Brownstein, 1997; Garrick & Requa, 1993; Hardaker, Erickson, & Myers, 1986; Liederbach & Compagno, 2001). In spite of the substantial research into dance-related injuries, injuries have become more prevalent and have affected the financial status or professional careers of dancers more seriously. Some researchers have begun to look elsewhere for injury risk factors (Hamilton, Hamilton, Meltzer, Marshall, & Molnar, 1989; Krasnow, Mainwaring, & Kerr, 1999; Liederbach & Compagno, 2001; Liederbach, Gleim, & Nicholas, 1994; Mainwaring, Kerr, & Krasnow, 1993; Patterson, Smith, Everett, & Ptacek, 1998; Smith, Ptacek, & Patterson, 2000).

In particular, dance researchers have begun to focus on psychosocial factors, such as

- stress,
- social support, and
- anxiety,

which have been studied in sport in relation to injury for 30 years. The previous research has given a broad description of the value of examining psychosocial variables, but the research has not explained the relationship between psychosocial factors and injury in dance (Noh, Morris, & Andersen, 2003). Much research is still needed to identify individuals at high risk of injury and explain various avenues/mechanisms by which psychosocial factors influence injury occurrence in dance.

Research on Psychosocial Stress and Injury in Sport and Dance

Although some research has demonstrated no significant relationship between psychosocial factors and injury, numerous studies have supported the stress-injury model (Williams & Andersen, 1998), which has provided a theoretical framework for the prediction and prevention of injury in sport, since Holmes (1970) conducted the first study of stress and injury in football players.

The most frequently repeated finding is that negative life events are associated with increased risk of injuries in athletes (Andersen & Williams, 1999; Petrie, 1992, 1993b; Smith et al., 1992; Smith, Smoll, & Ptacek, 1990). Many of the previous studies examined contact sports like football and high risk sports, such as gymnastics and skiing. These studies showed that athletes who experienced high levels of life stress were more likely to experience injury occurrence than athletes who experienced low levels of life stress (Blackwell & McCullagh, 1990; Bramwell, Masuda, Wagner, & Holmes, 1975; Coddington & Troxell, 1980; Kerr & Minden, 1988; Passer & Seese, 1983; Petrie, 1992, 1993a, 1993b). Relationships, however, between minor life events (daily hassles) and injury have not received consistent research support, due to methodological problems. A particular concern has been the approach of measuring daily hassles only once, either before the start of the season or at the end of the season (Blackwell & McCullagh, 1990; Hanson, McCullagh, & Tonymon, 1992). The study by Fawkner, McMurray, and Summers (1999) examined the relationship between daily hassles and athletic injuries, with a measure of minor stressful events administered on a weekly basis repeatedly over the course of a competitive season. Fawkner et al. found that a high rate of injury occurred among athletes who had increased minor life events for the week prior to injury. Fawkner et al. suggested that daily hassles should be measured frequently, for example, on a weekly basis, and hassles should be related to injuries incurred during the following week, because minor life events are changing continuously.

Recently, Maddison and Prapavessis (2005) examined prospective correlations between psychosocial factors and injury (the number of injuries and the time missed) among 470 rugby players. Maddison and Prapavessis found that psychosocial factors (i.e., social support, coping skills, and previous injury) interacted with the relationship between life stress and injury.

The different measures used to assess injury may have contributed to the varied results of research on psychosocial stress and injury in sport. Many researchers used the National Athletic Injury/Illness Reporting System (NAIRS), which records severity of injury. The NAIRS classifies injuries that disturbed athletes' training only by the amount of time-loss due to injury. When athletes have minor injuries, they might ignore them and practice or compete, because of differences in personality or pain tolerance levels. The measurement of injury severity might have added some confusion to examination of the stress-injury relationship.

A number of guidelines have been introduced for psychological interventions to enhance performance in sport. Psychological intervention for the prevention of injury, based on changing the levels of antecedents in the model or "inoculating" athletes against stress, has been limited, however (Cupal, 1998), even though researchers are aware that psychosocial factors play a role in injury occurrence.

Kerr and Goss (1996) examined the effect of stress inoculation training (SIT) on injury in 24 gymnasts (16 males, 8 females). Kerr and Goss monitored levels of stress and injury for 8 months, during which the gymnasts practiced SIT. Kerr and Goss randomly divided the gymnasts into SIT and control groups, according to sex, age, and performance. Kerr and Goss found that each gymnast had at least one injury during the 8-month period and most of the injuries were chronic or overuse. Kerr and Goss reported that the SIT group spent less time injured than the control group, but the difference was not statistically significant. Moreover, the SIT group had significantly lower levels of negative stress than the control group from mid-season to peak-season. Kerr and Goss concluded that the stress management program helped the gymnasts to cope with negative stress.

In a recent study, Kolt, Hume, Smith, and Williams (2004) examined the potential role of stress-management interventions to reduce injury risk among 20 gymnasts (17 girls, 3 boys). Kolt et al. divided participants into two groups (i.e., stress-management group and placebo). The stress-management group ($n = 10$) received a 12-session stress-management program, which focused on cognitive behavioral techniques over 24 weeks. The placebo group ($n = 10$) attended 12-session programs, which included nine lectures on nutrition and three anthropometric measurement sessions, over 24 weeks. Kolt et al. found that the stress-management group reported 25 injuries (4.8 injuries per 1,000 hours of training) and the placebo group had 32 injuries (5.7 injuries per 1,000 hours of training). The stress-management group and the placebo group, however, did not differ significantly on either stress (positive or negative general stress and gymnastic-related stress) or injuries (training hours lost to injury).

The Kerr and Goss (1996) and Kolt et al. (2004) studies showed that general stress management intervention programs had little effect on injury or stress. A key reason for these results is that the researchers used general stress management intervention programs to reduce injury rate or stress levels without any consideration of participants' situations or needs. There is no doubt that people are willing to do intervention programs, which are tailored for them with strong volition. Therefore, psychosocial intervention research needs to target injury reduction, based on research with well-defined instruments that identify specific psychosocial variables related to injury occurrence in that context.

In dance, some researchers have tried to explore aspects of the relationship between psychosocial factors and injury across a number of domains. There have been controlled studies on the relationship of injury in dance with stress, social support, and anxiety. Aside from the empirical studies by Hamilton et al. (1989), Krasnow et al. (1999), Mainwaring et al. (1993), Patterson et al. (1998), Smith et al. (2000), and Noh, Morris, and Andersen (2005), few studies have examined variables, such as

- daily hassles,
- life events,
- history of injury,
- performance anxiety,
- muscle tension,
- attention,
- coping skills, and
- social support,

all of which are predicted by the psychosocial stress-injury model in sport to be related to injury outcome. Only one study (Noh, Morris, & Andersen, 2005) has examined whether psychosocial factors, based on the stress-injury model in sport (Williams & Andersen, 1998), could predict dance injuries (frequency and duration) using a prospective research design. Noh et al. (2005) found that coping was the most important factor related to frequency of injury in Korean ballet dancers. Furthermore, except for the study by Noh, Morris, and Andersen (under review), there is no research on psychological interventions for reducing injuries in dance.

Recently, Noh and Morris (2004) proposed an approach to planning more efficient and effective intervention programs, using a combination of quantitative and qualitative research methods. Noh and Morris suggested that careful assessment of factors associated with stress in the specific context could help in the design of effective intervention programs for dancers. Differences from one context to another in the psychosocial stress variables that have the greatest influence on stress and injury mean that such assessment is always recommended to fine-tune interventions.

From Confirmatory Research to Efficient and Effective Practice

Much of the research on psychosocial variables and sports injury consists of confirmatory studies. As reflected in the previous sections, the largest body of research has focused on the relationship between life event stress and sport injury risk. Some of the early studies were criticized because researchers employed retrospective research designs. Athletes were asked to report on their life stress during a period of time, such as the previous year, and their injury history was examined for the same period. This research was criticized because the injuries sustained would have increased perception of life stress, producing a high correlation for the wrong reason. Researchers were interested in the impact of stress on injury, not the effect of injury on stress. Prospective studies followed in which researchers measured psychosocial variables and then monitored injuries over a period of months after the psychosocial variables had been recorded. The results of these more meaningful prospective studies have largely been positive (e.g., Williams & Andersen, 1998), as we, and others in this book, have discussed. Other studies have focused on daily hassles and some have targeted social support or coping resources.

The vast majority of this research has been directed at confirming elements of the psychosocial stress and sport injury model. Although most studies have provided support for the model, they offer only limited guidance for practitioners. One reason for this is that most studies have employed general measures of life stress, daily hassles, social support, and/or coping. Some measures of the psychosocial variables give us a hint at what might be the general issues that are of concern to performers in particular contexts, but most measures provide little information that is sufficiently specific to guide practice. For example, an instrument that has been used widely to measure coping resources is the Athletic Coping Skills Inventory–28 (ACSI-28; Smith, Schutz, Smoll, & Ptacek, 1995). The ACSI has seven subscales, which measure

- coping with adversity,
- peaking under pressure,
- goal setting/mental preparation,
- concentration,
- freedom from worry,
- confidence and achievement motivation, and
- coachability.

High and low scores on these subscales clearly provide information at a meaningful level about coping strengths and weaknesses of individuals, respectively, and indicate whether a clear pattern emerges from group data about the strengths and weaknesses of a group of athletes in a particular context.

Nonetheless, ACSI-28 scores alone do not provide sufficient information to design a targeted intervention. For example, if an especially low score is found on coping with adversity among players in a young, professional football team, this suggests that an intervention aimed at enhancing the footballers' coping skills should contain a substantial component that addresses coping with adversity. To this point, the use of a measure like the ACSI-28 helps by directing the focus of intervention strategies to coping skills and, more specifically, to coping with diversity. This is certainly more useful to practitioners (and, we would hope and expect, more effective for the footballers) than simply applying generalized stress management techniques, but it still doesn't identify the kinds of adversity that those footballers have to face. We might surmise that the main adversity faced by this team is losing. More precisely, we might look at the team and see that it has lost the last five games, so maybe the players in this team do not cope well with a series of consecutive losses. What we are not aware of is that, prior to the series of defeats, the team had lost several key players because of long-term, crippling injuries, and a couple of those injured players may never play high-level football again. The players in this tight-knit team are grieving for their teammates and, at the same time, the sudden spate of terrifying injuries, observed by the players in all its graphic horror, has shocked the players and made them fearful for their own careers and physical well-being. The players do not know how to cope with these adverse events; each is keeping his fears to himself, given the tough, "manly" culture of football, and the club has no idea that this represents an issue that is affecting performance, let alone psychological health. Armed with this information a psychologist might act quite differently in developing intervention strategies for the players. Specific aspects of the support the psychologist would give could include

- assuring the players that grieving about their friends and colleagues is a natural, if not essential, process;
- encouraging players to reflect on their personal reactions;
- addressing the fears about their own well-being raised by the traumatic events;
- explaining to the players that it is good to talk to other people about issues like the grieving, the shock, and the fear, especially to talk to each other, because their colleagues are likely to be going through similar experiences; and
- suggesting that the players might like to support their injured colleagues by maintaining contact with them, visiting them, and including them in social activities, where possible.

In addition, the psychologist should inform and educate the club coaching and administration staff, to ensure that they create a culture in which issues like grieving and fear are recognized and discussed in an open and positive atmosphere. We would expect that strategies like these would have a much bigger impact than a general coping skills intervention.

The position we are proposing does not glean a great deal of support from research, because there is little research in sport or other performance areas that has examined the application of targeted interventions, based on knowledge gleaned from the study of the key psychosocial variables in that specific context and the stressors that are preeminent in the context. As noted earlier in this chapter, the relatively few intervention studies in the sport injury literature mainly employed generalized stress management interventions. We have recently conducted a set of studies in the context of dance that we feel illustrates the approach we are advocating. More specifically, we carried out three studies with ballet dancers in Korea:

- In the first study, we explored the relationship between psychosocial variables and injury.
- The second study was an in-depth, qualitative examination of sources of stress and coping strategies in the same context.
- In the third study, we tested the effectiveness of an intervention designed on the basis of the knowledge we acquired in the preceding studies.

In the following section we describe the studies to show how we used findings from the first two studies to develop an intervention customized for elite ballet dancers in the Korean context. Although what we report in the following section represents a program of formal research, it is clear that practitioners could use equivalent procedures less formally in applied settings.

An Example: Dancers in Korea

Dancers are always concerned about injury, because serious injuries not only disturb their techniques, but they can also influence the opportunities they have during their limited careers. Many dance researchers have focused on the physical or environmental factors that are related to injuries, such as anatomical characteristics, overtraining, technique problems, and equipment failure (Hardaker et al., 1986; Kadel & Teitz, 1992; Kim, K., 1997; Liederbach & Compagno, 2001; Stephens, 1989; Teitz, 1991). Recently, however, some researchers have recognized that psychological factors play a role in dance injuries. In particular, research supporting this proposition has been conducted in Korea (Kim, E., 2001; Kim & Park, 2004; Kim, K., 1997; Lee, 1998; Noh, 1998).

Although psychological factors have been shown to have an impact on dance injury outcome, surprisingly, no psychosocial intervention research, which is aimed at reducing the risk of injury, has been reported in dance. There is vast potential for research to discover the roles of psychosocial factors through the combination of qualitative and quantitative research methods and research on the reduction of injury risk, using well-designed intervention programs. In this example, we describe a process for developing psychosocial interventions, extending application of the Williams and Andersen (1998) model of stress and injury from sport to dance, with the goal of reducing incidence of injury among ballet dancers in Korea.

- First, we examined whether psychosocial factors predict dance injuries (frequency and duration), based on the psychosocial stress-injury model in sport (Williams & Andersen, 1998), using a prospective, correlational research design, among Korean ballet dancers (Noh, Morris, & Andersen, 2005). In that quantitative study, we found that low levels of coping skills were associated with injury frequency and duration of injury, with dancers who had low levels of coping skills being injured more often and for longer periods of time.

- Second, we identified the major sources of stress associated with practice and performance in dance and explored the coping strategies used by performing dancers, based on a qualitative research method, using in-depth interviews (Noh, Morris, & Andersen, 2003). From the qualitative study, we found that Korean ballet dancers experienced substantial stress from many sources, such as their relationships with dance directors and with peers, weight and appearance issues, and the pressure of auditions and performances. The dancers used various coping strategies, including dysfunctional strategies like drinking alcohol or overeating.

- Finally, we conducted a study to examine the effects of two psychosocial interventions designed to reduce injury among dancers, based on the findings from the quantitative and qualitative studies integrated into the psychosocial stress-injury model (Noh, Morris, & Andersen, under review). The first two studies provided the information for designing interventions to focus the development of coping skills, perceived by performers. To illustrate this approach to the design of interventions, we now describe our recent research with dancers.

Psychosocial Factors Related to Ballet Injuries

To gain specific information about elite ballet dancers in Korea, based on the body of theoretical knowledge regarding whether and which psychosocial factors predicted dance injuries, we first conducted a prospective, correlational study, in which we examined 105 Korean ballet dancers (27 professional ballet dancers, 19 university ballet students, and 59 high school students specializing in ballet) with a mean age of 20.46 years ($SD = 5.50$), who participated in regular practice and performance. We selected psychosocial variables (i.e., life and dance stress, anxiety, coping skills, social support) to examine in this study, based on research on the model of stress and injury in sport (Williams & Andersen, 1998) and in dance (Mainwaring et al., 1993; Patterson et al., 1998; Smith et al., 2000). An injury was defined as any medical problem resulting from dance participation that restricted subsequent practice and performance for at least one day beyond the day the injury occurred.

In particular, quantitative measures of frequency and duration of injuries were recorded during the 10-month period after participants completed the psychosocial measures. The dancers completed a modified version of the Adolescent Perceived Event Scale (Compas, Davis, Forsythe, & Wagner, 1987) and the Sport Experiences Survey (Smith et al., 1992), which indicate whether stressors are major or minor and whether they are positive or negative; the Sport Anxiety Scale (Smith, Smoll, & Schutz, 1990) which has three subscales, namely somatic anxiety, cognitive anxiety, and concentration disruption; the Athletic Coping Skills Inventory-28 (Smith, Schutz, Smoll, & Ptacek, 1995), which has seven subscales, namely coping with adversity, peaking under pressure, goal setting/mental preparation, concentration, freedom from worry, confidence and achievement motivation, and coachability; and a social support scale (Patterson et al., 1998), which was developed specifically for research in dance.

From the matrix of correlations between all the psychosocial measures and injury frequency and duration, we found four psychosocial variables that had significant correlations with the injury measures. These were subscales of the ACSI-28, namely peaking under pressure, goal setting/mental preparation, freedom from worry, and confidence and achievement motivation. We entered participants' scores on these ACSI-28 subscales as predictor variables in separate regression analyses in which frequency and duration of injury, respectively, were the criterion variables.

In the regression analyses, we found that coping skills were the main factors that played a prominent role in the prediction of dance injury among ballet dancers in Korea. In particular, freedom from worry, confidence and achievement motivation, along with one specific stress measure, negative dance stress, accounted for 17–21% of variance in duration and frequency of injury in dance. The results of this study showed that, although stress played a role, lack of coping skills appeared to be the key predictor of increased frequency and duration of injury in the context of high-level dance in Korea.

Sources of Stress and Coping Strategies in Ballet Dancers

Of the psychosocial factors studied in the sport and dance research to date, stress has received the greatest amount of research attention. The evidence that stress is related to injury occurrence in athletes and dancers is, perhaps as a consequence, strongest, whereas there is not a great deal of information about the impact of coping skills on injury risk. One reason for this might be that in sport, at least at the elite level, athletes commonly have access to training in coping skills. To examine the details of stress experiences and coping skills of Korean ballet dancers through the dancers' own words, we conducted a qualitative, interview-based study. As well as investigating the major sources of stress perceived by Korean professional ballet dancers in the dance environment, we explored the main ways in which those dancers coped with the stress associated with practice and performance.

The participants in this qualitative study were female professional ballet dancers ($N = 20$), aged 25 to 32 (mean age = 28.25; $SD = 2.05$). Participants had trained in ballet for over 9 years (mean training period = 9.90; $SD = 3.55$) and had been professional dancers for a minimum of 5 years (mean professional careers = 5.10; $SD = 2.55$). We employed a semi-structured interview technique, starting with general questions about the dancers' background in terms of dance history (e.g., age, training duration, length of professional career). The interview became increasingly focused, to the point of inquiring about specific sources of stress and coping strategies. The in-depth interviews in this research revealed that ballet dancers experienced considerable stress, in particular associated with the demand as professional ballerinas to maintain low body weight. Efforts to lose weight are ubiquitous in dance, particularly in ballet. The perfect body image for ballet is tall, lean, narrow-hipped, and long-limbed (Ryan & Stephens, 1989), which is especially problematic for Korean dancers, given the typical Korean female body shape, which is relatively short in height and stocky in build.

Having an injury is problematic for professional dancers, because dancers perceive that dance directors, choreographers, or ballet companies expect them to practice and perform continually through the injury (Mainwaring, Krasnow, & Kerr, 2001). Most dancers continue to dance despite injuries, in particular when performances are scheduled.

Another stressor for Korean ballet dancers that emerged strongly from the interviews was dance directors' attitudes and behavior toward dancers. Ballet is a hierarchical profession. Dance directors, who are at the top of that hierarchy, often talked to dancers in what the dancers perceived to be an insulting or humiliating manner during practice or rehearsals. Further, dancers complained about experiencing negative feedback from directors regarding their performances, which were based on inconsistent requirements. Dancers found it particularly stressful when directors changed their minds, reversing their instructions/feedback to dancers on different occasions. Hamilton (1999) reported that dancers who experienced this kind of occupational stress had more performance anxiety and overuse injuries than those who did not report such experience.

Perhaps the most common stressor for dancers was performance demands. Despite their long hours of practice, it was common for dancers to perceive that they were not adequately prepared for a performance or for an audition. The perception of inadequate preparation might have been influenced by the practice requirements set by dance directors, which left limited time for dancers to work on their performance/audition pieces, leading them to experience stress because of the imbalance of performance demands and preparation resources.

Interviews also showed that the dancers used a range of coping strategies, such as
- seeking social interaction,
- hobby activities,
- individual cognitive and emotional strategies (e.g., screaming and crying, praying, positive thoughts),

- dance-related behavior (e.g., watching the best ballet company, analyzing their performance on video, dancing another kind of dance), and
- physical relaxation to deal with stress.

Even though some dancers used effective coping strategies, more than 60% of the dancers did not cope well with their circumstances, adopting dysfunctional behaviors, such as overeating or drinking alcohol, in response to the stressors. The substantial amount of dysfunctional coping is likely to add to the overall stress levels of the dancers or, at best, not to reduce it. Therefore, dancers experienced considerable stress, which the psychosocial stress-injury model suggests is likely to increase the risk of injury. The specific sources of stress and strategies used to cope with that stress that were revealed in the in-depth interviews corresponded to the general patterns found in the questionnaire study. These elite ballet dancers in Korea experienced stress from many sources, and most dancers reported that they possessed few coping resources to handle the stress they experienced.

Based on the findings of the questionnaire and interview studies together, we concluded that the development of coping skills to more effectively handle stressful circumstances should be an important area for intervention with Korean ballet dancers. This was a noteworthy finding, given that most studies of Western dancers and athletes have focused on stress and social support (Krasnow et al., 1999; Patterson et al., 1998). It is not clear whether this difference is based on cultural factors or is specific to the samples in our research. As noted, athletes in many cultures now receive training in stress management, including coping skills, and this trend is being transferred to dancers in countries like Australia. In contrast, the Korean ballet dancers we studied possessed few functional coping skills and seemed to have no access to resources to help them develop useful ways of managing the substantial stress they faced.

The ACSI-28 was valuable in helping to target general areas of coping that required particular attention in any intervention with Korean ballet dancers. The inductive analysis of the interview data provided guidance on the particular sources of stress that were not coped with well. This information is useful in contextualizing coping skills training. At the same time, both studies indicated that negative life and dance stress should be addressed directly.

Designing Psychosocial Interventions for Ballet Dancers

From the quantitative study, the results showed that low levels of coping skills were associated with injury frequency and duration of injury, with dancers who had low levels of coping skills being injured more often and for longer periods of time. In particular, peaking under pressure, goal setting/mental preparation, freedom from worry, and confidence and achievement motivation subscales of the Athletic Coping Skills Inventory-28 (Smith et al., 1995) were related to injury frequency. For duration of injury, freedom from worry, confidence, and achievement motivation, negative life stress and negative dance stress were associated with longer recovery times.

From the qualitative study, the results demonstrated that Korean ballet dancers had a lot of stress and used various coping strategies including dysfunctional strategies. In particular, the dance director's criticism was a major source of stress. Such criticisms, including insults, were made publicly about a specific dancer among the professional ballet dancers interviewed in that study. Typically, dancers reported that their relationship with the dance director was difficult, because the Korean culture prohibits disrespectful comments or any form of challenge to those in authority.

Based on the picture that emerged from the questionnaire study and the interviews with ballet dancers in Korea, it was clear that interventions should be directed at stress-management, in particular focusing on the development of coping strategies to reduce the effects of stress, with the aim of reducing injury incidence. An Autogenic Training (Schultz and Luthe, 1959) intervention was proposed to be an appropriate approach to address negative stress, as well as to provide a foundation of relaxation, which should help dancers to peak more effectively under pressure and remain free from or, at least, reduce worry. Autogenic Training (AT) is a relaxation technique based on self-suggestions, which has been called a "mind-to-muscle" relaxation technique (Morris, 1997) There are six stages of AT, which involve

- suggestions of warmth and heaviness in the arms and legs (Stages 1-2),
- suggestions of a slow, calm heartbeat (Stage 3),
- suggestions of slow, deep breathing (Stage 4),
- suggestions of a warm feeling in the solar plexus (Stage 5), and
- suggestions of a cool forehead (Stage 6).

The original training in AT took 10 to 12 weeks, with the introduction of a new stage every week or two weeks and practice of that stage every day thereafter. Recent research, however, has shown that a short version can be effective, in which the whole process is introduced in one session and then practiced for several days (Bhum, Morris, & Andersen, 1998).

To address coping directly with the issues identified by the studies of ballet dancers, it was proposed that positive self-talk and guided imagery, performed in a relaxed state could be used alongside AT, which provided a foundation of relaxation. Self-talk refers to all the thoughts we have about ourselves. Thus, specific statements must be devised to address each issue identified in Studies 1 and 2. In this case, the self-talk targeted the specific situations that dancers typically perceived to be stressful. For example, dancers practiced statements about their skill and commitment. We designed these statements to enhance the dancers' confidence and to counter common criticisms made by the dance director. Similarly, some statements reassured the dancers about performance at auditions. Imagery is another technique that has diverse uses. In this intervention, dancers imagined themselves performing well in training and during public performances, coping with the dance director's comments, and handling the stress of having other dancers around who were their friends and colleagues but also their competitors.

Imagery of emotion was also used to emphasize the relaxed and comfortable state that dancers experienced as they learned, buoyed by their self-talk and imagery, of the high levels of skill and commitment that they possessed. The knowledge of specific sources of stress and particular deficits in coping skills informed the development of the interventions, helping in the design of the specific content of the imagery and self-talk scripts.

We called the self-talk, imagery, and AT intervention a broad-based coping skills intervention because it was designed to address all the aspects of the ACSI-28, that is, all the areas of coping that were related to the frequency and duration of injury in the questionnaire study, namely confidence and achievement motivation, coachability, coping with adversity, and concentration associated with the goal setting/mental preparation aspect of coping skills. In addition, because AT was included, we proposed that the areas of coping under pressure and minimizing worries were also addressed by this intervention.

We examined the effects of these two psychological interventions, AT alone and the broad-based coping skills program designed to enhance coping skills of ballet dancers who reported low levels of coping skills. We investigated the effects of these interventions on the frequency and duration of injury over a 1-year period, following introduction of the intervention. Korean ballet dancers who had low levels of coping skills were assigned to one of three conditions:

- control (n = 12)
- Autogenic Training (n = 12)
- broad-based coping skills, including Autogenic Training, imagery, and self-talk (n = 11)

Participants, who were free from injury at the start of the study, completed a modified version of the Athletic Coping Skills Inventory-28 (ACSI-28) and a history of injury survey that was developed specifically for research in dance. Then those in the AT and broad-based conditions participated in a 12-week intervention program, followed by 12 weeks during which they were asked to continue doing the intervention activities. Throughout the 24-week period, they completed adherence logs as a record of the times they practiced the program. To log the practice of AT, participants in AT were asked to maintain a diary. Each diary entry included information regarding the date, the duration of the AT session, and time the session was performed (e.g., before going to bed, after practicing dance). In the broad-based coping skills condition, in addition to their AT sessions, participants were also asked to log self-talk and imagery. The diary entries consisted of the date, the frequency of the AT, self-talk, and imagery, the types of self-talk and imagery, and what time the participant conducted the session. In the control group, participants were asked to log their dancing in regular practice and performance. At the end of 24 weeks, participants completed the modified ACSI-28 again. Physiotherapists recorded injury frequency and duration for all the dancers each day for 24 weeks, using an injury form. Participants then recorded their injury occurrence for another 24 weeks after the intervention period, using self-report indices.

We checked level of adherence to the two coping skills interventions by examining frequency of use reported in adherence diaries, as a percentage of the instruction to practice three times a week. For the AT condition, average adherence was 83%, and for the broad-based coping skills condition average adherence was 82%, so no dancers were excluded and adherence rates were comparable.

Results indicated that all the improvements in coping skills were in the directions that we intended and the subscales that we proposed would be improved by each intervention. At the post-intervention coping skills manipulation check, the broad-based coping skills intervention increased confidence and achievement motivation, coachability, coping with adversity, and concentration associated with goal setting/mental preparation. Importantly, the broad-based coping skills intervention reduced the frequency and duration of injury. The relaxation function of AT was clearly supported by the results. For coping skills, the AT condition enhanced scores only on the peaking under pressure coping skill scale. Furthermore, AT did not significantly reduce injury frequency or duration. The importance of interventions that enhance coping skills, thus, helping dancers to manage stress and reduce injury occurrence, was a major outcome of this research.

In conclusion, here we have described two studies that explored stress, coping, and injury of elite ballet dancers in Korea. In a quantitative study we examined the relationship between psychosocial variables and injury frequency and duration in dance. Then, in a qualitative study, we examined in-depth the experiences of dancers low on coping skills. Next we explained the process by which we designed the interventions to increase ways of coping with the stress experienced by elite dancers. Finally, we described a third study, in which we examined the effect of tailored interventions on coping skills and injury. Even though it is impossible for dancers to avoid 100% of injuries, results of the broad-based intervention showed that dancers can benefit from a range of effective coping skills designed to help them deal with the demands of the ballet environment. We found that cognitive-behavioral intervention programs helped reduce injury incidence. It is hoped that the results reported in this research stimulate researchers to examine psychosocial factors in the model of stress and injury (Williams & Andersen, 1998) as they apply to dance, as well as to develop targeted interventions for decreasing or preventing dance injury.

Advice on Intervention Design for Practitioners

In an ideal world, the practice of psychology would be based only on the results of sound research, which has been repeated and repeated to show that techniques are effective or when, where, and why they are effective. In reality, practitioners are often faced with situations that must be managed, even if there is no body of research to direct their actions. Research on experts, including teachers and psychologists, has shown that their expertise develops through a number of stages from the novice, who tends to follow documented models and "recipes," to the expert, who works intuitively on the basis of past experience (Morris & Thomas, 2004). No doubt there are psychology practitioners working on sport and dance injuries who have intuitively adopted the approach described in the previous section. Nevertheless, the provision of research support for practice based on intuition is valuable and should be legally, as well as professionally, reassuring. Moreover, many sport psychology practitioners might not yet have hit on this approach, so they could still be using general stress management techniques, whereas present and future students can learn about the procedures used in our research as a way to work in their future practice. Thus, we will draw out some recommendations, based on our studies with ballet dancers in Korea, that we believe have relevance for applied work in many physical performance settings.

Recommendations for Applied Work

1. All individuals and group contexts are different, so it is important for practitioners to really understand what is happening in the specific context of their applied work. General intervention techniques are likely to have relatively low effectiveness compared with targeted interventions.

2. Although very experienced practitioners might identify subtle factors intuitively, in most cases it is recommended that practitioners employ systematic procedures to identify the major influences in each performance context. Such procedures include observation, interview with performers and those who guide and support them, and validated psychological tests. Nothing should be taken for granted in this phase. For example, in our work with ballet dancers in Korea, psychological tests revealed that low coping skills was the key area related to injuries, not life stress or social support, which had been widely observed as the preeminent psychosocial variables in much sport injury research and in the dance research in the USA by Patterson et al. (1998).

3. Psychological tests can be useful, but they should be chosen carefully and used sparingly. Tests of psychosocial variables, such as life event stress, daily hassles, social support, and coping resources, should be context specific where possible. For example, we found that the dance stress measure we used, which had been employed in only one previous study, was more informative than the well-validated and widely used general life stress scale we had chosen. Also, reliable and valid tests that consist of subscales measuring more specific aspects of the psychosocial variables can help practitioners to identify more precisely the psychological issues that need to be addressed. For instance, the ACSI-28, modified for dance, identified peaking under pressure, goal setting/mental preparation, freedom from worry, and confidence and achievement motivation as the significant predictors of frequency of injury, and freedom from worry and confidence and achievement motivation as the significant predictors of duration of injury in ballet dancers.

4. Practitioners will rarely identify the specific stressors that need to be addressed in their intervention work, solely on the basis of psychological tests. To seek out those aspects of individuals and their environments that create stress, practitioners should use observation and interview techniques. For example, although freedom from worry was a key factor in the frequency and duration of injury experienced by ballet dancers in Korea, information concerning what the dancers were worrying about is not evident in their responses to the ACSI-28. We found that worrying about factors like the unpleasant things that the dance director would and did say to them, having to compete with their closest colleagues and friends for lead roles, and maintaining the ballet dancer's body shape were most widely reported in our interviews.

5. Practitioners should always look for confirmation of conclusions drawn from the use of one exploratory method from the results derived from other techniques. This is akin to the process of triangulation, which is a foundation of trustworthiness in qualitative research (Patton, 1990). For instance, when we asked dancers about their coping skills, we found that over 60% of the ways they handled stress represented dysfunctional coping. We also discovered that, unlike many elite athletes in western countries in North America and Europe, most of the elite ballet dancers we worked with in Korea had received no training in coping with stress. These findings supported the results gleaned from the ACSI-28, which indicated that elite ballet dancers in Korea had low coping skills.

6. Practitioners should collate and review the information they obtain from psychological tests, interviews, and observation. Then they can use that knowledge as the basis for

devising targeted interventions to reduce injury risk. For example, in our work with dancers, although the areas of peaking under pressure, coping with adversity, confidence and achievement motivation, concentration, and coachability were not outstanding in the ACSI-28 profile that resulted from the first study, the specific sources of stress identified in the interviews indicated that these were the priority areas to address in the targeted intervention. In this way, the interviews moderated ACSI-28 findings in determining the elements of the targeted intervention.

7. In developing interventions practitioners should take into account the modes of delivery that are most fitting for the material to be delivered and the outcomes that the practitioners intend, as well as using techniques that they are confident will suit the performers. In developing the targeted intervention we developed for ballet dancers in Korea, we were aware, for example, that imagery has been shown to enhance confidence and motivation and can be used to reinforce the attainment of goals (Morris, Spittle, & Watt, 2005).

8. Practitioners must monitor the level of adherence of performers to the intervention that the practitioners devise for them. Through the development of rapport and an explanation of the expected benefits of the intervention, practitioners would expect to encourage adherence to the intervention, which will usually depend on the performers undertaking substantial amounts of practice on their own. If, however, performers do not practice very much, it is unlikely that the intervention will have a great deal of impact. Practitioners can take action to increase adherence, if they know that performers are not following instructions about practice. Logs or diaries can be used to check levels of adherence periodically. In research, like the interventions examined in the third study with ballet dancers in Korea, it is essential that levels of adherence are checked, for the same reason as in practice, namely that we could have attributed the absence of any effect to the intervention being ineffective, when it was actually a result of performers not practicing. We used an adherence diary, which dancers completed every time they had done a session of their intervention. We pre-determined that anyone whose adherence level was below 60% would be excluded from the study. In fact, every dancer maintained a level of adherence above 60%. The average across the two intervention conditions was actually 82.5%.

9. Practitioners should monitor the effectiveness of their interventions for changing the psychosocial variables that are being targeted, that is, they should not just wait to see if injuries are reduced. This is because it is possible that the intervention is not changing the psychosocial variables in the ways that were expected. If that is the case, then no effect on injury can be anticipated. This is the equivalent of the manipulation check that we included in our intervention study. By measuring coping skills before and again after the intervention, we were able to show that, as we expected, our Autogenic Training intervention increased dancers' reports of peaking under pressure after that intervention more than the control condition, whereas none of the other coping skills were shown to increase. The targeted intervention, on the other hand, as well as showing at least equivalent increases in peaking under pressure (not surprising because it also included an Autogenic Training component), showed increases in participants'

scores on coping with adversity, confidence and achievement motivation, concentration, and coachability.

10. Practitioners must monitor the impact of their interventions on injury occurrence. Given that the interventions are designed to reduce psychosocial stress, thus, lowering muscle tension and making people less distractible, based on the Andersen and Williams (1988) model, we would expect a reduction in the number of injuries that occur. If there is no such reduction, then it is not worth the effort of continuing to practice that intervention as an injury prevention strategy. One difficulty of doing applied work and research in the area of injury to people who perform physically is that it usually takes a substantial period of time to gather enough information to determine whether injuries have dropped or not. There is no substitute for the time needed to collect sufficient data, although variations in the frequency of injuries between sports has meant that researchers have often studied contact sports, like football, and high risk activities, such as gymnastics, where the frequency of injuries is higher than in low-risk, noncontact sports like badminton or swimming. Even compared with patterns in sport, injuries occur frequently in dance, largely through overuse, but a problem in doing research with dancers is that they often fail to report this kind of injury, continuing to practice until the injury deteriorates so much that they cannot perform. In our intervention study with ballet dancers in Korea, we hope we developed sufficient rapport to minimize this reporting problem. We did find reduction in the frequency and the duration of injury for the dancers in the targeted intervention condition, compared to those in the Autogenic Training intervention and the control condition, but that was after 8 months of injury monitoring.

Although the recommendations in this section are based on the Andersen and Williams (1988) model of psychosocial stress and injury and they are consistent with much of the research that has examined aspects of the model, ultimately, they are derived from one series of three studies. Thus, they must be viewed with some caution. We encourage other researchers to follow our lead by studying the psychosocial factors underpinning injury in other specific contexts and then devising and testing interventions based on the knowledge that emerges from the in-depth scrutiny of that context.

Summary

In this chapter, we have argued that substantial support has now accumulated for the relationship between psychosocial variables, such as life stress, daily hassles, social support, and coping skills, and the occurrence of injury in physical performance activities such as sport and dance. We observed that the volume of research confirming parts of the model is not matched by research testing the effectiveness of interventions based on the model. More particularly, we proposed that research should examine the key psychosocial variables in specific contexts so that interventions can be devised that target those psychological factors that have the greatest influence for performers in that context. We then reported a series of three studies we conducted on the context of ballet in Korea. This series of studies culminated in an intervention study in which we compared the impact of a targeted intervention, focused on developing coping skills to manage stressors prevalent in that context, with a standard stress management technique, Autogenic Training, and a control condition. We found that adherence was high in both interventions, the targeted intervention did enhance coping skills more than AT, and that frequency and duration of injuries was lower among performers in the targeted intervention than in the other conditions, over the next 9 months. We then made some recommendations for practitioners on the basis of our experience in that research program. At the end of the final section, we acknowledged that our recommendations were based only directly on the series of three studies we conducted, although some support can be argued from the model and from other research testing it. We called for further research of the sort we have conducted, where specific psychosocial issues are identified and used to develop interventions, which are then compared to more general stress management techniques to test their effectiveness in the prevention of injuries in performance activities. We acknowledge that this kind of research requires patience and perseverance because of the length of time that injuries must be monitored in most activities to get sufficient numbers for effects to become evident. It is our contention that, although research refining the role of specific variables still has a place, the relationship between the three classes of psychosocial variable and stress and injury is now well established. Practitioners need a larger evidence base for the use of targeted interventions in injury prevention. Thus, priority should shift to research on the impact of interventions designed to reduce the occurrence of injuries. We look forward to seeing a growth in this kind of research, and we hope that practitioners can see some useful advice in the story told and the argument unfolded in this chapter.

References

Andersen, M. B., & Williams, J. M. (1988). A model of stress and athletic injury: Prediction and prevention. *Journal of Sport & Exercise Psychology, 10*, 294-306.

Andersen, M. B., & Williams, J. M. (1999). Athletic injury, psychosocial factors and perceptual changes during stress. *Journal of Sports Sciences, 17*, 735-741.

Bhum, D. J., Morris, T., & Andersen, M. B. (1998, August). *Stress, stress management, and visual attention.* Paper presented at the 24th International Congress of Applied Psychology, San Francisco.

Blackwell, B., & McCullagh, P. (1990). The relationship of athletic injury to life stress, competitive anxiety and coping resources. *Athletic Training, 25*, 23-27.

Bond, J. W., Miller, B. P., & Chrisfield, P. M. (1988). Psychological prediction of injury in elite swimmers. *International Journal of Sports Medicine, 9*, 345-348.

Bowling, A. (1989). Injuries to dancers: Prevalence, treatment, and perceptions of causes. *British Medical Journal, 298*(6675), 731-734.

Bramwell, S. T., Masuda, M., Wagner, N. N., & Holmes, T. H. (1975). Psychosocial factors in athletic injuries: Development and application of the Social and Athletic Readjustment Rating Scale (SARRS). *Journal of Human Stress, 1*(2), 6-20.

Bronner, S., & Brownstein, B. (1997). Profile of dance injuries in a Broadway show: A discussion of issues in dance medicine epidemiology. *The Journal of Orthopaedic & Sports Physical Therapy, 26*, 87-94.

Coddington, R. D., & Troxell, J. R. (1980). The effect of emotional factors on football injury rates - A pilot study. *Journal of Human Stress, 6*(4), 3-5.

Compas, B. E., Davis, G. E., Forsythe, C. J., & Wagner, B. M. (1987). Assessment of major and daily stressful events during adolescence: The Adolescent Perceived Events Scale. *Journal of Consulting and Clinical Psychology, 55*, 534-541.

Cupal, D. D. (1998). Psychological interventions in sport injury prevention and rehabilitation. *Journal of Applied Sport Psychology, 10*, 103-123.

Davis, J. O. (1991). Sports injuries and stress management: An opportunity for research. *The Sport Psychologist, 5,* 175-182.

Fawkner, H. J., McMurrary, N. E., & Summers, R. J. (1999). Athletic injury and minor life events: A prospective study. *Journal of Science and Medicine in Sport, 2,* 117-124.

Finch, C., Valuri, G., & Ozanne-Smith, J. (1998). Sport and active recreation injuries in Australia: Evidence from emergency department presentations. *British Journal of Sports Medicine, 32,* 220-225.

Garrick, J. G., & Requa, R. K. (1993). Ballet injuries: An analysis of epidemiology and financial outcome. *American Journal of Sports Medicine, 21,* 586-590.

Hamilton, L. H. (1999). A psychological profile of the adolescent dancer. *Journal of Dance Medicine & Science, 3,* 48-50.

Hamilton, L. H., Hamilton, W. G., Meltzer, J. D., Marshall, P., & Molnar, M. (1989). Personality, stress, and injuries in professional ballet dancers. *American Journal of Sports Medicine, 17,* 263-267.

Hanson, S. J., McCullagh, P., & Tonymon, P. (1992). The relationship of personality characteristics, life stress, and coping resources to athletic injury. *Journal of Sport & Exercise Psychology, 14,* 262-272.

Hardaker, W. T. J., Erickson, L., & Myers, M. (1986). The pathogenesis of dance injury. In C. G. Shell (Ed.), *The dancer as athlete: The 1984 Olympic scientific congress proceedings* (Vol. 8, pp. 11-29). Champaign, IL: Human Kinetics.

Hardy, C. J., O'Connor, K. A., & Geisler, P. R. (1990). The role of gender and social support in the life stress injury relationship [Abstract]. *Proceedings of the Association for the Advancement of Applied Sport Psychology, fifth annual conference,* 51.

Holmes, T. H. (1970). Psychological screening. In *Football injuries: Papers presented at a workshop* (pp. 211-214). Washington, DC: National Academy of Sciences.

Kadel, N. J., & Teitz, C. C. (1992). Stress fractures in ballet dancers. *American Journal of Sports Medicine, 20,* 445-449.

Kerr, G., & Goss, J. (1996). The effects of s stress management program on injuries and stress levels. *Journal of Applied Sport Psychology, 8,* 109-117.

Kerr, G., & Minden, H. (1988). Psychological factors related to the occurrence of athletic injuries. *Journal of Sport & Exercise Psychology, 10,* 167-173.

Kim, E. (2001). *A study on social factors and dance injury of dancers.* Unpublished master's thesis, Chosun University, Gwangju.

Kim, E., & Park, J. (2004). The relationship between the participation in dancing, stress coping, psychological factors and dance injury. *Korea Sport Research, 15,* 199-208.

Kim, J., & Heo, J. (2003). The influence of dance injury on dance stage anxiety of ballet majoring students. *The Korean Journal of Physical Education, 42,* 643-650.

Kim, K. (1997). *A study on principles and applications of stretching in dance.* Unpublished master's thesis, Hanyang University, Seoul.

Kolt, G. S., Hume, P. A., Smith, P., & Williams, M. M. (2004). Effects of a stress management program on injury and stress of competitive gymnasts. *Perceptual and Motor Skills, 99,* 195-207.

Krasnow, D., Mainwaring, L., & Kerr, G. (1999). Injury, stress, and perfectionism in young dancers and gymnasts. *Journal of Dance Medicine & Science, 3,* 51-58.

Lee, M. (1998). *Relationship between professional dancer's life stress and dance injury with the intervening variable of coping skill and social support.* Unpublished master's thesis, Ewha Womans University, Seoul.

Liederbach, M., & Compagno, J. M. (2001). Psychological aspects of fatigue-related injuries in dancers. *Journal of Dance Medicine & Science, 5,* 116-120.

Liederbach, M., Gleim, G. W., & Nicholas, J. A. (1994). Physiologic and psychological measurements of performance stress and onset of injuries in professional ballet dancers. *Medical Problems of Performing Artists, 9,* 10-14.

Maddison, R., & Prapavessis, H. (2005). A psychological approach to the prediction and prevention of athletic injury. *Journal of Sport & Exercise Psychology, 27,* 289-311.

Mainwaring, L. M., Kerr, G., & Krasnow, D. (1993). Psychological correlates of dance injuries. *Medical Problems of Performing Artists, 8,* 3-6.

Mainwaring, L. M., Krasnow, D., & Kerr, G. (2001). And the dance goes on: Psychological impact of injury. *Journal of Dance Medicine & Science, 5,* 105-115.

Morris, T. (1997). *Psychological Skills Training in Sport: An Overview.* BASS Monograph No 3 (Revised Edition), Leeds, UK: British Association of Sports Sciences.

Morris, T., Spittle, M., & Watt, T. (2005). *Imagery in sport: The complete picture.* Champaign, IL: Human Kinetics.

Morris, T., & Thomas, P. (2004) Applied sport psychology. In T. Morris & J. Summers (Eds.) *Sport psychology: Theories, applications and issues (2nd ed.)* (pp. 236-277). Brisbane: Wiley.

Noh, Y. (1998). *The effect of life stress of dancers on dance injury.* Unpublished master's thesis, Chonnam National University, Gwangju.

Noh, Y., & Morris, T. (2004). Designing research-based interventions for the prevention of injury in dance. *Medical Problems of Performing Artists. 19,* 88-95.

Noh, Y., Morris, T., & Andersen, M. (2003). Psychosocial stress and injury in dance. *The Journal of Physical Education, Recreation & Dance, 74(4),* 36-40.

Noh, Y., Morris, T., & Andersen, M. (2005). Psychosocial factors and ballet injuries. *International Journal of Sport and Exercise Psychology, 3(1),* 7-25.

Noh, Y., Morris, T., & Andersen, M. (under review). Psychological intervention programs for reduction of injury in ballet dancer. *Research in Sports Medicine: An International Journal.*

Passer, M. W., & Seese, M. D. (1983). Life stress and athletic injury: Examination of positive versus negative events and three moderator variables. *Journal of Human Stress, 9(4),* 11-16.

Patterson, E. L., Smith, R. E., Everett, J. J., & Ptacek, J. T. (1998). Psychosocial factors as predictors of ballet injuries: Interactive effects of life stress and social support. *Journal of Sport Behavior, 21,* 101-112.

Patton, M. Q. (1990). *Qualitative evaluation and research methods* (2nd ed.). Newbury Park, CA: Sage.

Petrie, T. A. (1992). Psychosocial antecedents of athletic injury: The effects of life stress and social support on female collegiate gymnasts. *Behavioral Medicine, 18,* 127-138.

Petrie, T. A. (1993a). Coping skills, competitive trait anxiety, and playing status: Moderating effects on the life stress-injury relationship. *Journal of Sport & Exercise Psychology, 15,* 261-274.

Petrie, T. A. (1993b). The moderating effects of social support and playing status on the life stress-injury relationship. *Journal of Applied Sport Psychology, 5,* 1-16.

Petrie, T. A., & Perna, F. (2004). Psychology of injury: Theory, research, and practice. In T. Morris & J. Summers (Eds.), *Sport psychology: Theory, applications, and issues* (2nd ed., pp. 547-571). Brisbane, Australia: Wiley.

Ruibal, S. (2005, 05/12). Sports and exercise can put the hurt on. *USA TODAY,* p. 11.

Ryan, A. J., & Stephens, R. E. (Eds.) (1989). *The healthy dancer: Dance medicine for dancers: Selected articles from dance medicine: A comprehensive guide.* London: Dance Books.

Schultz, J., & Luthe, W. (1959). *Autogenic training: A psychophysiological approach to psychotherapy.* New York: Grune and Stratton.

Smith, R. E., Ptacek, J. T., & Patterson, E. (2000). Moderator effects of cognitive and somatic trait anxiety on the relation between life stress and physical injuries. *Anxiety, Stress, and Coping, 13,* 269-288.

Smith, R. E., Ptacek, J. T., & Smoll, F. L. (1992). Sensation seeking, stress, and adolescent injuries: A test of stress-buffering, risk-taking, and coping skills hypotheses. *Journal of Personality and Social Psychology, 62,* 1016-1024.

Smith, R. E., Schutz, R. W., Smoll, F. L., & Ptacek, J. T. (1995). Development and validation of a multidimensional measure of sport-specific psychological skills: The Athletic Coping Skills Inventory-28. *Journal of Sport & Exercise Psychology, 17,* 379-398.

Smith, R. E., Smoll, F. L., & Ptacek, J. T. (1990). Conjunctive moderator variables in vulnerability and resiliency research: Life stress, social support and coping skills, and adolescent sport injuries. *Journal of Personality and Social Psychology, 58,* 360-370.

Smith, R. E., Smoll, F. L., & Schutz, R. W. (1990). Measurement and correlates of sport-specific cognitive and somatic trait anxiety: The Sport Anxiety Scale. *Anxiety Research, 2,* 263-280.

Solomon, R., Micheli, L. J., Solomon, J., & Kelley, T. (1995). The "cost" of injuries in a professional ballet company: Anatomy of a season. *Medical Problems of Performing Artists, 10,* 3-10.

Stephens, R. E. (1989). The etiology of injuries in ballet. In A. J. Ryan & R. E. Stephens (Eds.), *The healthy dancer: Dance medicine for dancers: Selected articles from dance medicine: A comprehensive guide* (pp. 16-50). London: Dance Books.

Teitz, C. C. (1991). Gymnastic and dance athletes. In F. O. Mueller & A. J. Ryan (Eds.), *Prevention of athletic injuries: The role of the sports medicine team* (pp. 135-158). Philadelphia, PA: F. A. Davis.

Uitenbroek, D. G. (1996). Sports, exercise, and other causes of injuries: Results of a population survey. *Research Quarterly for Exercise and Sport, 67,* 380-385.

Weaver, N. L., Marshall, S. W., Spicer, R., Miller, T., Waller, A. E., & Mueller, F. O. (1999). Cost of athletic injuries in 12 North Carolina high school sports[Abstract]. *Medicine & Science in Sports & Exercise, 31*(Suppl.), S93.

Wiese-Bjornstahl, D., Smith, A., Shaffer, S., & Morrey, M. (1998) An integrated model of repsonse to sport injury: psychological and social dynamics. *Journal of Applied Sport Psychology, 10,* 46-69.

Williams, J. M., & Andersen, M. B. (1998). Psychosocial antecedents of sport injury: Review and critique of the stress and injury model. *Journal of Applied Sport Psychology, 10,* 5-25.

Preventing Sport Injuries: A Case for Psychology Intervention

Ralph Maddison
University of Auckland

Harry Prapavessis
University of Western Ontario

The role that psychology has to play in the prevention of sport injuries is discussed in this chapter. A brief discussion of pre-injury factors with a focus on theoretical perspectives for the prevention of injury is presented. This chapter will therefore focus on different applications of psychological based techniques to prevent athletic injury by providing an overview of the salient research of psychological interventions to prevent injury. Particular emphasis will be given to the impact of cognitive behavioral stress management interventions. Findings will be discussed and applied considerations given to the integration of psychology into injury prevention programs for sports.

Each year in the United States, an estimated 30 million children and adolescents participate in organized sports (Prevention CfDCa, 2003), and approximately 150 million adults participate in some type of nonworking-related physical activity (Conn, Annest, & Gilchrist, 2001). More sports-related nonfatal injuries are treated in hospital emergency departments than any other type of unintentional injury (Prevention CfDCa, 2003).

When one considers the imposing financial burden sporting- and recreation-related injuries place on society (Caine, Caine, & Linder, 1996) and the plethora of physical, social, and psychological implications for injured individuals (Evans & Hardy, 1995; A. M. Smith, 1996; Wiese-Bjornstal, Smith, Shaffer, & Morrey, 1998), then understanding the contribution of psychological factors in the prediction, prevention, and rehabilitation of sport-related injury warrants serious consideration. Indeed, sports medicine has traditionally focused on the physical factors that affect injury occurrence and rehabilitation, while the role psychological factors have in the prediction, prevention, and rehabilitation of sport-related injury has only emerged during the past 25 years (Brewer, 2001; Brewer, Andersen, & Van Raalte, 2001). The credibility of psycho-logical-based interventions to prevent injury is an area that is gaining greater research attention (Cupal, 1998).

In general, athletes still follow a course of injury prevention that concerns itself primarily with the physical aspects of injury (Cupal, 1998). These injury prevention programs typically focus on education to ensure adequate warm-up and stretching, correct alignment, adequate protective equipment, or safe footwear (Agre & Baxter, 1987; Bird, Waller, & Chalmers, 1995; Bird et al., 1998; Ekstrand & Gillquist, 1983; Petitpas & Danish, 1995). Moreover, some sports have investigated the nature of the game and playing conditions as a source of injury prevention (Chivers, Aldous, & Orchard, 2005; Orchard, Chivers, Aldous, Bennell, & Seward, 2005). Evolutions from this line of research have focused on rule changes, umpire involvement, etc. (Brunelle, Goulet, & Arguin, 2005).

The psychological dimensions of injury prevention are often overlooked, which is surprising considering the considerable research that has accumulated to implicate psychological and social factors (termed *psychosocial factors*) in the genesis of physical injuries (Bond, Miller, & Chrisfield, 1988; Bramwell, Masuda, Wagner, & Holmes, 1975; Coddington & Troxell, 1980; Crossman, 1985; Ford, Eklund, & Grove, 2000; Hanson, McCullagh, & Tonymon, 1992; C. J. Hardy, Richman, & Rosenfeld, 1991; C. J. Hardy & Riehl, 1988; L. Hardy, 1992; Junge, 2000; Kelley, 1990; Kerr & Fowler, 1988; Kerr & Minden, 1988; Passer & Seese, 1983; Petrie, 1992; R. E. Smith, Ptacek, & Smoll, 1992; Williams, Tonymon, & Wadsworth, 1986). The incorporation of psychosocial factors into understanding injury is important because of the effect that injury exerts on an athlete's psychological well-being, thereby directly influencing health, perform-ance, and the prevention of future injury (Heil, 1993).

To date, eight empirical injury prevention studies with a psychological foundation have been conducted (see Table 1). Hence, this field of research is still in its infancy with respect to understanding the interplay between psychological and physical vari-ables that contribute to the prevention of sport injury. The purpose of this paper is to

(a) provide an overview of the main theoretical models that have been used to guide psychological-based injury prevention research,

(b) critically review injury prevention research conducted to date,

(c) highlight and discuss important methodological issues for conducting future injury prevention research, and

(d) make recommendations for practice.

Theoretical/Conceptual Bases of Psychological Interventions to Prevent Injury

The focus of early research was on the effect major life event stress had on the predic-tion of athletic injury. For the most part, results from these early studies showed that injured athletes experienced greater life events or life stress in the preceding season (Holmes, 1970) compared to players who did not become injured (Bramwell et al., 1975; Coddington & Troxell, 1980; Cryan & Alles, 1983). These early studies provided important information about the role of psychosocial factors in injury, but were lim-

Table 1.

Psychological-based injury prevention intervention studies

Study	N	Participants	Intervention	Control group(s)	Method	Results	Statistical Comparison
DeWitt (1980)	12	Male Basketball players	Cognitive and biofeedback techniques	Yes	Quantitative/ Qualitative	Players self-reported noticeable decrease in the number of minor injuries	No
May & Brown (1989)	18	Olympic alpine skiers	Relaxation/ imagery/ counseling	No	Qualitative	Reduced injuries: increased self confidence and self-control	No
Schomer (1990)	10	Marathon runners	Attentional strategies	No	Qualitative	Facilitated heavy training without injury	No
Davis (1991)	21	Collegiate swimmers/ football players	Stress management	No	Quantitative	52% reduction in swimming injuries; 33% reduction in football injuries	No
Kerr & Goss (1996)	24	Elite gymnasts	Stress management	Yes	Qualitative/ Quantitative	Reduced injuries and stress levels	Yes
Perna, Antoni, Kumar, Cruess, & Schneiderman (2003)	34	Competitive rowers	Cognitive behavioral stress management	Yes	Quantitative	Reduced number of injury and illness days. Decreased cortisol and negative affect	Yes
Johnson, Ekengren, & Andersen (2005)	32	High injury-risk Swedish soccer players	Psychological skills training	Yes	Quantitative	Reduced number of injuries	Yes
Maddison & Prapavessis (2005)	48	High injury-risk New Zealand rugby players	Cognitive behavioral stress management	Yes	Quantitative	Reduced injury time missed: increased coping skills, decreased worry and concentration disruption	Yes

ited by an atheoretical approach and a singular focus on life stress. Therefore, a link between psychosocial variables and injury was not established (Petrie & Perna, 2004). As a result, Andersen and Williams (1988) developed a theoretical model that addressed these limitations and provided much of the direction for future research. This model and the revised Williams and Andersen (1998) stress injury model have been the most widely used theoretical frameworks for research into the prediction and prevention of athletic injury. (The diagrammed model is presented in Chapter 1.)

The core mechanism in this model is the stress response, a bidirectional relationship between athletes' cognitive appraisals of demands, consequences, and resources in the athletic situation and their physiological reactions (e.g., increased muscle tension) and attentional responses (e.g., increased distractibility, narrowing of the visual field). These variables may increase injury vulnerability by disrupting coordination and flexibility as well as interfering with the detection of important environmental cues.

Above the core of the model (e.g., stress response) are three major factors:
- personality
- history of stressors
- coping resources

which may operate alone or in combination to affect the stress response and, in turn, injury occurrence and severity. It is suggested through the model that these psychosocial variables influence how athletes respond under acutely stressful situations, but only the athlete's response itself directly affects injury susceptibility. In short, depending on the extent to which these psychosocial variables are present or absent, the athlete's stress responsivity is attenuated or exacerbated (Petrie & Perna, 2004). For example, it has been hypothesized that athletes with many life stressors, few coping resources, and certain personality dispositions (e.g., high competitive anxiety), will, when placed in a stressful situation, demonstrate a greater stress response (e.g., generalized muscle tension and disruption in attentional processes), and hence, be more at risk of injury. Athletes with this high-risk profile will have a greater likelihood of injury compared to those with the opposite profile (Andersen & Williams, 1988; Williams & Andersen, 1998).

The final component of the model refers to interventions. It is suggested that in order to prevent injuries caused by stress, the intervention should focus on
(a) altering the cognitive appraisal of potentially stressful events, and
(b) modifying the physiological and attentional aspects of the stress response (for a complete review see Williams, 2001).

It is important to acknowledge that other researchers (Perna & McDowell, 1995; Perna, Schneiderman, & LaPerriere, 1997) have characterized stress responses more broadly. Perna and colleagues argued that to fully understand the stress response, one must consider its effects on cognitive, emotional, behavioral, and physiological systems (Petrie & Perna, 2004). In addition to a wider range of stress responses, this conceptualization expands on the Andersen and Williams (1988) model in two distinct ways:
- First, stress responses are posited to be influenced not only by psychosocial factors, but also by their interaction with the extended and strenuous training performed by athletes. A central component of this conceptualization is that over and above the independent effects on health, psychosocially distressed derived (dis)stress may combine with exercise-related stress to widen the window of susceptibility to injury and illness (Petrie & Perna, 2004).
- Second, this conceptualization extends past psychosocial stress-induced injury outcomes to include other undesirable health outcomes such as physical symp-

toms, infections, and training maladaption. Petrie and Perna included multiple health outcomes because "each is affected by psychosocial stress and, ultimately, each affects athletes' availability to compete. Also, a complete understanding of potentially predisposing physiological factors to injury requires an understanding of the physiological systems and how stress may alter the normal functioning of these systems" (p.557).

Psychological Based Interventions to Reduce Injury Vulnerability: A Review

As previously mentioned, very few studies have specifically examined the role of psychological-based interventions in the prevention of injury (see Table 1). In an early review, Cupal (1998) argued that there was a paucity of empirical studies that have included control groups, standardized prevention protocols, and/or specific injury orientations, which blurred the issue of how significantly psychological interventions contributed to the prevention of injury. Although research has improved in the ensuing eight years, some of these observations may still hold true. This next section will review eight studies that have used a psychological-based approach to prevent injury.

In an early study, DeWitt (1980) exposed basketball and football players to an intervention aimed at stress reduction and performance enhancement using both cognitive and biofeedback techniques. Although no objective assessment of injury was used, players reported a notable decrease in minor injuries as a result of participating in the intervention. Utilizing a different approach and not specifically an injury prevention study, Murphy (1988) reported on the effectiveness of an intervention delivered at the 1987 US Olympic Festival. Specifically, relaxation sessions were provided after every workout for 12 athletes, 7 of whom were injured (2 seriously). Pain control techniques were also introduced for some individuals. Having participated in this intervention, all 12 athletes were able to compete at the festival. These early studies provided some initial anecdotal evidence for the inclusion of psychological-based interventions in the prediction of injury.

May and Brown (1989), conducted an intervention study and delivered a number of techniques such as attention control, imagery, and other mental skills to individuals, pairs, and groups of US alpine skiers at the Calgary Olympics. Skiers were also exposed to team building, relationship orientations, communication, and crisis interventions. The intervention was associated with a reduction in injuries, enhanced self-control, and an increase in self-confidence.

In a different approach, Schomer (1990) examined the role of associative versus disassociate strategies among 10 marathon runners. The intervention involved shaping associative thought processes during a 5-week training period using audiotapes of attentional strategies with a resulting convergence of increased associative thinking and perceptions of increased training effort. Athletes reported an ability to optimize training intensity without increasing injuries.

Davis (1991) introduced relaxation and guided imagery of sport skills to two cohorts, one with swimmers and the other with football players. Comparing injury rates after the intervention with previous archival data, Davis found a 52% reduction in injury rates in the swimmers and a 33% reduction in serious injuries for football players.

Despite the support provided by the preceding studies for the role of psychological interventions having an effect on injuries, methodological concerns exist. For example, none of the previous research utilized a randomized control design, nor was the assessment of injury prospective. Only a handful of studies (Johnson, Ekengren, & Andersen, 2005; Kerr & Goss, 1996; Maddison & Prapavessis, 2005; Perna, Antoni, Baum, Cordon, & Schneiderman, 2003) have used a randomized controlled methodology to offer experimental support for an intervention effect on injury and/or a reduction in life-stress—all using cognitive behavioral stress management (CBSM) interventions.

In one of the first studies to use a RCT design, Kerr and Goss (1996) examined the effect of a CBSM intervention based upon Meichenbaum's (1985) stress inoculation training in the reduction of life stress and injury among a group of national and international gymnasts. Participants were matched into pairs according to gender, age, and performance before being allocated to an intervention versus a control condition. Bimonthly sessions over an 8-month period addressed a plethora of psychological skills including thought stoppage, cognitive restructuring, relaxation, and imagery. At the end of the study participants in the intervention group reported significantly less negative athletic stress, less total negative stress, and a trend to more positive athletic stress toward the end of the program compared to the control group. Although a significant treatment effect occurred for decreased life stress, a nonsignificant (albeit robust $d = .67$) reduction was found for injury reduction. Kerr and Goss's (1996) explanation for the nonsignificant findings related to the late introduction (half-way) of relaxation and distraction control skills into the program. However, Andersen and Stoove (1998) argued that the small number of participants in each group and the resultant lack of power was the cause.

In a later study, Perna et al. (2003) also provided evidence supporting the efficacy of CBSM intervention in reducing injury and illness among collegiate athletes. Thirty-four competitive rowers were randomized to participate in the CBSM intervention using a stress inoculation training (SIT) format. For most of the intervention, athletes met for 35–40 minutes, twice a week for 3 weeks. Compared to the control group, athletes in the CBSM condition experienced significant reductions in the number of injury and illness days. In addition, the intervention was related to decreased cortisol and negative affect (indices of exercise training maladaption).

A criticism that might be directed at these previous studies is that the interventions were applied to a general population of athletes rather than to athletes with an "at-risk" psychological profile for injury. According to the Andersen and Williams' model, athletes most at risk of injury are those with high life stress, low coping resources, and high competitive anxiety. Two recent studies have addressed this limitation. The first by Johnson et al. (2005) examined the effect of a psychological-based injury prevention program to lower the incidence of injury among Swedish soccer players with at-risk psychological profiles. The psychological skills training intervention focused on
(a) somatic and cognitive relaxation,
(b) stress management skills,

(c) goal-setting skills,

(d) attribution and self-confidence training, and

(e) identification and discussion about critical incidents related to sport participation and everyday life situations,

and was applied over six to eight sessions. Compared to a control group, the intervention was found to be effective in reducing the number of injuries.

Most recently, Maddison and Prapavessis (2005) randomly assigned 48 New Zealand rugby players with a high-risk psychological profile for injury to either a CBSM intervention or a noncontact control condition. Participants completed psychological measures of coping and competitive anxiety at the beginning and end of the playing season. Results showed that those in the intervention condition reported missing less time due to injury compared to their nonintervention counterparts. Although statistically nonsignificant, a similar pattern of results was found for number of injuries. For the psychological variables, a significant condition effect was found for total coping resources and worry, whereas a nonsignificant trend for concentration disruption was also reported. Overall the intervention group reported a sharp increase in total coping resources and a decrease in worry and concentration disruption following the intervention. Unlike Perna et al. (2003), no support for mediation was found.

Taken together, these studies support the effect of a cognitive behavioral intervention to reduce injuries, and also highlight that athletes can be taught a variety of stress management skills. Furthermore, the data suggest that helping athletes acquire these techniques may help them avoid injury or better adapt to their training. Either of these outcomes could be useful in helping athletes improve their performance as well as their health (Petrie & Perna, 2004).

Methodological Issues for Future Injury Prevention Research

Measurement

An important issue relates to the assessment of injury. Both the original Andersen and Williams (1988) and the revised Williams and Andersen (1998) models propose a relationship between the stress response and injury occurrence, but do not specifically refer to time missed as an injury outcome. Andersen and Williams (1999) have also suggested a need to collect injury data that reflects minor as well as major injuries, including injury that requires modification to play (such as wearing protective head gear and strapping, etc.). They argued that collecting this type of injury data is more in line with the prediction of their model. Although we acknowledge the recommendation of Andersen and Williams with respect to injury occurrence, their assessment of injury is not the only one endorsed in the literature. Time missed has frequently been used as an injury variable (Petrie, 1992; R. E. Smith, Smoll, & Ptacek, 1990). For example, the National Athletic Injury Reporting System (Coddington & Troxell, 1980) uses number of days missed from athletic participation as an indication of injury severity. More recently, Hodgson-Phillips (Hodgson Phillips, 2000) recommended all injuries be recorded, including transient injury—that is, injuries that required treatment but did not necessarily result in time missed. Hodgson-Phillips also suggested that time lost from participation must be recorded accurately, using both training and game/competitive participation data. She suggested that failure to do so would see the loss of valuable data and the failure to portray the true injury picture of the sport. Injury occurrence and time missed are inexorably linked, thus both methods need to be considered when assessing this variable (injury).

Another related issue recently highlighted by Williams (2001) is that previous studies have not distinguished between the recurrence of an old injury and the occurrence of a new injury at a new site. Researchers need to delineate whether injuries sustained are an exacerbation of an existing injury or are sustained as a result of a new event. This point, although subtle, has implications for the effectiveness of injury prevention programs. For example, a psychological-based intervention is less likely to be effective in the prevention of injuries that are due to exacerbation of an existing condition. Injury researchers need to consider this important point in subsequent studies.

Statistics

An important methodological issue that warrants consideration is the analysis of injury data, because these data will always be skewed—some scores will equal zero (no injury). Despite applying transformation techniques, skewed data will still exist. Therefore, to overcome this problem some researchers have dichotomized injury into a binary variable (injured versus noninjured) (Rogers & Landers, 2005). This approach does not necessarily reflect the frequency of occurrence, nor does it provide any indication of injury severity. Thus, researchers need to consider a combination approach that indicates whether an athlete was injured (occurrence) and the severity of that injury (time missed). Alternate approaches to deal with these potentially skewed data are also needed. Consideration should therefore be given to the utilization of nonparametric statistical approaches, which are not subject to the same assumptions of normal distribution as parametric statistics (Johnson et al., 2005).

Finally, researchers need to consider the issue of clinical versus statistical significance. Specifically, the nonequivalence of statistical significance and clinical importance has long been recognized, but confusion over interpretation continues (Altman & Bland, 1995). A statistically significant difference may be real but not necessarily important. On the other hand, if a difference is not statistically different, it may be real and, furthermore, important (Bland, 2000; Hopkins, 2001).

Design of Injury-Prevention Interventions

What should intervention protocols look like and how should they be administered? Most of the prevention studies have incorporated multi-component intervention programs, thus there is limited information regarding the contribution of the individual components of these interventions. Moreover, most injury prevention studies have not used or presented standardized protocols.

The Williams and Andersen (1998) model suggests that in order to prevent injuries caused by stress, an intervention should focus on
(a) altering the cognitive appraisal of potentially stressful events, and
(b) modifying the physiological and attentional aspects of the stress response. A broader and probably more holistic approach is offered by Perna et al. (1998), who sug-

gested that interventions that facilitate health can prevent injury, illness, and in turn enhance performance. Perna et al. (1998) also suggested that if athletes are to achieve their performance goals, they require the ability to undertake many weeks and months of consistent training, without interruption by injury and illness. At times, increased training loads (e.g., high-intensity or prolonged bouts of exercise) are required to increase physical functioning. Therefore, arming athletes with strategies and skills to facilitate adaptation to exercise training and enhance recovery should be the focus of injury prevention interventions (Perna et al., 1998).

Components of an Intervention

Because of the importance of the stress-injury relationship, researchers have investigated the effect of various psychological intervention techniques on the stress response, concentration, and/or reducing injury. These interventions include the use of

- biofeedback (DeWitt, 1980),
- imagery, (Cupal & Brewer, 2001; Davis, 1991),
- relaxation (Davis, 1991),
- autogenics (Williams & Harris, 1998),
- various concentration techniques (Schmid & Peper, 1998; Schomer, 1990), and
- cognitive behavioral stress management training (e.g., stress inoculation training)

(Kerr & Goss, 1996; Mace & Carroll, 1985, 1989; Perna et al., 2003).

Specifically, a number of authors have provided detailed description of various relaxation techniques (progressive relaxation, meditation, autogenics, and breathing exercises) to decrease physiological arousal (Sherman & Poczwardowski, 2000; Zinsser, Bunker, & Williams, 2001). Schmid and Peper (1998) also provide a description of various concentration training strategies to increase focus and decrease distractibility.

Stress inoculation training (Meichenbaum, 1985), a set of techniques originally developed in clinical psychology for ameliorating the stress response, has also been found to be effective within the sporting context. Stress inoculation training involves three overlapping stages:

- conceptualization
- skills acquisition and rehearsal
- skill application

Mace and Carroll (1985) and Mace, Carroll, and Eastman (1986) found that participants given stress inoculation training had significantly lower psychological stress and anxiety levels before abseiling compared to a control condition receiving no such intervention. In a later study, Mace and Carroll (1989) also found that novice females exposed to stress inoculation techniques reported significantly less stress and performed better than a control group during a gymnastic test. Using a similar technique—**cognitive-affective stress management training** (SMT), Crocker, Alderman, Murray, and Smith (1988) found that the SMT intervention group reported significantly less negative thoughts in response to videotaped stressors and superior performance compared to the non-SMT control condition. However, no group differences were found for state or trait anxiety.

Interventions employing cognitive behavioral strategies such as relaxation training, imagery, and cognitive restructuring have also been effective in buffering psychological distress and immune function (Antoni et al., 1991; Esterling, Antoni, Fletcher, Margulies, & Schneiderman, 1994; Green, Green, & Santoro, 1988). Similar type interventions incorporating guided imagery and relaxation have been effective in decreasing stress and improving functional outcomes in injured athletes (Cupal & Brewer, 2001).

Practical Implications

Williams (2001) suggested that injuries contributed to by psychological variables need to be recognized as avoidable rather than unavoidable events. At a minimum, coaches, trainers, and so on need to be educated about the psychological factors that may contribute to injury so that these can be highlighted for possible prevention programs. Thus, providing athletes with a heightened awareness of factors in sport and everyday life that cause stress may be an important initial stage in the prevention of injury.

With respect to more structured psychological intervention prevention programs, sports might consider introducing group or individual sessions during a preseason period. These programs might consider incorporating the components of a CBSM program (relaxation, imagery, cognitive restructuring, etc.). Alternatively, psychological skills training programs might be incorporated with a sport injury prevention focus. The worst consequence of implementing such programs is that the athlete may merely experience performance benefits (Williams, 2001). Additional benefits of injury prevention programs may be realized by identifying players with an at-risk psychological profile for injury, which may take the form of a psychosocial risk assessment as part of the preseason physical exam.

Other important factors that might be considered in any injury prevention program might be to include components that might lessen the impact of preinjury factors. For example, an intervention may focus on improving coping resources. Coping, which refers both to the various coping skills and to the amount of social support an individual possesses, might be augmented by the introduction of coping skills or by promoting social support individually (e.g., coach-athlete relationship) or in a team environment (e.g., group cohesion). Richman, Hardy, Rosenfeld, and Callanan (1989) have offered various strategies for enhancing social support networks in sport. These were based on the six types of social support that individuals need to obtain from their environment:

(a) listening—characterized by active listening, that is, listening without giving advice or making judgments;

(b) emotional support—characterized by the willingness to be on the recipient's side in difficult situation, even if the supporter is not in total agreement with him or her;

(c) emotional challenge—characterized by challenges and questions to the recipient concerning whether she or he is doing her or his best to fulfill goals and overcome obstacles;

(d) shared social reality—characterized by the sharing of similar experiences, priorities, values, and views (the supporter serves as a social reality "touchstone" with whom perceptions of the social context are checked);

(e) technical appreciation—characterized by the acknowledgement of task effort;

(f) technical challenge—characterized by questions and challenge that keep the recipient from being stale or superficial by stretching, encouraging, and leading him or her to greater creativity, excitement, and involvement. (p. 150-152)

In their recommendations Richman et al. (1989) suggested that typical pep-talks and brief heart-to-heart talks are not sufficient to provide adequate social support; individuals need to extend their social support network by seeking appropriate support at different levels. Social support needs to be an essential part of the sport personnel's program. Moreover, social support needs to be seen as an integral part of any ongoing preventive program and should be purposely developed and nurtured in the sporting environment.

Prevention programs need to also incorporate strategies to improve coping skills. Interventions focused on developing and enhancing psychological skills that are known to influence performance, such as

- systematic goal setting (Gould, 2001),
- concentration, (Nideffer, 1989),
- imagery (Ievleva & Orlick, 1991), and
- stress management (Smith, 1989),

need to be integrated as part of an athlete's repertoire. These skills may not only help athletes cope more effectively with the demands of the athletic environment (Smith, 1999) and are effective in the prevention of injury (Johnson et al. 2005; Maddison & Prapavessis, 2005), but may also have an impact on athletes' ability to cope should they incur an injury (Albinson & Petrie, 2003).

Summary

This chapter has highlighted the importance of psychosocial factors in the prevention of athletic injury. Specifically, psychological frameworks such as the Williams and Andersen revised stress-injury model have informed injury prediction research and have provided a foundation for prevention empirical investigation. Petrie and Perna have extended the stress response model to consider its effects on cognitive, emotional, behavioral, and physiological systems.

Theoretically grounded randomized trials using cognitive behavioral stress management interventions have been found to be effective at reducing injuries. Based on these data we encourage athletes, coaches, trainers, and other sports personnel to incorporate psychological based interventions not only to improve performance, but also to help in the reduction of sport-related injury.

References

Agre, J. C., & Baxter, T. L. (1987). Musculoskeletal profile of male collegiate soccer players. *Archives of Physical Medicine and Rehabilitation, 68*, 147-150.

Altman, D. G., & Bland, J. N. (1995). Absence of evidence is not evidence of absence. *British Medical Journal, 311*, 485.

Andersen, M. B. (1988). *Psychosocial factors and changes in peripheral vision, muscle tension, and fine motor skills during stress.* Unpublished Dissertation Abstracts International, University of Arizona at Tucson.

Andersen, M. B., & Stoove, M. A. (1998). The sanctity of *p*< .05 obfuscates good stuff: A comment on Kerr and Goss. *Journal of Applied Sport Psychology, 10*, 168-173.

Andersen, M. B., & Williams, J. M. (1988). A model of stress and athletic injury: Prediction and prevention. *Journal of Sport & Exercise Psychology, 10*, 294-306.

Andersen, M. B., & Williams, J. M. (1999). Athletic injury, psychosocial factors and perceptual changes during stress. *Journal of Sport Sciences, 17*, 735-741.

Antoni, M., Baggett, L., G, I., August, S., LaPerriere, A., Klimas, N., et al. (1991). Cognitive behavioral stress management intervention buffers distress responses and elevates immunological markers following notification of HIV-1 seropositivity. *Journal of Consulting and Clinical Psychology, 59*(6), 906-915.

Bird, Y. N., Waller, A. E., & Chalmers, D. J. (1995). The rugby injury and performance project: Playing experience and demographic characteristics. *Journal of Physical Education New Zealand, 28*(2), 12-16.

Bird, Y. N., Wauer, A. E., Marshall, S. W., Alsop, J. C., Chalmers, D. J., & Gerrard, D. F. (1998). The New Zealand Rugby Injury and Performance Project: V. Epidemiology of a season of rugby injury. *British Journal of Sports Medicine 32*, 319-325.

Bland, M. (2000). *An introduction to medical statistics* (3rd ed.). Oxford: Oxford University Press.

Bond, J. W., Miller, B. P., & Chrisfield, P. M. (1988). Psychological prediction of injury in elite swimmers. *International Journal of Sports Medicine, 9*, 345-348.

Bramwell, S. T., Masuda, M., Wagner, N. N., & Holmes, T. H. (1975). Psychosocial factors in athletic injuries: Development and Application of the Social and Athletic Readjustment Rating Scale (SARRS). *Journal of Human Stress, 1*, 6-20.

Brewer, B. W. (2001). Psychology of sport injury rehabilitation. In R. N. Singer, H. A. Hausenblas & C. M. Janelle (Eds.), *Handbook of Sport Psychology* (pp. 787-809). New York: John Wiley & Sons, Inc.

Brewer, B. W., Andersen, M. B., & Van Raalte, J. L. (2001). Psychological aspects of sport injury rehabilitation: Toward a biopsychosocial approach. In D. I. Mostofsky & L. D. Zaichkowsky (Eds.), *Medical Aspects of Sport and Exercise*. Morgantown, WV: Fitness Information Technology.

Brunelle, J. P., Goulet, C., & Arguin, H. (2005). Promoting respect for the rules and injury prevention in ice hockey: evaluation of the fair-play program. *Journal of Science and Medicine in Sport, 8*(3), 294-304.

Caine, D. J., Caine, C. G., & Linder, K. J. (1996). *Epidemiology of sports injuries*. Champaign: Il: Human Kinetics.

Chivers, I., Aldous, D., & Orchard, J. (2005). The relationship of Australian Football grass surfaces to anterior cruciate ligament injury. *International Turfgrass Society Journal, 10*(1), 327-332.

Coddington, R., & Troxell, J. (1980). The effects of emotional factors on football injury rates: A pilot study. *Journal of Human Stress, 6*(4), 3-5.

Conn, J. M., Annest, J. L., & Gilchrist, J. (2001). *Sports and recreation related injury episodes in the US population, 1997-99*. Atlanta, Georgia: National Center for Injury Prevention and Control, Centers for Disease Control and Prevention.

Crocker, P. R., Alderman, R. B., Murray, F., & Smith, R. (1988). Cognitive-affective stress management training with high performance youth volleyball players: Effects on affect, cognition, and performance. *Journal of Sport and Exercise Psychology, 10*, 448-460.

Crossman, J. (1985). Psychosocial factors and athletic injury. *Journal of Sports Medicine and Physical Fitness, 25*, 151-154.

Cryan, P. D., & Alles, W. F. (1983). The relationship between stress and college football injuries. *Journal of Sports Medicine and Physical Fitness, 23*, 52-58.

Cupal, D. D. (1998). Psychological interventions in sport injury prevention and rehabilitation. *Journal of Applied Sport Psychology, 10*, 103-123.

Cupal, D. D., & Brewer, B. W. (2001). Effects of relaxation and guided imagery on knee strength, reinjury anxiety, and pain following anterior cruciate ligament reconstruction. *Rehabilitation Psychology, 46*(1), 28-43.

Davis, J. (1991). Sports injuries and stress management: An opportunity for research. *The Sport Psychologist, 5*, 175-182.

DeWitt, D. J. (1980). Cognitive and biofeedback training for stress reduction. *Journal of Sport Psychology, 2*, 288-294.

Ekstrand, J., & Gillquist, J. (1983). The avoidability of soccer injuries. *International Journal of Sports Medicine, 2*, 124-128.

Esterling, B. A., Antoni, M. H., Fletcher, M. A., Margulies, S., & Schneiderman, N. (1994). Emotional disclosure through writing or speaking modulates latent Epstein-Barr virus antibody titers. *Journal of Consulting and Clinical Psychology, 62*, 130-140.

Evans, L., & Hardy, L. (1995). Sport injury and grief responses: A review. *Journal of Sport and Exercise Psychology, 17*, 227-245.

Ford, I. W., Eklund, R. C., & Grove, R. J. (2000). An examination of psychosocial variables moderating the relationship between life stress and injury time-loss among athletes of a high standard. *Journal of Sport Sciences, 18*, 301-312.

Gould, D. (2001). Goal setting for peak performance. In J. M. Williams (Ed.), *Applied Sport Psychology: Personal Growth to Peak Performance*. Mountain View, California: Mayfield Publishing Company.

Green, R. G., Green, M. L., & Santoro, W. (1988). Daily relaxation modifies serum and salivary immunoglobulins and physiological symptom severity. *Biofeedback and Self-Regulation, 13*, 187-199.

Hanson, S. J., McCullagh, P., & Tonymon, P. (1992). The relationship of personality characteristics, life stress, and coping resources to athletic injury. *Journal of Sport and Exercise Psychology, 14*, 262-272.

Hardy, C. J., Richman, J. M., & Rosenfeld, L. B. (1991). The role of social support in the life stress/injury relationship. *Sport Psychologist, 5*, 128-139.

Hardy, C. J., & Riehl, R. E. (1988). An examination of the life stress-injury relationship among noncontact sport participants *Behavioral Medicine, 14*, 113-118.

Hardy, L. (1992). Psychological stress, performance, and injury in sport. *British Medical Bulletin, 48*, 615-629.

Heil, J. (1993). Mental training in injury management. In J. Heil (Ed.), *Psychology of sport injury* (pp. 151-174). Champaign: IL: Human Kinetics.

Hodgson Phillips, L. (2000). Sports injury incidence. *British Journal of Sports Medicine, 34*, 133-136.

Holmes, T. H. (1970). Psychological screening. In *Football injuries: Papers presented at a workshop* (pp. 211-214). Washington, DC: National Academy of Sciences.

Hopkins, W. G. (2001). Clinical vs statistical significance. *Sportscience, 5*, 1-2.

Ievleva, L., & Orlick, T. (1991). Mental links to enhanced recovery: An exploratory analysis. *The Sport Psychologist, 5*, 25-40.

Johnson, U., Ekengren, J., & Andersen, M. B. (2005). Injury prevention in Sweden: Helping soccer players at risk. *Journal of Sport and Exercise Psychology, 27*, 32-38.

Junge, A. (2000). The influence of psychological factors on sports injuries. *The American Journal of Sports Medicine, 28*(5), S-10-28.

Kelley, M. J. J. (1990). Psychological risk factors and sports injuries. *Journal of Sports Medicine, Science and Physical Fitness, 30*, 202-221.

Kerr, G., & Fowler, B. (1988). The relationship between psychological factors and sports injuries. *Sports Medicine, 6*, 127-134.

Kerr, G., & Goss, J. (1996). The effects of a stress management program on injuries and stress levels. *Journal of Applied Sport Psychology, 8*, 109-117.

Kerr, G., & Minden, H. (1988). Psychological factors related to the occurrence of athletic injuries. *Journal of Sport and Exercise Psychology, 10*, 167-173.

Mace, R. D., & Carroll, D. (1985). The control of anxiety in sport: stress inoculation training prior to abseiling. *International Journal of Sport Psychology, 16*, 165-175.

Mace, R. D., & Carroll, D. (1989). The effect of stress inoculation training on self-reported stress, observer's rating of stress, heart rate and gymnastics performance. *Journal of Sport Sciences, 7*, 257-266.

Mace, R. D., Carroll, D., & Eastman, C. (1986). Effects of stress inoculation training on self-report, behavioural and physiological reactions to abseiling. *Journal of Sport Sciences, 4*, 229-236.

Maddison, R., & Prapavessis, H. (2005). A psychological approach to the prediction and prevention of athletic injury. *Journal of Sport and Exercise Psychology, 27*, 289-310.

May, J. R., & Brown, L. (1989). Delivery of psychological services to the U.S. alpine ski team prior to and during the Olympics in Calgary. *The Sport Psychologist, 3*, 320-329.

Meichenbaum, D. (1985). *Stress inoculation training*. New York: Permagon Press.

Murphy, S. M. (1988). The on-site provision of sport psychology services at the U.S. Olympic Festival. *The Sport Psychologist, 2*, 337-350.

Nideffer, R. M. (1989). Psychological aspects in sports injuries: Prevention and treatment. *International Journal of Sport Psychology, 20*, 241-255.

Orchard, J. W., Chivers, I., Aldous, D., Bennell, K., & Seward, H. (2005). Rye grass is associated with fewer noncontact anterior cruciate ligament injuries than Bermuda grass. *British Journal of Sports Medicine, 39*(10), 704-709.

Passer, M. W., & Seese, M. D. (1983). Life stress and athletic injury: Examination of positive and negative events and three moderator variables. *Journal of Human Stress 9*, 11-16.

Perna, F. M., Antoni, M. H., Baum, A., Cordon, P., & Schneiderman, N. (2003). Cognitive behavioral stress management effects on injury and illness among competitive athletes: A randomized clinical trial. *Annals of Behavioral Medicine, 25*(1), 66-73.

Perna, F. M., & McDowell, S. L. (1995). Role of psychological stress in cortisol recovery from exhaustive exercise among elite athletes. *International Journal of Behavioral Medicine, 2*, 13-26.

Perna, F. M., Schneiderman, N., & LaPerriere, A. (1997). Psychological stress, exercise, and immunity. *International Journal of Sports Medicine, 18*(Suppl. 1), S78-S83.

Petitpas, A. J., & Danish, S. J. (1995). Caring for injured athletes. In S. M. Murphey (Ed.), *Sport Psychology Interventions* (pp. 225-282). Champaign IL: Human Kinetics.

Petrie, T. (1992). Psychosocial antecedents of athletic injury: The effects of life stress and social support on female collegiate gymnasts. *Behavioral Medicine, 18*, 127-138.

Petrie, T., & Perna, F. (2004). Psychology of injury: theory, research, and practice. In T. Morris & J. Summers (Eds.), *Sport psychology: Theory, applications, and issues.* (2nd Edition). Australia: John Wiley & Sons.

Prevention CfDCa. (2003). Nonfatal sports- and recreation-related injuries treated in emergency departments - United States, July 2000 - June 2001. *CDC Morbidity and Mortality Weekly Report, 51*, 736-740.

Richman, J. M., Hardy, C. J., Rosenfeld, L. B., & Callanan, R. A. E. (1989). Strategies for enhancing social support networks in sport: A brainstormimg experience. *Applied Sport Psychology, 1*, 150-159.

Rogers, T. J., & Landers, D. M. (2005). Mediating effects of peripheral vision in the life event stress-athletic injury relationship. *Journal of Sport and Exercise Psychology, 27*, 271-288.

Schmid, A., & Peper, E. (1998). Strategies for training concentration. In J. M. Williams (Ed.), *Applied sport psychology: Personal growth to peak performance* (pp. 316-328). Mayfield: Mountain View: CA.

Schomer, H. H. (1990). A cognitive strategy training programme for marathon runners: ten case studies. *South African Journal for Research in Sport, Physical Education and Recreation, 13*, 47-48.

Sherman, C. P., & Poczwardowski, A. (2000). Relax!...It ain't easy (or is it?). In M. B. Andersen (Ed.), *Doing Sport Psychology* (pp. 47-60). Champaign IL: Human Kinetics.

Smith, A. M. (1996). Psychological impact of injuries in athletes. *Sports Medicine, 22*(6), 391-405.

Smith, R. E. (1999). Generalization effects in coping skills training. *Journal of Sport and Exercise Psychology, 21*, 189-204.

Smith, R. E., Ptacek, J. T., & Smoll, F. L. (1992). Sensation seeking, stress, and adolescent injuries: A test of stress-buffering, risk-taking, and coping skills hypotheses. *Journal of Personality and Social Psychology, 62*, 1016-1024.

Smith, R. E., Smoll, F. L., & Ptacek, J. T. (1990). Conjunctive moderator variables in vulnerability and resiliency research: Life stress, social support and coping skills and adolescent sport injuries. *Journal of Personality and Social Psychology, 58*, 360-370.

Tabachnick, B. G., & Fidell, L. S. (2001). *Using Multivariate Statistics* (Fourth ed.). New York: Allyn & Bacon.

Wiese-Bjornstal, D. M., Smith, A. M., Shaffer, S. M., & Morrey, M. A. (1998). An integrated model of response to sport injury: Psychological and sociological dimension. *Journal of Applied Sport Rehabilitation, 5*, 214-223.

Williams, J. M. (2001). Psychology of injury risk and prevention. In R. N. Singer, H. A. Hausenblas & C. M. Janelle (Eds.), *Handbook of Sport Psychology* (2nd ed., pp. 766-786). New York: John Wiley & Sons, Inc.

Williams, J. M., & Andersen, M. B. (1998). Psychosocial antecedents of sport injury: Review and critique of the stress and injury model. *Journal of Applied Psychology, 10*, 5-25.

Williams, J. M., & Harris, D. V. (1998). Relaxation and energizing techniques for regulation of arousal. In J. M. Williams (Ed.), *Applied sport psychology: Personal growth to peak performance* (3rd ed., pp. 219-236). Mayfield: Mountainview: CA.

Williams, J. M., Tonymon, P., & Wadsworth, W. A. (1986). Relationship of life stress to injury in intercollegiate volleyball. *Journal of Human Stress, 12*, 38-43.

Zinsser, N., Bunker, L., & Williams, J. M. (2001). Cognitive techniques for building confidence and enhancing performance. In J. M. Williams (Ed.), *Applied sport psychology: Personal growth to peak performance* (Fourth ed., pp. 284-311). Mayfield Publishing Company: Mountain View: CA.

Chapter Three

Psychosocial Antecedents to Sport Injury Prevention: A Case Study of Competitive Soccer Players at Risk

Urban Johnson
Halmstad University

Psychology offers different intervention actions in order to prevent the occurrence of injury. In the domain of sport psychology different psychological risk variables and models have been outlined to explain potential links between psychosocial antecedents and sport injury. However, few studies in sport psychology have used the findings in applied settings.

Thus, this chapter has two objectives:

(1) to provide a conclusive review of important issues related to psychosocial antecedents and preventive actions of injury in sport settings,

(2) to describe and discuss a specific prevention intervention program for competitive soccer players at risk of injuries.

The Risk and Occurrence of Injury in Sport Settings

It is widely known that high-level sport is associated with elevated risk of suffering injury. For instance, epidemiological studies from Finland and the United Kingdom report that the injury risk for elite soccer players is between 65% (Lüthje, et al., 1996) and 91% (Lewin, 1989) during one season.

Researchers studying athletes at risk of injury have attempted to identify physical factors (e.g., muscle mass or physical status) that could be involved in the pathogenesis of an injury in order to explain why certain individuals are more frequently injured than others (MacIntosh, Skrien, & Shephard, 1971). However, there has been only very modest evidence to support the assumption that acute injury is directly related to an athlete's physical characteristics (Williams, 2001). This line of research has led to general acceptance that there are two types of interrelated risk factors:

(a) extrinsic, related to the type of sport, the way it is practiced, contextual factors, and equipment;

(b) intrinsic, related primarily to an individual's physical and psychological features.

It is still not clear, however, how certain physical and psychological factors or combinations of these predispose some athletes to greater risk of injury.

Psychosocial Factors Influencing the Onset of Injury in Sport

Over the last few decades, a growing number of researchers have tried to determine which psychosocial variables influence injury vulnerability and resistance to injuries (e.g. Williams, 2001). Researchers have found that individuals who have experienced many recent stressors and who did not have the personal resources and skills to cope with the stressors were most at risk for injury. A substantial body of research has been directed at identifying mechanisms that might explain why the stress-injury relationship occurs and what interventions will reduce injury risk. The most influential and best known model, based on the before-mentioned risk factors, is outlined by Williams & Andersen (1998) and has formed the theoretical base of some recent studies. (See Figure 1 in Chapter 1.)

Personality Variables

Personality characteristics may dispose individuals to perceive fewer situations and events as stressful, or to be more susceptible to the effects of stressors such as major life events and daily hassles. Relationships are often found between injury outcome and risk factors such as internal or external locus of control (Pargman & Lunt, 1989), competitive trait anxiety (Lavallee & Flint, 1996), low self-esteem (Kolt & Roberts, 1998), and low mood state early in the season (Williams, Hogan, & Andersen, 1993). Most of this research was conducted on male, elite, or competitive athletes.

History of Stressors

Since Holmes' study in 1970, many others have examined the relationship of life stress to athletic injury. The vast majority of these studies have found a positive relationship between injury and high life stress (Patterson, Smith, & Everett, 1998), daily hassles (Fawkner, McMurray, & Summer, 1999), and life changes (Hardy & Riehl, 1988). These findings suggest that preoccupation with life change may affect concentration on training and competition and increase the likelihood of injury. However, researchers have also found contrasting results showing no relation between previous injury and frequency or severity of injury (Hanson, McCullagh, & Tonymon, 1992) and showing that even positive life events can be related to injury outcome (Petrie, 1993).

Coping Resources

Several studies have supported the link between general coping resources and athletic injury. Williams, Tonymon, and Wadsworth (1986) reported a relationship between athletes low in coping resources and prediction of injury. Hanson et al. (1992) found that coping resources were the best discriminator for both severity and number of injuries. Research about the effect of social support on injury occurrence has not provided consistent findings. Some studies have shown a direct effect, with athletes low in social support exhibiting more injuries (e.g., Hardy, Richman, & Rosenfeld, 1991).

Others have found a relationship between negative life events and injury outcome only for athletes low in both social support and coping skills (Smith, Smoll, & Ptacek, 1990).

Psychological Prevention Intervention Studies in Sport

Injury Prevention

In contrast to the rich body of empirical studies investigating psychological factors in sport injury occurrence, there are but few controlled intervention studies examining relationships among psychological risk variables, prevention treatments, and injury outcomes (Cupal, 1998). Moreover, little attention has been given to those brief interventions that occur frequently when working with athletes in the field, often referred to as brief contact interventions (see Giges & Petitpas, 2000). In the field of clinical psychology, there has been interest in brief or focused interventions, especially in the cognitive-behavioral therapies, and particularly for clients diagnosed with anxiety and somatic disorders (Bergin & Garfield, 1994). Most brief therapies typically range from 5 to 15 sessions (Pinkerton & Rockwell, 1994) and are commonly organized with close spacing of initial sessions and gradually increasing inter-session intervals with a planned follow-up or booster session (Budman & Gurman, 1983). Such brief therapy models seem well suited for sport interventions and have been used, in various forms, in the past.

In the following review some significant prevention intervention studies using brief therapy models will be reported. Schomer (1990) investigated the effects of associative (monitoring bodily functions and feelings such as heart and breathing rate) versus dissociative thought patterns (distraction and tuning out) on injuries with marathon runners. Schomer (1990) reported an ability to optimize training intensity without increasing injury using associative strategies. The intervention involved shaping associative thought processes over a 5-week training period using audiotapes of attentional strategies. Associative thinking was related to perceptions of increased training effort. Through the use of light-weight recorders worn on the body during training, this study used a simple yet effective method to shape attentional strategies to produce optimal, injury-free performance.

Davis (1991) used imagery and relaxation with college-level swimmers and football players to reduce injuries. The program was composed of progressive relaxation combined with imagined rehearsal of swimming and football skills and related content during the competitive season. Relaxation instructions usually required 10 minutes and included the guided imagery techniques of Suinn (1982). Davis reported a 52% reduction in swimming injuries and a 33% reduction in football injuries.

Kerr & Goss (1996) conducted a stress-management intervention with 24 elite gymnasts based on Meichenbaum's (1985) stress inoculation training program. The gymnasts were matched into pairs according to sex, age, and performance. One member of each pair was randomly assigned to the intervention group and received the stress management program. The other member of each pair acted as a control, completing the stress and injury measures without exposure to the training program. The training consisted of 16 sessions covering skills such as cognitive restructuring, thought control, imagery, and mental rehearsal. The gymnasts were responsible for maintaining training logs that contained homework assignments for the skills in the program. A trend for reduced injury in the stress management group was reported.

In a recent piece of research Maddison and Prapavessis (2005) conducted two interrelated studies examining the role psychological factors play in the prediction and prevention of sport-related injuries among competitive rugby players in New Zeeland:

- In the first study 470 rugby athletes completed several measures corresponding to variables in William & Andersen stress and injury model from 1998. Result showed that social support, the type of coping, and previous injury interacted in a conjunctive fashion to maximize the relationship between life stress and injury.

- Study 2 examined the effectiveness of a six-session cognitive behavioral stress management (CBSM) intervention in reducing injury among 48 athletes from study 1 who were identified as having an at-risk psychological profile for injury. Result indicated that those in the intervention condition reported missing less time due to injury compared to the nonintervention group. The intervention group also had an increase in coping resources and a decrease in worry following the program (Maddison & Prapavessis, 2005).

Injury Prevention in Competitive Soccer

As mentioned earlier the occurrence of injuries in competitive soccer is fairly high, especially injuries connected to lower extremities and of acute nature. An example of injury frequency is shown in Table 1. This table clearly demonstrates the occurrence of injuries in a population of male-female elite soccer players in Sweden.

My background as a former professional trainer in team sport involves frequent meetings with injured players during all phases of the competitive season. Working close to competitive athletes in team sport has prompted the question as to why some athletes were able to be free of injury while others were more prone. Previous research (e.g. Johnson 1997; 2000) has concluded that some psychological feature, such as lack

Table 1.

Frequency of injuries among male-female elite soccer players in Sweden during one season, (Adapted from Engström, Johansson, & Törnkvist, 1991; Hägglund, Waldén, & Ekstrand, 2003.)

Amount of injuries	Occurrence of injuries	Type of injury	Division of injuries
33 female players á 78 injuries	88% lower extremities	72% acute 36% moderate	49% minor 15% severe
49 male players á 85 injuries	93% lower extremities	65% acute 39% moderate	27% minor 34 % severe

Minor = less than 1 week of physical rehabilitation time
Moderate = 1 week to 1 month of physical rehabilitation time
Severe = More than 1 month of physical rehabilitation time (Lysens et al., 1991)

of social network and future plans, seems to distinguish those injured athletes faced with prolonged rehabilitation time or even questionable return to sport from those who have faced no problems. This finding is in line with contemporary research about psychological characteristics of athletes faced with problems during rehabilitation (see e.g. Crossman, 2001). However, as the review has shown, rather few studies have used the findings from the above-mentioned studies in order to test an intervention program for athletes at risk of gaining injury. It is especially important to integrate scientific knowledge from factors affecting rehabilitation outcome as well as those related to injury occurrence in order to construct the best possible preventive intervention strategy. What follows is a description of an attempt to identify competitive soccer players at risk for injury, and also to test a short-term intervention program designed to reduce the incidence of their sport-related injuries during the forthcoming soccer season (see Johnson, Ekengren & Andersen, 2005a).

Background information

At the very beginning of the soccer season 235 male and female players representing different teams in southwest Sweden were tested on selected psychological variables. Sport-specific pencil and paper instruments were used because of their potential to screen for psychosocial risk factors outlined in the stress and injury model by Williams and Andersen (1998):

- Personality variables of athletes were assessed by application of the Sport Anxiety Scale (SAS; Smith, Smoll, & Schutz, 1990).
- Psychological variables connected to history of stressors were examined by the Life Event Scale for Collegiate Athletes (LESCA; Petrie, 1992).
- Coping resources were examined through use of the Athletic Coping Skills Inventory 28 (ACSI –28; Smith, Schutz, Smoll, & Ptacek, 1995).

In the screening process the strategy was to use the above-mentioned test in such a way that it was possible to sort out a potentially at-risk player. Reference data (e.g. Maddison & Prapavessis, 2005; Johnson, 1997) pointed to the fact that at least 10–20% of the competitive population could be at risk of sport injury. In a previous study Smith, Smoll, and Ptacek (1990) found that athletes who rated lower in psychosocial variables such as social support and coping resources, and had experienced many stressful life events, were the ones more likely to be injured. Those athletes who received scores representing the highest 50 % of the LESCA and the highest 50% of SAS (total) were considered to have high-injury-risk profiles. With regard to the ACSI-28, high scores on five subscales (coping with adversity, peaking under pressure, goal setting/mental preparation, concentration, and confidence and achievement motivation) were considered to be indicative of adaptive coping responses. Moreover, low scores on two subscales (freedom from worry, and coachability) indicated adaptive coping responses. Soccer players who received scores representing the lowest 50% on the five ACSI-28 subscales and highest 50% on two ACSI-2 subscales were labelled high-injury-risk. Participants had to be in the "risk" 50% on all variables.

Risk screening resulted in identification of 32 players with high injury-risk profiles. This risk group was then randomly divided into control and experimental groups:

- The control group consisted of 16 soccer players with eight male and eight female players.
- The experimental group comprised 16 soccer players and included seven male and nine female athletes.

During the intervention, three male soccer players in the experimental group declared their inability to continue for various reasons and therefore withdrew. Thirteen participants remained throughout the entire protocol.

Injury recording

On six occasions during the protocol (approximately every third to fourth week) the head coach, physiotherapist, or team doctor for every participating team was asked to record each injury that occurred for their soccer players and indicate the number of days that each recorded injury interfered with regular training and match game on a structured Sport Injury Frequency Form.

Intervention program

The intervention program consisted of six different personal interactions with one of the researchers, in addition to two telephone contacts between weeks 6 and 26. Each athlete in the treatment group was met with twice a month for the first two months and again in the middle and end of the intervention. The intervention involved five distinct treatments:

1. *Somatic and cognitive relaxation.* For every player, two different prerecorded compact discs were created by the researchers and distributed in the beginning (session 1) (somatic relaxation) and in the middle (session 4) of the intervention period (somatic and cognitive relaxation). The somatic relaxation was centered on the principles underlying autogenic training (Linden, 1994). Participants were told to imagine walking down a 10-step staircase into a comfortable practice situation. They were told to imagine being successful when competing and were advised to practice every second to third day throughout the intervention period.

2. *Stress management skills.* During the second session, the players learned how to cope effectively with stressors, using the problem- and emotion-focused coping strategies of Folkman and Lazarus (1984). They were taught to take responsibility for their actions and actively confront potential stressors through a cognitive reappraisal strategy that included trying to see stressors from a more positive point of view or as a challenge instead of a threat (problem-focused coping).

3. *Goal-setting skills.* At the third session, the players actively learned how to develop a goal-setting model. After an initial education in the basic tenets of goal setting, they were provided with the rationale behind the "target approach for goal setting" adapted from Smith (1991). Participants were encouraged to continually integrate long-term (dream and season) goals, intermediate (monthly) goals, short-term (weekly) goals, and daily goals into the daily training. They were told to make the goals as specific, measurable, achievable, realistic, and time-phased as possible.

4. *Attribution and self-confidence training.* During the fifth session, two separate but still connected topics were covered. During the attribution training, players were taught a sport attribution model based on Weiner's classification (1992). The self-confidence training was aimed toward a brief orientation about the nature of optimal self-confidence compared to lack of confidence, as well as toward understanding how expectation influences performance from self and others (e.g. coach) (Jones, Hanton & Swain, 1994).

5. *Identification and discussion about critical incidents* related to their soccer participation and situations in everyday life. This last treatment, named "critical incident diary" (CID), was used as a base for discussion all through sessions 2 to 6 in combination with the main focus for each session.

All sessions lasted between 45 to 90 minutes and were mostly situated at the homes of the athletes or in rooms close to the training venues. Each player received a folder at the first session with written materials, carefully designed with easy-to-read descriptions for every meeting, including homework and a general time-table over the intervention period. The sequence for the intervention is presented in Table 2.

Table 2.
Intervention program for the experimental group (n=13).

Session	Topic
Session 1	Somatic (autogenetic) relaxation (1)
Session 2	Stress management (2)
Session 3	Goal setting skills (3)
Telephone contact (1)	Follow up feedback (1-3)
Session 4	Somatic and cognitive relaxation (4)
Session 5	Attribution/self-confidence (5)
Telephone contact (2)	Follow up feedback (4-5)
Session 6	Summary, feedback, and future directions (6).

Athletes were responsible for maintaining separate training logs for the relaxation training and preparing a monthly summary of their participation on a preprinted paper. They were also told to continuously redefine their goal setting as well as evaluate their latest competitive performance. Logbooks and homework assignments were reviewed and discussed at a following meeting and used to monitor the progress. In the last session, a summary was made and discussions were held about the different notes in the logbooks, including plans for future directions.

Injury prevention in competitive soccer: Some interesting results

At the time of pretest all participants were free from physical injuries according to their head coaches. During the intervention period, several injuries occurred, particularly in the control group. Control group members received 21 injuries (1.31 injuries per person) distributed across 13 different players. The experimental group incurred altogether three injuries (0.22 injuries per person) distributed across three different players (see also Johnson et al., 2005a). During the first and second test athletes in the experimental group were higher in confidence and achievement motivation and lower in coachability than the control group (Johnson et al., 2005b).

In the Maddison & Prapavessis study (2005), the experimental group also showed an increase in general coping resources and a decrease in worry compared to the control group. Kerr and Goss (1996) reported significantly less negative athletic stress at the third measure than the control group.

There are several potential explanations for the experimental group having significantly fewer injuries during the intervention period than the control group. One probable contributing factor is that the experimental group received training in somatic relaxation and stress management early in the intervention period. This intervention strategy, used in a systematic and planned way, has the potential to buffer stress (Jones, 1993) and may have prepared the players to handle potentially stressful situations in a more adaptive way. Kerr and Goss (1996), as well, highlighted the usefulness of early training in specific skills, such as relaxation, in order to prevent injury outcome. Another possible explanation was the weekly note taking in the CID, which may have contributed to the athlete's attentiveness to potential effects of negative events related to soccer and everyday life. Avoiding stressful situations when possible or interpreting them more positively may be conducive to enhanced levels of both mental and physical well-being. In an applied perspective, it turned out to be a successful approach to let the players keep a diary during the intervention period since it made it possible to come close to their "real life" thinking and to discuss potential stressors and uplifts in life.

The lowered coachability (e.g., ability to handle criticism from coach or manager) at the termination of the intervention speaks for an effect that could be related to the intervention training period. The training was done with the aim of understanding the importance of making internal and stable attributions in game-related situations in order to enhance self-confidence and motivation and to lower worry in competitive games. It is possible that this training might have had some immediate effect on the player's self-confidence. May and Brown (1989), using a combination of intervention strategies, were also able to report increased self-confidence in the athletes in their study.

Conclusion, practical implications, and future research

An overall conclusion to be drawn from data collected in this study is that by using combinations of psychological intervention techniques in a brief therapy model, injury reduction may be achieved in soccer players identified as having high-injury-risk profiles.

Major life event stress and daily hassles seem to have a direct or indirect effect on injury resiliency and vulnerability. Soccer coaches and trainers should thus understand the effect these factors have on injury outcome. Because of their close relationships with players, coaches, trainers, and therapists are in a unique position to recognize players at risk and to help them. They are able to teach players how to expand their range of coping skills and thus to meet troublesome life events and daily hassles. Moreover, it might be advisable to include a psychosocial risk assessment that focuses on life event stressors as part of the general physical examination at the start of the soccer season in order to identify at-risk players. Appropriate intervention would then follow.

Another practical implication of findings obtained in this study relates to prevention techniques and skills. Relaxation techniques, especially those that emphasize breathing and/or progressive muscle relaxation, have the potential to lower injury incidence for competitive soccer players. This is particularly true for players who have a tendency to worry or exhibit signs of competitive state anxiety before games. Soccer coaches and sport psychologists should consider implementing intervention programs for athletes with a high-injury-risk profile. Optimally, such programs would combine physiological and psychological skills and techniques in an integrated design.

An additional suggestion would be to study psychosocial background variables as they relate to overuse injuries. For instance, repeated microtrauma of the knee and elbow due to overload training is likely to activate different sets of coping resources and thus different sets of social support systems to handle the injury situation than traditional acute injuries. In many sports such as swimming (McMaster, 1996), tennis (Bylak & Huchinson, 1998) and long-distance running and triathlon (Burns, Keenan, & Redmond, 2003), the dominant injury pattern is overuse injuries.

Another interesting avenue for future applied work involves separation of intervention studies conducted on men and women soccer athletes. A body of evidence demonstrates that female soccer players are overrepresented in terms of sport-related injuries (Kontos, 2000), especially knee-related ones (Soderman, Pietila, Alfredson, & Werner, 2002). At the same time, it is well known that women tend to activate other coping strategies, such as seeking social support and venting emotions, to a greater extent than men do when faced with potential difficulties (e.g., Wingerhoets & Van Heck, 1990). More knowledge into the psychosocial mechanisms that seem to make female players more vulnerable to injury will most likely yield valuable information about how to structure an adaptive preventive intervention design.

References

Bergin, A. E., & Garfiled, S. L. (1994). *Handbook of psychotherapy and behavior change* (4th ed.). New York: Wiley.

Budman, S. H., & Gurman, A. S. (1983). The practice of brief therapy. *Professional Psychology: Research and Practice, 14*, 277-292.

Burns, J., Keenan, A. M., & Redmond, A. C. (2003). Factors associated with triathlon-related overuse injuries. *The Journal of Orthopaedic & Sports Physical Therapy, 33(4)*, 177–184.

Bylak, J., & Huchinson, M. R. (1998). Common sports injuries in young tennis players. *Sports Medicine, 26(2)*, 119–132.

Crossman, J. (2001). *Coping with sport injuries. Psychological strategies for rehabilitation*. Oxford, University Press.

Cupal, D. D. (1998). Psychological interventions in sport injury prevention and rehabilitation. *Journal of Applied Sport Psychology, 10*, 103–123.

Davis, J. O. (1991). Sport injuries and stress management. An opportunity for research. *The Sport Psychologist 5*, 175-182.

Engström, B., Johansson, C., & Törnkvist, H. (1991). Soccer injuries among female players. *American Journal of Sports Medicine, 19*, 273-275.

Fawkner, H. J., McMurray, N., & Summer, J. J. (1999). Athletic injury and minor life events: A prospective study. *Journal of Science and Medicine in Sport 2*, 117-124.

Folkman, S., & Lazarus, R. S. (1984). *Stress, appraisal and coping*. New York: Springer Publishing Company.

Giges, B., & Petitipas, A. (2000). Brief contact interventions in sport psychology. *The Sport Psychologist, 14*, 176-187.

Hägglund, M., Waldén, M., & Ekstrand, J. (2003). Exposure and injury risk in Swedish elite football: A comparison between season 1982 and 2001. *Scandinavian Journal of Medicine and Science in Sports, 13,* 364-370.

Hanson, S. J., McCullagh, P., & Tonymon, P. (1992). The relationship of personality characteristics, life stress, and coping resources to athletic injury. *Journal of Sport & Exercise Psychology, 14,* 262-272.

Hardy, C. J., & Riehl, M. A. (1988). An examination of the life stress-injury relationship among noncontact sport participants. *Behavioral Medicine, 14,* 113-118.

Hardy, C. J., Richman, J. M., & Rosenfeld, L. B. (1991). The role of social support in the life stress/injury relationship. *The Sport Psychologist, 5,* 128-139.

Johnson, U. (1997). *The long-term injured competitive athlete: A study of psychosocial risk factors.* Almqvist Wiksell, Sweden.

Johnson, U. (2000). Short-Term Psychological Intervention: A Study of Long-Term Injured Competitive Athletes. *Journal of Sport rehabilitation, 9, 207-218.*

Johnson, U., Ekengren, J., & Andersen, M. B. (2005a). Injury Prevention in Sweden. Helping Soccer Players at Risk. *Journal of Sport and Exercise Psychology, 1, 32-38.*

Johnson, U., Ekengren, J., & Andersen, M. B. (2005b). Injury Prevention in Sweden: Effect of a brief intervention program for at-risk soccer player on sport anxiety and coping. *Proceedings of the 11th World Congress of Sport Psychology*, Sydney 15-19 of August; ISSP.

Jones, G. (1993). The role of performance profiling in cognitive behavioral interventions in sport. *The Sport Psychologist, 7,* 160-172.

Jones, G., Hanton, S., & Swain, A. (1994). Intensity and interpretation of anxiety symptoms in elite and non-elite sports performers. *Personality and Individual Differences 17(5),* 657-663

Kerr G., & Goss, J. (1996). The effects of a stress management program on injuries and stress levels. *Journal of Applied Sport Psychology 8,* 109-117.

Kolt, G., & Roberts, P. D. T. (1998). Self-esteem and injury in competitive field hockey players. *Perceptual and Motor Skills, 87(1),* 353-354.

Kontos, A. P. (2000). *The effects of perceived risk, risk-taking behaviors, and body size on injury in youth sport.* Unpublished doctoral thesis, Michigan State University.

Lavallee, L., & Flint, F. (1996). The relationship of stress, competitive anxiety, mood state, and social support to athletic injury. *Journal of Athletic Training 31,* 296-299.

Lewin, G. (1989). The incidence of injury in an English professional soccer club during one competitive season. *Physiotherapy, 75,* 601-605.

Linden, P. (1994). Somatic literacy: bringing somatic education into physical education. *The Journal of Physical Education, Recreation & Dance 65(9),* 15-21

Lüthje, P., Nurmi, I., Kataja, M., Belt, E., Helenius, P., & Kaukonen, J. P. (1996). Epidemiology and traumatology of injuries in elite soccer: A prospective study in Finland. *Scandinavian Journal of Medicine and Science in Sport, 6,* 180-185.

MacIntosh, D. L., Skrien, T., & Shephard, R. J. (1971). Athletic injuries at the University of Toronto. *Medicine and Science in Sports, 3(4),* 195-199.

Maddison, R., Prapavessis, H. (2005). A psychological approach to the prediction and prevention of athletic injury. *Journal of Sport & Exercise Psychology, 27,* 289-310.

May, J. R., & Brown, L. (1989). Delivery of psychological service to the U.S. Alpine ski team prior to and during the Olympics in Calgary. *The Sport Psychologist, 3,* 320-329.

McMaster, W. C. (1996). Swimming injuries: An overview. *Sports Medicine, 22(5),* 332–336.

Meichenbaum, D. (1985). *Stress inoculation training.* New York: Pergamon Press.

Pargman, D., & Lunt, S. D. (1989). The relationship of self-concept and locus of control to the severity of injury in freshman collegiate football players. *Sports Medicine, Training and Rehabilitation, 1,* 201-208.

Patterson, E. L., Smith, R. E., & Everett, J. J. (1998). Psychosocial factors as predictors of ballet injuries: Interactive effects of life stress and social support. *Journal of Sport Behavior, 21,* 101-112.

Petrie, T. A. (1992). Psychosocial antecedents of athletic injury: The effects of life stress and social support on female collegiate gymnasts. *Behavioral Medicine, 18,* 127-138.

Petrie, T. A. (1993). Coping skills, competitive trait anxiety, and playing status: Moderation effects of the life stress-injury relationships. *Journal of Sport & Exercise Psychology, 5,* 1-16.

Pinkerton, R. S., & Rockwell, W .J .K. (1994). Very brief psychological interventions with university students. *Journal of American College Health, 13,* 344-357.

Schomer, H. H. (1990). A cognitive strategy training program for marathon runners: Ten case studies. *South African Journal of Research in Sport, Physical Education and Recreation, 13,* 47-78.

Smith, R. E., Smoll, F. L., & Ptacek, J. T. (1990). Conjunctive moderator variables in vulnerability and resiliency research: Life stress, social support and coping skills, and adolescent sport injuries. *Journal of Personality and Social Psychology, 58,* 360–369.

Smith, R. E., Smoll, F. L., & Schutz, R. W. (1990). Measurement and correlates of sport-specific cognitive and somatic trait anxiety: The Sport Anxiety Scale. *Anxiety Research, 2*, 263-280.

Smith, R. E., Schutz, R. W., Smoll, F. L., & Ptacek, J. T. (1995). Development and validation of a multidimensional measure of sport-specific psychological skills: The Athletic Coping Skills Inventory-28. *Journal of Sport & Exercise Psychology, 17*, 379-398.

Soderman, K., Pietila, T., Alfredson, H., & Werner, S. (2002). Anterior cruciate ligament injuries in young females playing soccer at senior levels. *Scandinavian Journal of Medicine and Science in Sports, 12(2)*, 65-668.

Suinn, R. M. (1982). Imagery and sport. In A. Sheikh (Ed.), *Imagery, current theory, research and application* (pp. 507-534). New York: John Wiley.

Weiner, B. (1992). *Human motivation: Metaphors, Theories, and Research.* Sage Publications, Inc.

Williams, J. M. (2001). Psychology of injury risk and prevention. In R. N. Singer, H. A. Hausenblas & C. M. Janelle (Eds.), *Handbook of sport psychology* (pp 766-786). New York: John Wiley.

Williams, J. M., & Andersen, M. B. (1998). Psychosocial antecedents of sport injury: Review and critique of the stress and injury model. *Journal of Applied Sport Psychology, 10*, 5-25.

Williams, J. M., Hogan, T. D., & Andersen, M. B. (1993). Positive states of mind and athletic injury risk. *Psychosomatic Medicine, 55*, 468-472.

Williams, J. M., Tonymon, P., & Wadsworth, W. A. (1986). Relationship of stress to injury in intercollegiate volleyball. *Journal of Human Stress, 12*, 38-43.

Wingerhoets, J. J. M., & Van Heck, G. L. (1990). Gender, coping and psychosomatic symptoms. *Psychological Medicine, 20*, 125-135.

Section Two | Rehabilitating the Injured Athlete

All contributions to this section address sport injury rehabilitation perspectives.

In the section's first chapter, J. Robert Grove and Scott Cresswell discuss aspects of personality that may relate to injury recovery. They suggest that various personality dispositions require specific rehabilitative strategies.

In the section's second chapter, Britton Brewer, Judy Van Raalte, and Albert Petipas write about the importance of interventions and communications between rehabilitating athletes and various health professionals. They also discuss patient and practitioner perceptions about the injury and recovery process.

In chapter 6, the third in this section, Frances A. Flint presents a creative strategy for motivating rehabilitating athletes. She posits that an athlete/model who has succeeded in rehabilitating from the same or a similar trauma may demonstrate that recovery is possible.

In their chapter (7), Leslie Podlog and Robert C. Eklund discuss the various psychological stressors associated with return to sport. They remind the reader that physical readiness alone does not provide a sufficient platform for re-entry.

The last chapter in Section 2 (chapter 8), written by Lance B. Green and Kimberlee Bethany Bonura, addresses a widely used approach to the rehabilitation of injury athletes, namely imagery.

Chapter Four

Personality Correlates of Appraisal, Stress, and Coping during Injury Rehabilitation

J. Robert Grove and Scott L. Cresswell
The University of Western Australia

Psychological theory suggests a link between personality and the thoughts, feelings, and behaviors of athletes during rehabilitation. Research on the personality correlates of appraisal processes, stress perceptions, and coping behaviors indicates that neuroticism, explanatory style, optimism, perfectionism, and hardiness might be particularly important dispositional factors in this regard. Knowledge about these traits may therefore help sports medicine personnel to anticipate, understand, and deal with undesirable rehabilitation responses. For that reason, formal and informal assessment approaches are examined, and behavior management strategies are discussed in relation to these personality traits.

Introduction

Psychological factors have been examined as contributors to both injury occurrence and the response to injury. Historically, the literature provides evidence of an initial emphasis on the psychological antecedents of injury (e.g., Andersen & Williams, 1988) followed by an emphasis on psychological factors influencing post-injury reactions and rehabilitation progress. Conceptual models developed specifically to address rehabilitation issues point to a variety of situational and personal factors that might influence an injured athlete's thoughts, feelings, behaviors, and rehabilitation outcomes (Brewer, 1994, 1998, 2001; Evans & Hardy, 1995; Grove, 1993; Wiese-Bjornstal & Smith, 1993). Situational factors within these models include injury-related variables (e.g., type, severity, rehabilitation progress, recovery status) as well as treatment-related variables (e.g., facilities, time demands, pain, medical personnel) and various external influences (e.g., life stress, social support, pressure to return). Personal factors include general demographic variables (e.g., age) as well as injury history, coping resources, psychological skills, and personality traits.

In this chapter, we focus specifically on personality traits as mediators of the athlete's psychological response to injury, his or her rehabilitation behaviors, and the eventual rehabilitation outcomes. Our treatment of this issue is guided by a situation-specific adaptation of Lazarus and Folkman's (1984) transactional model of stress and coping that acknowledges an empirical link between personality traits and relevant psychological processes. This injury-specific model, which is similar in many ways to the more general "integrated model of coping" proposed by Hardy, Jones, and Gould (1996), is shown in Figure 1. It suggests that injury-related appraisals, perceived stress, and coping tendencies are all influenced to some extent by personality factors. These three processes, in addition to having reciprocal effects on each other, subsequently influence rehabilitation behaviors which, in turn, influence rehabilitation outcomes. The importance of personality in this series of events has been addressed from a theoretical perspective by Bolger and Zuckerman (1995) as well as Holahan, Moos, and Schaefer (1996). It is also supported by empirical findings linking personality to appraisal processes, stress perceptions, and coping tendencies (e.g., Anderson, 1995; Shewchuk, Elliott, MacNair-Semands, & Harkins, 1999; Wearing & Hart, 1996). Clues to the specific personality factors that may have the most relevance for sport injury research and practice can be gleaned from the broader literature on personality and health.

Personality and Health

Reviews of the personality and health literature suggest that a number of traits are potential correlates of health status (Eysenck, 1988; Friedman, 1990; Rodin & Salovey, 1989; Scheier & Bridges, 1995; Taylor, 1990). Five of these personality factors (neuroticism, explanatory style, dispositional optimism, perfectionism, and hardiness) are

Figure 1.

Relationship of personality traits to psychological processes, rehabilitation behaviors, and rehabilitation outcomes.

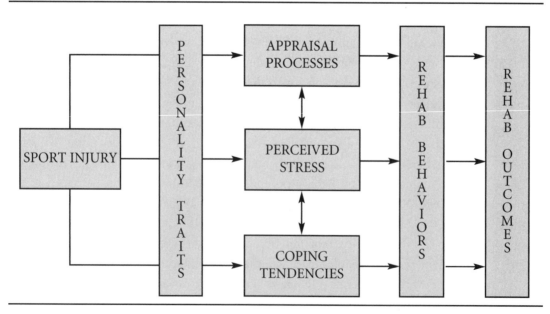

examined here. These particular factors have been selected because their documented connection to appraisal processes, stress reactions, and/or coping behaviors indicates they are likely to influence the athlete's psychological and behavioral responses during injury rehabilitation.

Neuroticism

Neuroticism is a basic dimension of personality that reflects a general tendency toward emotional lability and negative affect (McCrae & John, 1992; Eysenck & Eysenck, 1985). This trait has logical and empirical links to recovery-relevant constructs such as stress reactivity, distress proneness, and symptom reports (Bolger & Schilling, 1991; Ormal & Wohlfarth, 1991; Watson & Pennebaker, 1989). For example, Bolger and Zuckerman (1995) reported that students high in neuroticism experienced more conflict in their daily lives than did those low in neuroticism. In addition, those high in neuroticism used more confrontive coping which, in turn, contributed to more interpersonal problems. Thus, neuroticism contributed to both greater stress exposure and greater reactivity to stress. Further, researchers have reported that neuroticism is a common feature of anxiety and depressive disorders (Weinstock & Whisman, 2006) and, in combination with rumination, is associated with increases in susceptibility to depression (Roberts, Gilboa, & Gotlib, 1998).

Although there is limited evidence linking neuroticism with cognitive, emotional, or behavioral responses to sport injuries, there is abundant evidence that such injuries produce generalized negative affect, especially when they are severe (Daly, Brewer, Van Raalte, Petitpas, & Sklar, 1995; McDonald & Hardy, 1990; Meyers, Sterling, Calvo, Marley, & Duhon, 1991; Pearson & Jones, 1992; Smith, Scott, O'Fallon, & Young, 1990; Weinstock & Whisman, 2006). In a study of elite skiers who had sustained serious sport injuries, for example, Bianco (1999) reported that typical emotional responses included disappointment, frustration, confusion, and depression. One athlete who suffered a career-ending injury summarized it this way: "There was pain because I had the surgery; pain because I knew my career was over. It was probably the moment I suffered the most in my life, mentally and physically. There was pain all over" (p. 163).

If high levels of neuroticism are associated with selective attention to (or an exaggeration of) these negative emotions in response to injury, then various types of maladaptive behavior and rehabilitation difficulties could ensue (cf. Sanderson, 1981). Inappropriate displays of anger could be one form of maladaptive behavior exhibited by individuals with strong neurotic tendencies. Impatience, irritability, and hostility are known to correlate positively with neuroticism (Costa & McCrae, 1992), and the stressful nature of the rehabilitation process increases the likelihood of these sorts of negative reactions. Hostile outbursts can also contribute to relationship strain between the patient and health professional, thereby resulting in withdrawal of support. Silver, Wortman, and Crofton (1990) have shown that communicating a need for social support by showing distress often led to rejection rather than eliciting support. Similarly, Ford and Gordon (1993) reported that injured athletes who exhibited distress were rated as least desirable to treat by sport physiotherapists. Unfortunately, the distress of injury can frequently cause athletes to direct negative emotional reactions toward health-care professionals: "I was not a nice person to be around. I just wasn't easy to get along with. I'd be moody and was just not happy a lot of the time. I was kind of frustrated, and I got into arguments with my doctor" (Bianco, 1996, cited in Grove & Bianco, 1999, p. 91).

Another form of maladaptive behavior among highly neurotic athletes could be a tendency to rely on inefficient coping strategies. Neurotic tendencies have been reliably linked to the use of certain types of coping strategies, and these same strategies appear to be negatively related to coping effectiveness in the health domain. More specifically, various measures of neuroticism have exhibited positive correlations with avoidance-oriented and emotion-oriented coping strategies such as

- denial,
- escapist fantasy,
- withdrawal, passivity,
- selfblame,
- wishful thinking,
- indecisiveness,
- emotional focus/venting,
- sedation, and
- mental/behavioral disengagement

(Costa & McRae, 1989; Endler & Parker, 1990; Kardum & Hudek-Knezevic, 1996; Scheier, Carver, & Bridges, 1994; Wearing & Hart, 1996). At the same time, neuroticism has been shown to correlate negatively with problem-focused coping strategies involving direct action and active coping (Endler & Parker, 1990; Parkes, 1986; Rim, 1986; Scheier et al., 1994). These relationships between neurotic tendencies and coping behaviors could have important consequences for injury rehabilitation because the medical literature shows that patients who use passive/avoidant, emotion-focused coping strategies often have more difficulty adjusting to health problems than those who use more active, problem-focused strategies (Maes, Leventhal, & de Ridder, 1996; Zeidner & Saklofske, 1996).

Explanatory Style

Explanatory style is the way an individual typically accounts for significant events in his or her life. In other words, it is a relatively permanent tendency to explain things in a certain way. Individuals who exhibit a pessimistic explanatory style tend to explain negative events as personally caused (e.g., "It's my own fault I got injured"), stable over time (e.g., "I'm never going to get back all my mobility"), and global in nature (e.g., "It's going to affect my entire life"). At the same time, these individuals tend to explain positive events as externally caused (e.g., "Healing just takes time"), unstable over time (e.g., "My progress is likely to be up and down"), and specific in nature (e.g., "My recovery depends on this particular therapist and treatment").

Researchers investigating the links between explanatory style and health have demonstrated a connection between pessimistic explanatory style and negative health consequences. Simply put, individuals who attribute bad events to internal, stable, and global causes experience poorer health than their more optimistic counterparts who explain bad events with external, unstable, and specific causes (Peterson, 1995). Kamen and Seligman (1987) suggested that links between pessimism and immune system function might underlie this relationship, and, in a study investigating this hypothesis, they found that older adults with a pessimistic explanatory style did indeed exhibit lowered immunocompetence (Kamen-Siegel, Rodin, Seligman, & Dwyer, 1991). Mundane passivity in the face of disease could be another possible mechanism contributing to the relationship between pessimistic explanatory style and poor health (Lin & Peterson, 1990). Kamen and Seligman (1987) noted that pessimists are passive with regard to self-help, self-care, and life challenges. Finally, it is also possible that pessimistic explanatory style increases the chances of social isolation, loneliness, and/or depression (Peterson & Seligman, 1984). Interestingly, all three of these factors have been observed to be indicators of poor psychological adjustment among injured athletes (Gordon, Milios, & Grove, 1991a). Consideration of explanatory style also has important ramifications for rehabilitation interventions. Specifically researchers have demonstrated that depressive symptoms decrease significantly as explanatory style becomes more optimistic during treatment (Barber et al., 2005).

Dispositional Optimism

Scheier and Carver (1985, 1987, 1992) have discussed the health-related consequences of a personality variable that bears some resemblance to explanatory style. They call this variable dispositional optimism and define it simply as a general expectancy for good rather than bad outcomes to occur. It has been suggested that these positive expectancies might influence health via physiological and behavioral/interpersonal pathways (Peterson & Bossio, 1991; Scheier & Carver, 1987). Investigations of the proposed physiological mechanisms have not obtained consistent results, but some studies have found differences in susceptibility to stress and depression, cardiovascular reactivity, and immunological functioning to be associated with individual differences in optimism. For example, dispositional optimism has been identified as a significant predictor of future depressive symptoms (Vickers & Vogeltanz, 2000). In addition, Van Treuren and Hull (1986) found that optimists were less reactive than pessimists when blood pressure and pulse rate responses were monitored during exposure to positive and negative events. There is also some evidence that an optimistic orientation is positively related to natural killer cell activity (Bachen et al., cited in Scheier & Carver, 1992; Levy & Wise, 1987), while a pessimistic orientation is associated with disease progression (Goodkin, Antoni, & Blaney, 1986).

Studies of the proposed behavioral mechanisms have been more consistent in their findings. Taylor and Aspinwall (1996) summarize these findings by suggesting that optimism may mitigate the stress-illness relationship by facilitating successful coping efforts, preventing stressful events from intruding into other aspects of life, and/or encouraging better health practices. Coping appears to be a particularly important behavioral mechanism, and it has been repeatedly shown that optimists tend to cope by accepting the reality of negative situations, seeking social support, engaging in positive reinterpretation, and using direct, problem-focused coping strategies (Grove & Heard, 1997; Scheier & Carver, 1987, 1992). At the same time, they tend not to deny the reality of negative situations, disengage from their coping efforts, and become pre-occupied with their emotional distress:

> "As soon as you can start moving your toes, you move your toes. As soon as you can start moving your leg, you move your leg. As soon as you can walk, you walk... I think you have highs and lows. But I always say to myself, no matter how bad it gets, it always gets better. So even if I was really down, I didn't worry about it. I just looked on ahead and knew that it would get better."
> (Bianco, 1996, cited in Grove & Bianco, 1999, p. 91)

> "The best feeling is when you can put down one crutch, and then two."
> (Bianco, 1999, p.164)

A compelling demonstration of the potential link between optimism and health was provided in a study of recovery from coronary artery bypass surgery (Scheier et al., 1989). In that investigation, optimists and pessimists were compared on mood states and coping strategies prior to surgery, physiological reactions during surgery, and recovery progress after surgery. The findings indicated that optimism had positive consequences at all three points in time. Specifically, optimists reported less hostility and depression than pessimists immediately prior to surgery. They also made plans and set goals for recovery prior to the operation to a greater extent than pessimists, and they exhibited fewer adverse physiological reactions during surgery than the pessimists. In addition, optimists tended to recover faster than pessimists, both in terms of objective recovery indices and in terms of subjective ratings of improvement by members of the rehabilitation team. Finally, there was a strong relationship ($r = .57$, $df = 1.39$) between presurgery optimism and self-reported quality of life six months after the operation. [1]

The importance of an optimistic outlook has also been demonstrated in relation to sport injury rehabilitation. More specifically, Ievleva and Orlick (1991) found that such an outlook correlated negatively ($r = -.21$, $df = .44$) with the time needed for athletes to recover from Grade II ankle and knee injuries. Bianco (1996, 1999) obtained additional evidence for the central role of an optimistic orientation during sport injury rehabilitation in her interviews with elite skiers experiencing long and difficult recovery periods:

> "I knew I would be 100% after 6 months. Many other racers had gone through it and returned to ski racing and had been successful again. So, I didn't really let it get me down." (Bianco, 1999, p.162)

> "The more positive you keep, the more you can really believe that you can come back full strength to compete as good, or better, than you did before the injury. That's what really keeps you driving and working through the pain and the setbacks....I'm a pretty positive person. I see the good in everything. You've got to turn everything into good. Sometimes when bad things happen, I just remember that in a month or two, I'll look back at the situation and laugh—so that makes it a lot easier." (Bianco, 1996, cited in Grove & Bianco, 1999, p. 94)

Perfectionism

Perfectionists have a tendency to set extremely high standards for their own behavior and/or to believe that others are setting extremely high standards that they must meet (Hewitt & Flett, 1996). Such beliefs are associated with a heightened stress responses due, in part, to associated tendencies toward

- constant striving,
- self-doubt,
- excessive concern about mistakes,
- all-or-none thinking, and
- overgeneralization of failure

(Frost, Martens, Lahart, & Rosenblate, 1990; Hewitt & Flett, 1993). Various aspects of perfectionism have also been linked to

- heightened anger responses,
- obsessive compulsive behavior,
- depression, and
- psychosomatic distress

(Dunkley & Blankstein, 2000; Flett, Hewitt, Blankstein, & Mosher, 1995; Mor, Day, Flett, & Hewitt, 1995; Saboonchi & Lundh, 2003; Schweitzer & Hamilton, 2002). From an appraisal perspective, perfectionists typically hold stringent criteria for success, and also tend to equate their self-worth with their performance. Thus, minor setbacks can be perceived as major failures leading to fears about losing control, looking foolish, and being criticized which, in turn, can increase anxiety and have negative effects on self-concept and self-esteem (Blankstein, Flett, Hewitt, & Eng, 1993; Flett, Hewitt, Blankstein, & O'Brien, 1991; Hall, Kerr, & Matthews, 1998; Hewitt & Genest, 1990; Koivula, Hassmen, & Fallby, 2002). In addition, there is evidence to suggest that high levels of perfectionism may be associated with an increased incidence of injury among dancers (Liederbach & Compagno, 2001).

In terms of coping processes, it appears that high personal standards are sometimes associated with the use of active, task-oriented coping strategies such as planned action and suppression of competing activities (Dunkley, Blankstein, Halsall, Williams, & Winkworth, 2000; Flett, Hewitt, Blankstein, Solnick, & Van Brunschot, 1996; Flett, Russo, & Hewitt, 1994; Grove, 2004). However, this same aspect of perfectionism has also shown a relationship to less positive forms of coping such as

- denial,
- avoidance,
- self-blame,
- emotional preoccupation, and
- behavioral disengagement

(Flett, Russo, & Hewitt, 1994; Grove, 2004; Hewitt, Flett, & Endler, 1995). These less positive forms of coping appear to be particularly prevalent when high personal standards exist alongside high levels of concern over mistakes and/or socially prescribed perfectionism (Dunkley & Blankstein, 2000; Dunkley et al., 2000; Flett et al., 1994, 1996; Hewitt et al., 1995).

Finally, perfectionistic tendencies have shown an association with unfavorable outcomes from therapeutic interventions (Blatt, 1995). Although most of this work has focused on psychological treatment for depression, the processes underlying these negative outcomes may have implications for practitioners who work in the injury rehabilitation area. More specifically, Zuroff and colleagues (2000) found that the negative relationship between perfectionism and therapeutic outcomes was partially explained by a general failure on the part of perfectionistic clients to develop strong alliances with members of the treatment team. In subsequent research, Shahar, Blatt, Zuroff, Krupnick, and Sotsky (2004) discovered that pretreatment perfectionism was also associated with poor development of social support networks. This combination of weak therapeutic alliances and poor social support networks was highly predictive of poor treatment outcomes for perfectionistic individuals.

Hardiness

Hardiness is another personality trait believed to moderate appraisal processes, perceived stress, coping strategies, and health outcomes. Hardiness represents a "constellation of personality characteristics that function as a resistance resource in the encounter with stressful life events" (Kobasa, Maddi & Kahn, 1982, p. 169). It is composed of three interrelated elements:

- commitment
- challenge
- control

Commitment refers to a strong belief in one's own value and self-worth as well as a sense of purpose and involvement in whatever one is doing. Challenge refers to a tendency to view difficulties and change as problems to be overcome rather than threats to one's personal security. Individuals scoring high in challenge exhibit a high degree of cognitive flexibility that permits effective appraisal of potentially threatening events. Control involves a sense of personal power over the events in one's life. Individuals with a strong sense of control assume responsibility for their actions and are able to avert feelings of helplessness through the use of effective thinking, decision making, and coping strategies. Simply put, hardy people are committed to what they are doing in their lives, they believe they have personal control over the solutions to life problems, and they view adaptation and change as opportunities for growth rather than as threats.

Research conducted by Kobasa and colleagues has linked hardiness to physical health both retrospectively and prospectively. Kobasa (1979), for example, measured various elements of the hardiness construct and self-reported illness among executives from a utility company. Groups of executives experiencing low rather than high levels of illness over the previous 3 years were characterized by a high level of commitment (vs. alienation), a perception of meaningfulness in their activities, and an internal locus of control. These findings were viewed as consistent with the three-dimensional model of hardiness outlined above. In another study, Kobasa et al. (1982) collected data on personality and previous illness from a group of middle-aged male executives. These individuals were then followed for two years, with illness data recorded at the end of each 12-month period. Results once again supported the importance of the hardiness construct within the health domain. Specifically, the executives who were low in hardiness experienced high levels of illness when exposed to stressful environments, but the executives who were high in hardiness had self-reported illness scores that were close to baseline under these conditions.

The mechanisms underlying the connection between hardiness and health have been debated (cf. Hull, Van Treuren, & Virnelli, 1987), but it has been suggested that both appraisal and coping processes contribute to this relationship (Gentry & Kobasa, 1984; Florian, Mikulincer, & Taubman, 1995). More specifically, individuals high in hardiness seem to evaluate and interpret potentially stressful experiences in a way that minimizes their negative impact (Allred & Smith, 1989; Wiebe, 1991). Even when stress is perceived, however, hardy individuals have a tendency to rely on adaptive rather than maladaptive coping strategies (Blaney & Ganellen, 1990; Nowack, 1989). This tendency is nicely illustrated by the findings of Williams, Wiebe, and Smith (1992), who examined relationships between hardiness and coping in a group of university undergraduates. They observed significant negative correlations between avoidance-oriented coping and three hardiness variables (commitment, control, total hardiness score) as well as significant positive correlations between problem-focused coping, seeking of social support, and the commitment component of hardiness.

Studies of Injured Athletes

Personality traits have not been extensively examined in connection with appraisal processes, perceived stress, and coping among injured athletes. However, there is some evidence that neuroticism, explanatory style, dispositional optimism, perfectionism, and hardiness are related to these psychological processes. Grove, Stewart, and Gordon (1990), for example, investigated emotional reactions among 21 sport performers who underwent knee reconstruction surgery because of anterior cruciate ligament (ACL) damage. The athletes completed questionnaire measures of hardiness and dispositional optimism, and they provided periodic explanations for their rehabilitation progress that were transformed into an index of explanatory style. The athletes also responded to a mood state inventory once a week for 3 months following surgery. The mood state inventory assessed seven moods (tension, depression, anger, fatigue, confusion, vigor, and esteem-related affect), which were then correlated with scores on the personality measures. The results are summarized in Table 1.

Several aspects of the data in Table 1 deserve comment:

- First, all three personality factors exhibited potentially meaningful relationships to mood during the first 3 months of recovery from knee reconstruction surgery.
- Second, the direction of these relationships was generally consistent with expectations based on a conceptual understanding of the hardiness, optimism, and explanatory style constructs. More specifically, negative emotions such as tension, depression, and anger exhibited inverse relationships with hardiness and optimism but direct relationships with explanatory pessimism. Positive emotions such as vigor and esteem-related affect, on the other hand, exhibited mostly direct relationships with hardiness and optimism but inverse relationships with explanatory pessimism.

Table 1.

Personality and mood state relationships in the 3 months following knee reconstruction surgery (Grove, Stewart, & Gordon, 1990)

Time Period and Mood Variable	Hardiness Total	Optimism Total	Explanatory Pessimism
First Month			
Tension	-.22 *	-.30 *	+.46 **
Depression	-.24 *	-.27 *	+.37 **
Anger	-.06	-.12	+.26 *
Fatigue	-.38 **	-.32 *	+.47 **
Confusion	-.22 *	-.32 *	+.37 **
Vigor	-.03	+.04	-.44 **
Esteem	-.17	+.01	-.34 *
Second Month			
Tension	-.08	-.04	+.44 **
Depression	-.25 *	-.28 *	+.42 **
Anger	-.04	-.13	+.36 **
Fatigue	-.20	+.01	+.35 *
Confusion	-.16	-.25 *	+.50 **
Vigor	-.03	+.26 *	-.41 **
Esteem	-.08	+.16	-.28 *
Third Month			
Tension	-.15	+.04	+.30 *
Depression	-.24 *	-.35 *	+.19
Anger	-.15	-.35 *	+.13
Fatigue	-.31 *	-.21	+.38 **
Confusion	-.23 *	-.33 *	+.37 **
Vigor	+.22 *	+.48 **	-.39 **
Esteem	+.16	+.39 **	-.20

* Moderate effect size (d > .45 but d < .75) 1
** Large effect size (d > .75)

- Third, depression, fatigue, confusion, and vigor were the most consistent correlates of the personality factors assessed in this study, with 25 of the 36 possible relationships exhibiting effect sizes of .50 or more.
- Finally, the findings related to explanatory style are generally consistent with those obtained by other investigators who assessed this construct in relation to sport injury rehabilitation. More specifically, Laubach, Brewer, Van Raalte, and Petitpas (1996) found that athletes who were recovering relatively quickly from knee surgery had a tendency to attribute their rehabilitation progress to internal and personally controllable factors. This finding was replicated by Brewer et al. (2000), who also found that attendance at rehabilitation sessions was predicted by attributional style.

Neuroticism was investigated in relation to coping behavior during rehabilitation by Grove and Bahnsen (1997). In that study, 72 athletes who had recently received 4-

6 weeks of treatment for a sport-related injury completed a neuroticism scale and also supplied information about the strategies they had used to cope with the stress of the injury and its rehabilitation. Relationships were then examined between neuroticism, injury severity, coping strategies, and the amount of time needed for full physical recovery. Selected findings from this study are summarized in Table 2. These findings indicate that the use of certain coping strategies during rehabilitation was more closely linked to neuroticism than to injury severity. The coping strategies exhibiting the strongest relationships to neuroticism were primarily emotion-focused and/or avoidant in nature, and they included emotional focus/venting, denial, mental disengagement, and alcohol/drug use. Importantly, several of these same coping strategies also exhibited positive correlations with the length of the recovery period. That is, increased use of emotional focus/venting, denial, and mental disengagement was associated not only with higher levels of neuroticism but also with longer recovery periods. It is noteworthy that these relationships occurred in the absence of a direct association between neuroticism and recovery time ($r = -.02$, $d = .04$).

More recently, Ford, Gordon, and Eklund (2000) examined selected personality traits as potential moderators of the relationship between life stress and injury recovery. While Ford et al. did not address rehabilitation processes per se, their use of total time lost due to injury as a dependent variable makes their findings potentially relevant to practitioners working in rehabilitation settings. These findings included evidence

Table 2.

Correlations of neuroticism, injury severity, and recovery time with self-reported use of coping strategies by injured athletes (Grove & Bahnsen, 1997)

Coping Strategies	Neuroticism	Injury Severity	Recovery Time (Weeks)
Focus on and Vent Emotions	+.42**	+.02	+.30*
Positive Reinterpretation	+.36**	+.17	+.32*
Denial	+.34*	-.04	+.27*
Mental Disengagement	+.33*	+.01	+.36**
Behavioral Disengagement	+.32*	-.01	+.14
Turning to Religion	+.28*	+.14	+.13
Alcohol and Drug Use	+.28*	+.01	+.08
Restraint Coping	+.20	-.02	-.01
Emotional Social Support	+.18	+.07	+.05
Active Coping	-.16	-.13	-.13
Instrumental Social Support	-.14	-.14	-.32*
Suppress Competing Activities	+.11	+.03	-.02
Planning	-.10	-.03	-.01
Humor	+.02	+.12	-.03
Acceptance	-.01	+.11	-.11

* Moderate effect size (d > .45 but d < .75) 1

** Large effect size (d > .75)

for a moderating role of dispositional optimism and hardiness in the relationship between life stress and recovery. More specifically, athletes who experienced high levels of life stress lost more time to injury when they were low in dispositional optimism and when they were low in hardiness. Although it was unclear whether these relationships were due to more frequent injury occurrence or less effective progress during rehabilitation, the authors speculated that appraisal processes related to the injury itself and ineffective coping during rehabilitation may have been responsible. They further speculated that various personality factors might operate conjunctively to influence time lost due to injury (cf., Smith, Smoll, & Ptacek, 1990). In other words, athletes who possess more than one undesirable trait might be particularly vulnerable to negative appraisals, exaggerated stress perceptions, and maladaptive coping tendencies.

Overall then, the findings from these sport-specific studies are consistent with our model (Figure 1) and with the more general literature on psychological correlates of neuroticism, explanatory style, optimism, perfectionism, and hardiness in the health domain. More importantly, however, they strongly suggest that these dispositional constructs are related to the cognitive and behavioral responses of injured athletes during rehabilitation. Individuals who interact with injured athletes will therefore be in a better position to understand their rehabilitation behaviors and facilitate positive rehabilitation outcomes if they know how to obtain information about these personality traits.

Obtaining Personality Information

There are basically two ways that personality information can be collected by practitioners. These two procedures are best used in a complementary fashion, but they will be discussed separately here for ease of exposition. A formal approach to personality assessment involves the use of written scales. The advantage of this approach is that it is time-efficient and quantifiable. At the same time, however, it can sometimes be perceived as impersonal by the athlete. The alternative method, informal personality assessment, involves an analysis of statements and/or behaviors that arise spontaneously in face-to-face interactions. This approach is less directive and allows therapists considerable latitude to pursue issues that they think are meaningful. It does tend to be less precise than the formal approach, however, and for that reason may require more experience on the part of the therapist.

Formal Assessment Procedures

All of the personality factors discussed in this chapter can be measured with relatively brief pen-and-paper scales, and sports medicine personnel can obtain this information with very little inconvenience to the athlete. Relevant scales can be administered in the waiting area prior to treatment, during periods of passive treatment (e.g., icing), or as part of a post-treatment debriefing. If the athlete is presented with one or two scales per visit, practitioners can obtain a reasonably comprehensive personality profile in just three or four treatment sessions.

Neuroticism. Because neuroticism is recognized as a basic dimension of personality in numerous theoretical models, many different scales are available to assess this trait. The classic measure, however, is the 23-item neuroticism subscale from the

Eysenck Personality Questionnaire (EPQ-N; Eysenck & Eysenck, 1975). This subscale requires simple yes or no responses to questions like "Does your mood often go up and down?" and "Are your feelings easily hurt?", and scores range from 0-23 according to the number of yes responses. Similar items appear in the form of statements on the 48-item neuroticism subscale of the Revised NEO Personality Inventory (NEO PI-R; Costa & McCrae, 1992), with responses made on a five-point scale ranging from "strongly disagree" to "strongly agree." Although longer than the EPQ-N scale, the NEO PI-R neuroticism scale offers the advantage of providing separate scores for six different aspects of neuroticism rather than just a single neuroticism score. Information about these subcomponents (anxiety, angry hostility, depression, self-consciousness, impulsiveness, and vulnerability) could be useful to sports medicine personnel in some circumstances. A shortened, 12-item version of the NEO PI-R neuroticism scale is also available, but it is less reliable than the 48-item scale and does not provide scores for the subcomponents (Costa & McCrae, 1992). Nevertheless, this briefer scale could be useful if time constraints are a problem.

Explanatory style. Scales that measure explanatory style typically list a series of positive and/or negative events and ask respondents to indicate what the most likely cause of each event would have been if it had happened to them. The causal statements are then categorized along several different dimensions, and conclusions are drawn about the person's typical ways of interpreting good and bad events. A number of general explanatory style scales could be used to measure explanatory pessimism among injured athletes in this fashion. These general scales include several versions of the Attributional Style Questionnaire (ASQ; Peterson, Semmel, von Baeyer, Abramson, Metalsky, & Seligman, 1982; Peterson & Villanova, 1988; Whitley, 1991), the Balanced Atttributional Style Questionnaire (BASQ; Feather & Tiggemann, 1984), and the Attributional Style Assessment Test (ASAT; Anderson, Horowitz, & French, 1983; Anderson & Riger, 1991). The Revised Causal Dimension Scale (CDSII; McAuley, Duncan, & Russell, 1992) could also be used, but its standard format specifies a single event rather than multiple events. Two sport-specific instruments are also available: the Wingate Sport Achievement Responsibility Scale (WSARS; Tenenbaum, Furst, & Weingarten, 1984) and the Sport Attributional Style Scale (SASS; Hanrahan & Grove, 1990a; Hanrahan, Grove, & Hattie, 1989). The SASS allows athletes to generate their own causal statements in an open-ended response format, while the WSARS uses forced-choice responses. A short form of the SASS has also been developed (Hanrahan & Grove, 1990b), and it may be the instrument of choice in sport medicine settings.

Dispositional optimism. A variety of instruments are available to measure trait optimism. These instruments include the Expected Balance Scale (EBS; Staats, 1989), the Optimism and Pessimism Scale (OPS; Dember, Martin, Hummer, Howe, & Melton, 1989), and the Life Orientation Test (LOT; Scheier & Carver, 1985). The LOT offers the advantages of being brief and well researched. It is also easily accessed via published papers, and it has been used in sport injury studies (e.g., Ford et al., 2000). These characteristics probably make it the instrument of choice for assessing dispositional optimism in sport medicine settings. The most recent version of this instrument (Revised LOT; Scheier et al., 1994) contains just 10 items, with three of them worded in a positive direction and three of them worded in a negative direction. The remaining four statements are filler items and do not contribute to the score on the scale (Scheier et al., 1994). Respondents are simply asked to indicate the extent to which they agree or disagree with each of the statements. Response categories and their numerical equivalents are as follows: strongly agree (4); agree (3); neutral (2); disagree (1); strongly disagree (0). A total score for dispositional optimism is obtained by reverse-scoring the ratings for the negatively worded items and then totalling the numerical values for the six relevant items. Scores can range from 0 to 24, and higher scores indicate more optimsim on the part of the athlete. Separate scores can also be calculated for optimism and pessimism if that is preferred.

Perfectionism. The most widely used measures of perfectionism were developed by Frost et al. (1990) and Hewitt, Flett, Turnbull-Donovan, and Mikail (1991). Both measures have the same name (i.e., Multidimensional Perfectionism Scale or MPS), but they are based on different theoretical models and therefore measure different aspects of perfectionism. The instrument developed by Frost and colleagues contains 35 statements reflecting six aspects of perfectionism: personal standards, doubts about actions, concern over mistakes, need for organization, parental expectations, and parental criticism. Responses are made on five-point Likert-type scales to indicate the extent of agreement with each statement. Subscale scores can be used if desired, or a total perfectionism score can be obtained by summing the scores for all of the dimensions except organizational needs. The organizational needs subscale tends not to correlate with the other subscales and is therefore excluded when calculating the total.

Hewitt et al.'s (1991) scale consists of 45 items designed to assess three dimensions of perfectionism: self-oriented perfectionism, other-oriented perfectionism, and socially prescribed perfectionism. Respectively, these dimensions reflect unrealistic standards and perfectionistic motivations for oneself and for others as well as a belief that others expect one to be perfect. The scale requires a grade 6 or 7 reading level, and responses are made on seven-point, Likert-type scales to indicate the extent of agreement with each statement. The three dimensions of perfectionism assessed by this instrument are not typically combined with each other. More recently, scales measuring positive as well as negative aspects of perfectionism have appeared in the literature (e.g., Terry-Short, Owens, Slade, & Dewey, 1995). These two forms of perfectionism appear to have differential influences on attitudes toward the physical self among athletes (Haase, Prapavessis, & Owens, 2002), and it is therefore logical to assume that they would also have differential influences on appraisal processes related to physical recovery from injury. Although no research has specifically addressed this issue, the measurement tools are available to do so (e.g., Haase & Prapavessis, 2004).

Hardiness. Numerous hardiness scales have appeared in the psychological literature during the past two decades. The original Hardiness Scale (HS; Kobasa et al., 1982) contained 71 items drawn from preexisting scales believed to measure constructs related to commitment, challenge, and control. An abbreviated, 36-item version of this original instrument, the Revised Hardiness Scale (RHS), subsequently became available. Two additional hardiness scales were also developed in an effort to overcome measurement problems associated with the HS and the RHS. These "third generation" scales are the 50-item Personal Views Survey (PVS; Hardiness Institute, 1985) and the 45-item Dispositional Resilience Scale (DRS; Bartone, Ursano, Wright, & Ingraham, 1989). Despite the relatively large item pools in the third generation scales, we recommend their use in sports medicine settings because they appear to possess better psychometric properties than the earlier scales (Funk, 1992). Applications of the PVS have supported the usefulness of this measure in investigations of athletic injury (e.g., Ford et al., 2000).

Informal Assessment Procedures

Some sports medicine personnel may decide that informal assessment procedures are more appropriate than formal ones. This decision could arise because the desired personality scales are unavailable, because the practitioner is uncomfortable with written scales, or because the athlete indicates that he or she is uncomfortable with such scales. For purposes of this discussion, adopting an informal approach to personality assessment means

(a) talking to the injured athlete on a one-to-one basis in an effort to gain insight into his or her character and

(b) paying attention to comments made by the athlete either spontaneously or in response to others in the rehabilitation setting (including other injured athletes).

Effective use of this approach requires a thorough understanding of the personality factors that may influence rehabilitation behavior as well as good communication skills. The practitioner must be able to establish trust and rapport with the athlete, ask appropriate questions at appropriate times, listen attentively to statements made by the athlete, and draw logical inferences about his or her character and behavior based on these statements.

A tendency to experience negative emotions such as fear, sadness, embarrassment, guilt, and anger is the core feature of neuroticism (Costa & McCrae, 1992). Although some degree of negative emotionality is to be expected during rehabilitation, practitioners should be alert for comments or behaviors that suggest inappropriate amounts of anxiety or hostility for a given injury. Persistent feelings of guilt, rapid discouragement, and/or obvious withdrawal and isolation from teammates could also indicate neurotic tendencies, as could hypersensitivity and strong feelings of inferiority. Neurotic individuals may also be prone to experience and/or express feelings of being overwhelmed with the demands of rehabilitation and being unable to cope. They may also exhibit very low frustration tolerance and engage in impulsive behaviors such as experimenting with unconventional treatments or attempting to perform physical actions that they are clearly not well enough to perform.

Insight into the athlete's explanatory style will be obtained most directly by paying attention to "why" statements. These statements might refer to events that have actually occurred or to hypothetical events. For example, if actual recovery has been either slower than expected or faster than expected, the athlete could be asked why he or she believes this has occurred. Similarly, he or she could be asked to generate a likely cause for a hypothetical setback during rehabilitation. Although athletes generally tend to view the causes of these events in a realistic and productive manner (Grove, Hanrahan,

& Stewart, 1990), there might be occasions when this is not the case. If, for example, explanations for positive rehabilitation events tend to be external, unstable, and specific (e.g., "I had a different therapist for those two weeks where I did really well") or explanations for negative events tend to be internal, stable, and global (e.g., "I never have been able to handle pain and discomfort too well"), then a pessimistic explanatory style may be indicated. In order to confirm such an impression, it is essential that the practitioner obtain several explanations and carefully consider both their dimensional properties and their legitimacy. If, for example, one of the therapists really *is* much more competent than another, then such an attribution may reflect accurate perception more than pessimistic style.

Dispositional optimism could be assessed informally by asking specific questions at opportune times during treatment. An athlete who is handling a particular phase of treatment in a positive manner could be asked something like "Are you always so positive about things?" or "Do you approach everything with such a bright outlook?" Similarly, an athlete who has experienced a setback could be asked "I tend to believe that every cloud has a silver lining; how do you feel about that?" If responses to several of these questions and/or other comments made by the athlete indicate a consistently positive or negative outlook, then the practitioner may be able to make an inference about the degree of general optimism possessed by the individual.

Perfectionists set very high standards for themselves, and they tend to believe that others hold similarly high expectations for their performance. They also have a tendency to be overly concerned about making mistakes and to be extremely self-critical. By being aware of these tendencies and also being observant, rehabilitation professionals should be able to recognize potentially problematic levels of perfectionism among athletes. Athletes who are never satisfied with their own efforts, who refuse to undertake rehabilitation activities unless they can do them well, or who sabotage their progress by repeatedly trying to work beyond their current capabilities are exhibiting perfectionistic tendencies. If these behaviors are also accompanied by constant worries about what others might think of them and excessive negative self-talk, then high levels of perfectionism are indicated.

The defining characteristics of the hardy personality are:
- a tendency to view obstacles as challenges rather than threats (challenge);
- a tendency to become absorbed in what one is doing rather than just "going through the motions" (commitment); and
- a tendency to believe that one's outcomes are self-determined rather than determined by external forces (control).

Statements and behaviors that occur in response to setbacks during rehabilitation can provide valuable information about the athlete's perceptions of challenge versus threat. Similarly, comments or actions indicating a lack of enthusiasm for studies, sport, work, or life in general could indicate low levels of commitment, and, if pronounced, could suggest the need for psychological intervention. The therapist should note such comments and discuss them with other members of the rehabilitation team. Statements or behaviors that reflect a denial of personal responsibility during rehabilitation are also noteworthy. Refusing to set recovery goals or blaming the therapist and/or rehabilitation program for lack of progress may reflect such an attitude. Placing responsibility for recovery primarily in the hands of an external spiritual entity could also indicate a low level of perceived control, although one must be cautious in this regard because of the central role of religion in some people's lives.

When evaluating information obtained through either formal or informal assessment procedures, it is very important to bear in mind that, regardless of their personality traits, athletes are likely to cycle between denial, distress, and determined coping throughout the recovery process (Heil, 1993).

- Denial refers to a sense of disbelief about the seriousness of the injury, which can range from mild to profound and may vary across time and circumstances.
- Distress often includes anxiety, anger, depression, and feelings of helplessness.
- Determined coping implies acceptance of the injury and is characterized by the purposeful use of coping resources in working through the process of recovery.

Denial and distress will tend to be at their peak in the early stages of injury, while determined coping will usually prevail as rehabilitation proceeds. It is important to assess the magnitude of distress and how appropriate it is relative to the severity of the injury and the phase of recovery. Similarly, denial can sometimes be advantageous in that it allows athletes to maintain a positive outlook and mobilize their coping resources, but it can also become problematic if it allows the athlete to avoid the emotional work of recovery.

Implications for Practice

Effective provision of sports medicine services involves more than the facilitation of physical recovery. Indeed, if practitioners do not also take steps to help athletes cope with the psychological stress of injury and rehabilitation, then physical recovery may be delayed. Members of the sports medicine team are in an excellent position to help athletes cope with the stress of rehabilitation, and, as observed in Bianco's (2001) study of elite skiers, injured athletes often look to them for this type of support:

"We had the best relationship ever. He knew what I was thinking. He knew what I was going through. He was my moral supporter, a helper and a psychologist. He was pretty much everything for me." (p. 382)

Personality information can help rehabilitation personnel to provide a more complete (and therefore more effective) service by enabling them to recognize interrelated patterns of thought, emotion, and behavior during recovery. Although we have limited information about the effects of neuroticism, explanatory style, dispositional optimism, perfectionism, or hardiness on the thoughts, emotions, and behaviors of *injured athletes*, the research literature does offer some clues about what we can expect from individuals who differ substantially on these traits. Since maladaptive rehabilitation responses are likely to concern sports medicine personnel more than adaptive ones, a summary of probable responses from individuals at the negative extremes of these traits will be presented.

Highly neurotic athletes are prone to over-reactions, negative emotions, quick frustration, and impulsive actions. They also have a tendency to exaggerate physical symptoms and to use denial, disengagement, and emotional venting as injury-related coping mechanisms (Costa & McCrae, 1992; Grove & Bahnsen, 1997). Practitioners may need to make a conscious effort to model rational behavior when dealing with this type of athlete. At the same time, they should be prepared for emotional reactions and questioning of what might seem like well-planned and thoughtful treatment regimens. Maintaining precise records of progress and making even the smallest gains known to the athlete may be beneficial. Within limits, a tolerance may also need to be exhibited for impatience with conventional treatment modalities. At the same time, the athlete should be encouraged to develop skills in stress management (e.g., Greenberg, 2006), thought management (e.g., Zinsser, Bunker & Williams, 2001), and problem-focused coping strategies such as goal setting (e.g., Evans & Hardy, 2002a, 2002b; Potter & Grove, 1999).

Injured athletes with a highly pessimistic attributional style may be predisposed to feelings of helplessness and depression. Therefore, they may tend to isolate themselves from coaches and teammates and/or feel overwhelmed by the adjustments necessary because of their incapacitation. These adjustments could include such things as retaining a job during convalescence, scheduling time for treatments, depending on others for transportation, and handling unexpected medical expenses (Gordon, Milios, & Grove, 1991b). Athletes with pessimistic attributional styles may also fail to follow recommended treatment programs (especially the unsupervised aspects of their programs) and may exhibit a lack of persistence in the face of poor progress or setbacks (Brewer et al., 2000; Laubach et al., 1996; Shaffer & McAuley, 1993). Therapists should take steps to short-circuit such responses if they detect a highly pessimistic orientation on the part of the athlete. Encouraging continued attendance at training sessions and offering advice about how to cope with the extra demands of injury may prevent the athlete from feeling isolated and overwhelmed. In addition to providing such pragmatic advice, medical personnel may also need to provide emotional social support to these athletes (cf. Bianco, 2001).

Scheier and Carver (1987, 1992) have noted a number of similarities between the concepts of explanatory pessimism and dispositional optimism. They went on to say that pessimistic attributions may influence behavior primarily through their effect on generalized expectancies (i.e., optimism). Thus, therapists might expect to see many of the same reactions from athletes high in explanatory pessimism and those low in dispositional optimism. This similarity would seem especially relevant for depressive emotions, absence of self-initiated behavior change, and lack of persistence in times of difficulty. Because individuals low in dispositional optimism tend to use avoidance-oriented and emotion-oriented strategies to cope with stress (Grove & Heard, 1997; Scheier et al., 1994), therapists might also expect these athletes to deny the seriousness of their injuries and/or express anger during the course of rehabilitation. Denial tendencies might be diminished somewhat by providing the athlete with objective evidence about the extent of damage. In most cases, anger can be defused by listening empathetically, confronting the athlete in a calm and rational manner if expressions of anger become disruptive, and/or providing information on thought management techniques (Novaco, 1995). In cases where anger persists, Faulkner, Maguire, and Regnard (1994) suggest that individuals should first be asked to consider whether there are "hidden" reasons for their anger. A situation-specific assessment should then be made of the anger's causes, focus, and rationality. Finally, the athlete should be given "space" to recover before addressing further rehabilitation issues.

High levels of perfectionism present unique challenges for individuals working in sport injury rehabilitation. In general, athletes are goal-oriented individuals with a strong work ethic, a desire to master the tasks they undertake, and a tendency to hold themselves accountable for their outcomes. These characteristics can help them to succeed, but when exaggerated, they can also be counter-productive in therapeutic settings. Indeed, perfectionists can undermine the therapeutic process by placing unrealistic demands on themselves, the therapists, the treatment modalities, or significant others such as family, coaches, and teammates (cf. Lundh, 2004). At the same time, they are likely to be unaware that they are doing so, because these attitudes and behaviors have produced positive results for them in the past. When confronted with this type of client, it is sometimes beneficial to draw attention first to the nature of the demands that are being placed on an impersonal process (e.g., the treatment) or other people (e.g., family members or the therapist). Because these aspects of the situation are either prescribed or beyond the athlete's control, they are, unfortunately, likely to remain imperfect no matter what the athletes does (Ellis, 2002). If athletes' thinking can be shifted toward *desiring* perfection from the procedures and other people rather than *demanding* it, then it may be easier for them to accept that their own interests are best served by personally striving for perfection while still being able to accept imperfection (Lundh, 2004). To the extent that this occurs, the therapeutic relationship will be more congenial, and there will be less risk of noncompliance due to dissatisfaction with results.

Individuals low in hardiness (particularly the commitment and control dimensions of hardiness) share several common tendencies. Specifically, these individuals tend to worry about their public image, over-generalize negative aspects of their character, and experience depressive moods (Hull et al., 1987). They also tend to view potentially stressful events as threatening, suffer high levels of anxiety and apprehension about their ability to cope, and make infrequent use of social support resources (Florian et al., 1995; Maddi & Khoshaba, 1994). Thus, practitioners might expect injured athletes who are low in hardiness to ruminate about the way others view them and their injury, become nervous and tense when faced with stressful treatment procedures, and, perhaps, get depressed about their incapacities. In addition, they might be inclined to isolate themselves from coaches and teammates and may fail to adhere to recommended treatment regimens. Therapists should take care to communicate clearly with these athletes about the severity of the injury, and they should also consider the need for supplying information on stress management (e.g., Greenberg, 2006). Contacts with coaches, teammates, and other recovering athletes should be actively encouraged, and steps should be taken to reinforce personal initiative in relation to rehabilitation. Active involvement in the determination of rehabilitation goals and self-monitoring of rehabilitation progress via charts or graphs may also be desirable for these athletes in order to enhance feelings of personal commitment and control.

Summary

Personality is one of several factors that influence an athlete's appraisal processes, perceived stress levels, and coping behaviors during rehabilitation. Research indicates that neuroticism, explanatory style, dispositional optimism, perfectionism, and hardiness have health-related consequences, and it was suggested that these traits might also influence thoughts, feelings, and behaviors during recovery from injury. Studies of injured athletes indicate that this is indeed the case. More specifically, mood states, coping behaviors, and time lost due to injury have been shown to be correlated with several of these personality factors in predictable ways. Knowledge of an athlete's personality may therefore help sports medicine personnel to anticipate, understand, and deal with undesirable rehabilitation responses. For that reason, formal and informal approaches to personality assessment were examined, and problems that could arise during rehabilitation were discussed with reference to specific personality characteristics. Effective resolution of these problematic responses will require knowledge, awareness, compassion, and creativity on the part of the practitioner.

Chapter Note

[1] We provide Cohen's d as an estimate of effect size rather than the more traditional p-value because of the disparate sample sizes in the studies cited. Unlike significance levels, this statistic is independent of sample size, with small, moderate, and large effect sizes indicated by ds of approximately .20, .50, and .80, respectively (Cohen, 1988).

References

Allred, K. D., & Smith, T. W. (1989). The hardy personality: Cognitive and physiological responses to evaluative threat. *Journal of Personality and Social Psychology, 56,* 257-266.

Andersen, M. B., & Williams, J. M. (1988). A model of stress and athletic injury: Prediction and prevention. *Journal of Sport & Exercise Psychology, 10,* 294-306.

Anderson, C. A., Horowitz, L. M., & French, R. (1983). Attributional style of lonely and depressed people. *Journal of Personality and Social Psychology, 45,* 127-136.

Anderson, C. A., & Riger, A. L. (1991). A controllability attributional model of problems in living: Dimensional and situational interactions in the prediction of depression and loneliness. *Social Cognition, 9,* 149-181.

Anderson, S. E. H. (1995). Personality, appraisal, and adaptational outcomes in HIV seropositive men and women. *Research in Nursing & Health, 18,* 303-312.

Barber, J. P., Abrams, M. J., Connolly-Gibbons, M. B., Crits-Christoph, P., Brarett, M. S., Rynn, M. & Siqueland, L. (2005). Explanatory style change in supportive-expressive dynamic therapy *Journal of Clinical Psychology, 61,* 257-268.

Bartone, P. T., Ursano, R., Wright, K., & Ingraham, L. (1989). The impact of military air disaster on the health of assistance workers. *Journal of Nervous and Mental Disease, 177,* 317-328.

Bianco, T. (1996). *Social support influences on recovery from sport injury.* Unpublished master's thesis. School of Human Kinetics, University of Ottawa, Ottawa, Ontario, Canada.

Bianco, T. (1999). Sport injury and illness: Elite skiers describe their experiences. *Research Quarterly for Exercise and Sport, 70,* 157-169.

Bianco, T. (2001). Social support and recovery from sport injury: Elite skiers share their experiences. *Research Quarterly for Exercise and Sport, 72,* 376-388.

Blaney, P. H., & Ganellen, R. J. (1990). Hardiness and social support. In I. G. Sarason, B. Sarason, & G. Pierce (Eds.), *Social support: An international view* (pp. 297-318). New York: Wiley.

Blankstein, K. R., Flett, G. L., Hewitt, P. L., & Eng, A. (1993). Dimensions of perfectionism and irrational fears: An examination with the Fear Survey Schedule. *Personality and Individual Differences, 15*, 323-328.

Blatt, S. J. (1995). The destructiveness of perfectionism: Implications for the treatment of depression. *American Psychologist, 50*, 1003-1020.

Bolger, N., & Schilling, E. A. (1991). Personality and the problems of everyday life: The role of neuroticism in exposure and reactivity daily stressors. *Journal of Personality, 59*, 355-386.

Bolger, N., & Zuckerman, A. (1995). A framework for studying personality in the stress process. *Journal of Personality and Social Psychology, 69*, 890-902.

Brewer, B. W. (1994). Review and critique of models of psychological adjustment to athletic injury. *Journal of Applied Sport Psychology, 6*, 87-100.

Brewer, B. W. (1998). Adherence to sport injury rehabilitation programs. *Journal of Applied Sport Psychology, 10*, 70-82.

Brewer, B. W. (2001). Psychology of sport injury rehabilitation. In R. N. Singer, H. A. Hausenblas, & C. M. Janelle (Eds.), *Handbook of sport psychology (2nd ed.)* (pp. 787-809). New York: Wiley.

Brewer, B. W., Cornelius, A. E., Van Raalte, J. L., Petitpas, A. J., Sklar, J. H., Pohlman, M. H., et al. (2000). Attributions for recovery and adherence to rehabilitation following anterior cruciate ligament reconstruction: A prospective analysis. *Psychology & Health, 15*, 283-291.

Cohen, J. (1988). *Statistical power analysis for the behavioral sciences (2nd ed.).* Hillsdale, NJ: Erlbaum.

Costa, P. T., & McCrae, R. R. (1989). Personality, stress, and coping: Some lessons from a decade of research. In K. S. Markides & C. L. Cooper (Eds.), *Aging, stress, and health* (pp. 269-285). New York: Wiley.

Costa, P. T., & McCrae, R. R. (1992). *Professional manual: Revised NEO Personality Inventory and NEO Five-Factor Inventory.* Odessa, FL: Psychological Assessment Resources.

Daly, J. M., Brewer, B. W., Van Raalte, J. L., Petitpas, A. J., & Sklar, J. H. (1995). Cognitive appraisal, emotional adjustment, and adherence to rehabilitation following knee surgery. *Journal of Sport Rehabilitation, 4*, 23-30.

Dember, W. N., Martin, S., Hummer, M. K., Howe, S., & Melton, R. (1989). The measurement of optimism and pessimism. *Current Psychology: Research & Reviews, 8*, 102-119.

Dunkley, D. M., & Blankstein, K. R. (2000). Self-critical perfectionism, coping, hassles, and current distress: A structural equation modeling approach. *Cognitive Therapy and Research, 24*, 713-730.

Dunkley, D. M., & Blankstein, K. R., Halsall, J., Williams, M., and Winkworth, G. (2000). The relation between perfectionism and distress: Hassles, coping, and perceived social support as mediators and moderators. *Journal of Counseling Psychology, 47*, 437-453.

Ellis, A. (2002) The role of irrational beliefs in perfectionism. In G. L. Flett & P. L. Hewitt (Eds.), *Perfectionism: Theory, research, and treatment* (pp. 217-229). Washington, DC: American Psychological Association.

Endler, N. S., & Parker, J. D. A. (1990). Multidimensional assessment of coping: A critical evaluation. *Journal of Personality and Social Psychology, 58*, 844-854.

Evans, L., & Hardy, L. (1995). Sport injury and grief responses: A review. *Journal of Sport & Exercise Psychology, 17*, 227-245.

Evans, L., & Hardy, L. (2002a). Injury rehabilitation: A goal-setting intervention study. *Research Quarterly for Exercise and Sport, 73*, 310-319.

Evans, L., & Hardy, L. (2002b). Injury rehabilitation: a qualitative follow-up study. *Research Quarterly for Exercise and Sport, 73*, 320-329.

Eysenck, H. J. (1988). Personality, stress and cancer: Prediction and prophylaxis. *British Journal of Medical Psychology, 61*, 57-75.

Eysenck, H. J., & Eysenck, M. W. (1985). *Personality and individual differences.* New York: Plenum.

Eysenck, H. J., & Eysenck, S. B. G. (1975). *Manual of the Eysenck Personality Questionnaire.* London: Hodder & Stoughton.

Faulkner, A., Maguire, P., & Regnard, C. (1994). Dealing with anger in a patient or relative: A flow diagram. *Palliative Medicine, 8*, 51-57.

Feather, N. T., & Tiggemann, M. (1984). A balanced measure of attributional style. *Australian Journal of Psychology, 36*, 267-283.

Flett, G. L., Hewitt, P. L., Blankstein, K. R., & Mosher, S. W. (1995). Perfectionism, life events, and depressive symptoms: A test of a diathesis-stress model. *Current Psychology: Research & Reviews, 14*, 112-137.

Flett, G. L., Hewitt, P. L., Blankstein, K. R., & O'Brien, (1991). Perfectionism and learned resourcefulness in depression and self-esteem. *Personality and Individual Differences, 12*, 61-68.

Flett, G. L., Hewitt, P. L., Blankstein, K. R., Solnick, M., & Van Brunschot, M. (1996). Perfectionism, social problem-solving ability, and psychological distress. *Journal of Rational-Emotive and Cognitive-Behavior Therapy, 14*, 245-274.

Flett, G. L., Russo, F., & Hewitt, P. L. (1994). Dimensions of perfectionism and constructive thinking as a coping response. *Journal of Rational-Emotive and Cognitive-Behavior Therapy, 12*, 163-179.

Florian, V., Mikulincer, M., & Taubman, O. (1995). Does hardiness contribute to mental health during a stressful real-life situation? The roles of appraisal and coping. *Journal of Personality and Social Psychology, 68*, 687-695.

Ford, I. W., & Gordon, S. (1993). Social support and athletic injury: The perspective of sport physiotherapists. *Journal of Sports Sciences, 18*, 301-312.

Ford, I. W., Gordon, S., & Eklund, R. C. (2000). An examination of psychosocial variables moderating the relationship between life stress and injury time-loss among athletes of a high standard. *The Australian Journal of Science and Medicine in Sport, 25*, 17-25.

Friedman, H. S. (Ed.). (1990). *Personality and disease.* New York: Wiley.

Frost, R. O., Marten, P., Lahart, C., & Rosenblate, R. (1990). The dimensions of perfectionism. *Cognitive Therapy and Research, 14*, 449-468.

Funk, S.C. (1992). Hardiness: A review of theory and research. *Health Psychology, 11*, 335-345.

Gentry, W. D., & Kobasa, S. C. (1984). Social and psychological resources mediating stress-illness relationships in humans. In W.D. Gentry (Ed.), *Handbook of behavioral medicine* (pp. 87-116). New York: Guilford Press.

Goodkin, K., Antoni, M. H., & Blaney, P. H. (1986). Stress and helplessness in the promotion of cervical intraepithelial neoplasia to invasive squamous cell carcinoma of the cervix. *Journal of Psychosomatic Research, 50*, 67-76.

Gordon, S., Milios, D., & Grove, J. R. (1991a). Psychological aspects of the recovery process from sport injury: The perspective of sport physiotherapists. *Australian Journal of Science and Medicine in Sport, 23*, 53-60.

Gordon, S., Milios, D., & Grove, J. R. (1991b). Psychological adjustment to sports injuries: Implications for athletes, coaches, and family members. *Sports Coach, 14 (2)*, 40-44.

Greenberg, J. S. (2006). *Comprehensive stress management (9th ed.).* New York: McGraw-Hill.

Grove, J. R. (1993). Personality and injury rehabilitation among sport performers. In D. Pargman (Ed.), *Psychological bases of sport injuries* (pp. 99-120). Morgantown, WV: Fitness Information Technology.

Grove, J. R. (2004). Performance slumps in sport: Prevention and coping. In C. D. Spielberger (Ed.), *Encyclopedia of applied psychology – volume 2* (pp. 833-841). New York: Elsevier.

Grove, J. R., & Bahnsen, A. (1997). *Neuroticism, injury severity, and coping with rehabilitation.* Unpublished manuscript, School of Human Movement & Exercise Science, The University of Western Australia.

Grove, J. R., & Bianco, T. (1999). Personality correlates of psychological processes during injury rehabilitation. In D. Pargman (Ed.), *Psychological bases of sport injuries (2nd ed.)* (pp. 89-110). Morgantown, WV: Fitness Information Technology.

Grove, J. R., & Heard, N. P. (1997). Optimism and sport-confidence as correlates of slump-related coping among athletes. *The Sport Psychologist, 11*, 400-410.

Grove, J. R., Hanrahan, S. J., & Stewart, R. M. L. (1990). Attributions for rapid or slow recovery from sports injuries. *Canadian Journal of Sport Sciences, 15*, 107-114.

Grove, J. R., Stewart, R. M. L., & Gordon, S. (1990, October). *Emotional reactions of athletes to knee rehabilitation.* Paper presented at the annual meeting of the Australian Sports Medicine Federation, Alice Springs.

Haase, A. M., & Prapavessis, H. (2004). Assessing the factor structure and composition of the Positive and Negative Perfectionism Scale. *Personality & Individual Differences, 36*, 1725-1740.

Haase, A. M., & Prapavessis, H., & Owens, R. G. (2002). Perfectionism, social physique anxiety, and disordered eating: A comparison of male and female elite athletes. *Psychology of Sport and Exercise, 3*, 209-222.

Hall, H. K., Kerr, A. W., & Matthews, J. (1998). Precompetitive anxiety in sport: The contribution of achievement goals and perfectionism. *Journal of Sport & Exercise Psychology, 20*, 194-217.

Hanrahan, S. J., & Grove, J. R. (1990a). Further examination of the psychometric properties of the Sport Attributional Style Scale. *Journal of Sport Behavior, 13*, 183-193.

Hanrahan, S. J., & Grove, J. R. (1990b). A short form of the Sport Attributional Style Scale. *Australian Journal of Science and Medicine in Sport, 22*, 97-101.

Hanrahan, S. J., Grove, J. R., & Hattie, J. A. (1989). Development of a questionnaire measure of sport-related attributional style. *International Journal of Sport Psychology, 20*, 114-134.

Hardiness Institute. (1985). *Personal Views Survey.* Arlington Heights, IL: Author.

Hardy, L., Jones, G., & Gould, D. (1996). *Understanding psychological preparation for sport: Theory and practice of elite performers.* New York: Wiley.

Heil, J. (1993). A psychologist's view of the personal challenge of injury. In J. Heil (Ed.), *Psychology of sport injury* (pp. 34-46). Champaign, IL: Human Kinetics.

Hewitt, P. L., & Flett, G. L. (1993). Dimensions of perfectionism, daily stress, and depression: A test of the specific vulnerability hypothesis. *Journal of Abnormal Psychology, 102,* 58-65.

Hewitt, P. L., & Flett, G. L. (1996). Personality traits and the coping process. In M. Zeidner & N. S. Endler (Eds.), *Handbook of coping: Theory, research, applications* (pp. 410-433). New York: Wiley.

Hewitt, P. L., Flett, G. L., & Endler, N. S. (1995). Perfectionism, coping, and depression symptomatology in a clinical sample. *Clinical Psychology and Psychotherapy, 2,* 47-58.

Hewitt, P. L., Flett, G. L., Turnbull-Donovan, W., & Mikail, S. F. (1991). The Multidimensional Perfectionism Scale: Reliability, validity, and psychometric properties in psychiatric samples. *Psychological Assessment: A Journal of Consulting and Clinical Psychology, 3,* 464-468

Hewitt, P. L., & Genest, M. (1990). Ideal self: Schematic processing of perfectionistic content in dysphoric university students. *Journal of Personality and Social Psychology, 102,* 802-808.

Holahan, C. J., Moos, R. H., & Schaefer, J. A. (1996). Coping, resistance, and growth: Conceptualizing adaptive functioning. In M. Zeidner & N. S. Endler (Eds.), *Handbook of coping* (pp. 24-43). New York: Wiley.

Hull, J. G., Van Treuren, R. R., & Virnelli, S. (1987). Hardiness and health: A critique and alternative approach. *Journal of Personality and Social Psychology, 53,* 518-530.

Ievleva, L., & Orlick, T. (1991). Mental links to enhanced healing: An exploratory study. *The Sport Psychologist, 5,* 25-40.

Kamen, L., & Seligman, M. E. (1987). Explanatory style and health. *Current Psychology: Research & Reviews, 6,* 207-218.

Kamen-Siegel, L., Rodin, J., Seligman, M. E., & Dwyer, J. (1991). Explanatory style and cell-mediated immunity in older men and women. *Health Psychology, 10,* 229-235.

Kardum, I., & Hudek-Knezevic, J. (1996). The relationship between Eysenck's personality traits, coping styles and moods. *Personality and Individual Differences, 20,* 341-350.

Kobasa, S. C. (1979). Stressful life events, personality, and health: An inquiry into hardiness. *Journal of Personality and Social Psychology, 37,* 1-11.

Kobasa, S. C., Maddi, S. R., & Kahn, S. (1982). Hardiness and health: A prospective study. *Journal of Personality and Social Psychology, 42,* 168-177.

Koivula, N., Hassmen, P., & Fallby, J. (2002). Self-esteem and perfectionism in elite athletes: Effects on competitive anxiety and self-confidence. *Personality & Individual Differences, 32,* 865-875.

Laubach, W. J., Brewer, B. W., Van Raalte, J. L., & Petitpas, A. J. (1996). Attributions for recovery and adherence to sport injury rehabilitation. *Australian Journal of Science and Medicine in Sport, 28,* 30-34.

Lazarus, R. S., & Folkman, S. (1984). *Stress, appraisal, and coping.* New York: Springer.

Levy, S. M., & Wise, B. D. (1987). Psychosocial risk factors, natural immunity, and cancer progression: Implications for intervention. *Current Psychology: Research & Reviews, 6,* 229-243.

Liederbach M., & Compagno, J. M. (2001). Psychological aspects of fatigue-related injuries in dancers. *Journal of Dance Medicine & Science, 5,* 116-120.

Lin, E. H., & Peterson, C. (1990). Pessimistic explanatory style and response to illness. *Behavior Research & Therapy, 28,* 243-248.

Lundh, L-G. (2004). Perfectionism and acceptance. *Journal of Rational-Emotive & Cognitive-Behavior Therapy, 22,* 255-269.

Maddi, S. R., & Khoshaba, D. M. (1994). Hardiness and mental health. *Journal of Personality Assessment, 63,* 265-274.

Maes, S., Leventhal, H., & de Ridder, D. T. (1996). Coping with chronic diseases. In M. Zeidner & N. S. Endler (Eds.), *Handbook of coping: Theory, research, applications* (pp. 221-251). New York: Wiley.

McAuley, E., Duncan, T. E., & Russell, D. W. (1992). Measuring causal attributions: The Revised Causal Attribution Scale (CDSII). *Personality and Social Psychology Bulletin, 18,* 566-573.

McCrae, R. R., & John, O. P. (1992). An introduction to the five-factor model and its applications. *Journal of Personality, 60,* 175-215.

McDonald, S. A., & Hardy, C. J. (1990). Affective response patterns of the injured athlete: An exploratory analysis. *The Sport Psychologist, 4,* 261-274.

Meyers, M. C., Sterling, J. C., Calvo, R. D., Marley, R., & Duhon, T. K. (1991). Mood state of athletes undergoing orthopaedic surgery and rehabilitation: A preliminary report [Abstract]. *Medicine and Science in Sports and Exercise, 23*(Suppl.), S138.

Mor, S., Day, H. I., Flett, G. L., & Hewitt, P. L. (1995). Perfectionism, control, and components of performance anxiety in professional artists. *Cognitive Therapy and Research, 19,* 207-225.

Novaco, R. W. (1995). Clinical problems of anger and its assessment and regulation through a stress coping skills approach. In W. O'Donohue & L. Krasner (Eds.), *Handbook of psychological skills training: Clinical techniques and applications* (pp. 320-338). Boston: Allyn & Bacon.

Nowack, K. M. (1989). Coping style, cognitive hardiness, and health status. *Journal of Behavioral Medicine, 12,* 145-158.

Ormal, J., & Wohlfarth, T. (1991). How neuroticism, long-term difficulties, and life situation change influence psychological distress: A longitudinal model. *Journal of Personality and Social Psychology, 60,* 744-755.

Parkes, K. R. (1986). Coping in stressful episodes: The role of individual differences, environmental factors, and situational characteristics. *Journal of Personality and Social Psychology, 51,* 1277-1292.

Pearson, L., & Jones, G. (1992). Emotional effects of sports injuries: Implications for physiotherapists. *Physiotherapy, 78,* 762-770.

Peterson, C. (1995). Explanatory style and health. In G. M. Buchanan & M. P. Seligman (Eds.), *Explanatory style* (pp. 233-246). Hillsdale, NJ: Erlbaum.

Peterson, C. & Bossio, L. M. (1991). *Health and optimism.* New York: Free Press.

Peterson, C. & Seligman, M. E. P. (1984). Causal explanations as a risk factor for depression: Theory and evidence. *Psychological Review, 91,* 347-374.

Peterson, C., Semmel, A., Von Baeyer, C., Abramson, L. Y., Metalsky, G. I., & Seligman, M. E. P. (1982). The Attributional Style Questionnaire. *Cognitive Therapy and Research, 6,* 287-299.

Peterson, C., & Villanova, P. (1988). An Expanded Attributional Style Questionnaire. *Journal of Abnormal Psychology, 97,* 87-89.

Potter, M., & Grove, J. R. (1999). Mental skills training during rehabilitation: Case studies of injured athletes. *New Zealand Journal of Physiotherapy, 27,* 24-31.

Rim, Y. (1986). Ways of coping, personality, age, sex and family structure variables. *Personality and Individual Differences, 7,* 113-116.

Roberts, J. E., Gilboa, E., & Gotlib, I. H. (1998). Ruminative response style and vunerability to episodes of dysphoria: Gender, neuroticism, and episode duration. *Cognitive Therapy and Research, 22,* 401-423.

Rodin, J., & Salovey, P. (1989). Health psychology. *Annual Review of Psychology, 40,* 533-579.

Saboonchi, F., & Lundh, L. G. (2003). Perfectionism, anger, somatic health, and positive affect. *Personality & Individual Differences, 35,* 1585-1599.

Sanderson, F. H. (1981). The psychological implications of injury. In T.P. Reilly (Ed.), *Sports fitness and sports injuries* (pp. 37-41). London: Faber & Faber.

Scheier, M. F., & Bridges, M. W. (1995). Person variables and health: Personality predispositions and acute psychological states as shared determinants for disease. *Psychosomatic Medicine, 57,* 255-268.

Scheier, M. F., & Carver, C. S. (1985). Optimism, coping, and health: Assessment and implications of generalized outcome expectancies. *Health Psychology, 4,* 219-248.

Scheier, M. F., & Carver, C. S. (1987). Dispositional optimism and physical well-being: The influence of generalized outcome expectancies on health. *Journal of Personality, 55,* 169-210.

Scheier, M. F., & Carver, C. S. (1992). Effects of optimism on psychological and physical well-being: Theoretical overview and empirical update. *Cognitive Therapy and Research, 16,* 201-228.

Scheier, M. F., Carver, C. S., & Bridges, M. W. (1994). Distinguishing optimism from neuroticism (and trait anxiety, self-mastery, and self-esteem): A reevaluation of the Life Orientation Test. *Journal of Personality and Social Psychology, 67,* 1063-1078.

Scheier, M. F., Matthews, K. A., Owens, J. F., Magovern, G. J., Lefebvre, R. C., Abbott, R. A., & Carver, C. S. (1989). Dispositional optimism and recovery from coronary artery bypass surgery: The beneficial effects on physical and psychological well-being. *Journal of Personality and Social Psychology, 57,* 1024-1040.

Schweitzer, R. D., & Hamilton, T. K. (2002). Perfectionism and mental health in Australian university students: Is there a relationship? *Journal of College Student Development, 43,* 684-695.

Shaffer, S., & McAuley, E. (1993). Attributions and self-efficacy as predictors of rehabilitative success [Abstract]. *Journal of Sport & Exercise Psychology, 15*(Suppl.), S71.

Shahar, G., Blatt, S. J., Zuroff, D. C., Krupnick, J. L., & Sotsky, S. M. (2004). Perfectionism impedes social relations and response to brief treatment for depression. *Journal of Social & Clinical Psychology, 23,* 140-154.

Shewchuk, R. M., Elliott, T. R., MacNair-Semands, R. R., & Harkins, S. (1999). Trait influences on stress appraisal and coping: An evaluation of alternative frameworks. *Journal of Applied Social Psychology, 29,* 685-704.

Silver, R. C., Wortman, C. B., & Crofton, C. (1990). The role of coping in support provision: The self-representational dilemma of victims of life crisis. In B. R. Sarason, I. G. Sarason, & G. R. Pierce (Eds.), *Social support: An interactional view* (pp. 397-426). New York: Wiley.

Smith, A. M., Scott, S. G., O'Fallon, W. M., & Young, M. L. (1990). Emotional responses of athletes to injury. *Mayo Clinic Proceedings, 65,* 38-50.

Smith, R. E., Smoll, F. L., & Ptacek, J. T. (1990). Conjunctive moderator variables in vulnerability and resiliency research: Life stress, social support and coping skills, and adolescent sport injuries. *Journal of Personality and Social Psychology, 58,* 360-370.

Staats, S. (1989). Hope: A comparison of two self-report measures for adults. *Journal of Personality Assessment, 53,* 366-375.

Taylor, S. E., & Aspinwall, L. G. (1996). Mediating and moderating processes in psychosocial stress: Appraisal, coping, resistance, and vulnerability. In H. B. Kaplan (Ed.), *Psychosocial stress: Perspectives on structure, theory, life-course, and methods* (pp. 71-110). San Diego, CA: Academic Press.

Taylor, S. E. (1990). Health psychology: The science and the field. *American Psychologist, 45,* 40-50.

Tenenbaum, G., Furst, D., & Weingarten, G. (1984). Attribution of causality in sport events: Validation of the Wingate Sport Achievement Responsibility Scale. *Journal of Sport Psychology, 6,* 430-439.

Terry-Short, L. A., Owens, R. G., Slade, P. D., & Dewey, M. E. (1995). Positive and negative perfectionism. *Personality & Individual Differences, 18,* 663-668.

Van Treuren, R. R., & Hull, J. G. (1986, October). *Health and stress: Dispositional optimism and psychophysiological responses.* Paper presented at the annual meeting of the Society for Psychophysiological Research, Montreal, Canada.

Vickers, K. S. & Vogeltanz, N. D. (2000). Dispositional optimism as a predictor of depressive symptoms over time. *Personality and Individual Differences, 28,* 259-272.

Watson, D., & Pennebaker, J. W. (1989). Health complaints, stress, and distress: Exploring the central role of negative affectivity. *Psychological Review, 96,* 234-254.

Wearing, A. J., & Hart, P. M. (1996). Work and non-working coping strategies: Their relation to personality, appraisal, and life domain. *Stress Medicine, 12,* 93-103.

Weinberg, R. S. (1996). Goal setting in sport and exercise: Research to practice. In J. L. Van Raalte & B. W. Brewer (Eds.), *Exploring sport and exercise psychology* (pp. 3-24). Washington, DC: American Psychological Association.

Weinstock, L. M., & Whisman, M. A. (2006). Neuroticism as a common feature of the depressive and anxiety disorders: A test of the revised integrative hierarchical model in a national sample. *Journal of Abnormal Psychology, 115,* 64-74.

Whitley, B. E. (1991). A short form of the Expanded Attributional Style Questionnaire. *Journal of Personality Assessment, 56,* 365-369.

Wiebe, D. J. (1991). Hardiness and stress moderation: A test of proposed mechanisms. *Journal of Personality and Social Psychology, 60,* 89-99.

Wiese-Bjornstal, D. M., & Smith, A. M. (1993). Counseling strategies for enhanced recovery of injured athletes within a team approach. In D. Pargman (Ed.), *Psychological bases of sport injuries* (pp. 149-182). Morgantown, WV: Fitness Information Technology.

Williams, P. G., Wiebe, D. J., & Smith, T. W. (1992). Coping processes as mediators of the relationship between hardiness and health. *Journal of Behavioral Medicine, 15,* 237-255.

Zeidner, M., & Saklofske, D. (1996). Adaptive and maladaptive coping. In M. Zeidner & N. S. Endler (Eds.), *Handbook of coping: Theory, research, applications* (pp. 505-531). New York: Wiley.

Zinsser, N., Bunker, L. & Williams, J. M. (2001). Cognitive techniques for building confidence and enhancing performance. In J. M. Williams (Ed.), *Applied sport psychology: Personal growth to peak performance* (pp. 284-311). Mountain View, CA: Mayfield.

Zuroff, D. C., Blatt, S. J., Sotsky, S. M., Krupnick, J. L., Martin, D. J., Sanislow, C. A., & Simmens, S. (2000). Relation of therapeutic alliance and perfectionism to outcome in brief outpatient treatment of depression. *Journal of Consulting and Clinical Psychology, 68,* 114-124.

Chapter Five | Patient-Practitioner Interactions in Sport Injury Rehabilitation

Britton W. Brewer, Judy L. Van Raalte, and Albert J. Petitpas
Springfield College

Interactions between athletes with injuries and their sports medicine providers can exert an important influence on the athletes' psychological state, treatment adherence, and rehabilitation outcome. In this chapter, research on patient-practitioner interactions in the context of sport injury rehabilitation is reviewed. Topics such as patient-practitioner communication, patient and practitioner perceptions, and adherence to sport injury rehabilitation programs are addressed. Guidelines for referring patients for psychological services and recommendations for enhancing patient-practitioner interactions are presented.

Introduction

Enhancement of physical well-being is the primary focus in sports medicine settings. It is abundantly clear, however, that sport injury rehabilitation occurs within broader social context comprised of patient interactions with orthopedic surgeons, physical therapists, athletic trainers, support staff, other patients, family members, and friends. The nature and quality of these interactions may have a profound impact on both processes (e.g., emotional adjustment, adherence) and outcomes (e.g., satisfaction, recovery of physical function) in sport injury rehabilitation.

Arguably the most important interactions in sport injury rehabilitation are those between patients and the sports medicine practitioners (i.e., physical therapists and athletic trainers) who direct their rehabilitation efforts on a day-to-day basis. In addition to facilitating physical recovery following injury, sport injury rehabilitation professionals can be an important source of social support for athletes with injuries (Ford & Gordon, 1993; Hardy, Burke, & Crace, 1999; Johnston & Carroll, 1998; Udry, 1996; Udry, Gould, Bridges, &

Tuffey, 1997). In a study of competitive and recreational athletes undergoing rehabilitation following knee surgery, physical therapists/athletic trainers were identified as second only to parents as providers of social support (Izzo, 1994). Similarly, intercollegiate athletes undergoing rehabilitation expressed greater satisfaction with the social support provided by athletic trainers than that given by their head and assistant coaches (Robbins & Rosenfeld, 2001). Along with coaches, medical practitioners have been identified as the most frequent providers of technical and informational support to athletes with injuries (Johnston & Carroll, 1998; Udry et al., 1997). Social support is particularly important in rehabilitation because it has implications for the psychological distress (Brewer, Linder, & Phelps, 1995; Manuel et al., 2003), rehabilitation adherence (Byerly, Worrell, Gahimer, & Domholdt, 1994; Duda, Smart, & Tappe, 1989; Fisher, Domm, & Wuest, 1988; Johnston & Carroll, 2000) and treatment outcome (Tuffey, 1991) of patients with sport injuries.

Given the central importance ascribed to physical therapists and athletic trainers in sport injury rehabilitation, this chapter focuses on the interactions that these practitioners have with their patients. After presenting an overview of patient-practitioner communication in sport injury rehabilitation settings, empirical research exploring patient and practitioner perceptions in sport injury rehabilitation is examined, issues in patient adherence to rehabilitation regimens prescribed by sports medicine practitioners are discussed, and guidelines for referral of patients with sport injuries for counseling or psychotherapy are provided. The chapter concludes with recommendations for enhancing patient-practitioner interactions in sport injury rehabilitation.

Patient-Practitioner Communication

By definition, interactions between patients with sport injuries and the professionals supervising their rehabilitation involve communication. Although the importance of effective patient-practitioner communication in sport injury rehabilitation has been acknowledged by athletes (DeFrancesco, Miller, Larson, & Robinson, 1994; Fisher & Hoisington, 1993), sport rehabilitation professionals (Fisher, Mullins, & Frye, 1993; Gordon, Milios, & Grove, 1991; Larson, Starkey, & Zaichowsky, 1996; Wiese, Weiss, & Yukelson, 1991), and sport psychologists (e.g., Danish, 1986; Nideffer, 1983), it has received little empirical attention. The topic has, however, been examined extensively in the general medical literature, where a number of barriers to effective patient-practitioner communication have been identified. Patient characteristics that may interfere with communication include

- anxiety,
- inexperience with the medical disorder, and
- a lack of intelligence.

Practitioner behaviors that may contribute to poor communication include

- not listening,
- using jargon and technical language,
- providing overly simplistic explanations,
- depersonalizing the patient,
- displaying worry, and
- holding pejorative stereotypes of patients (Taylor, 1995).

Poor patient-practitioner communication can discourage the future use of medical services (Taylor, 1995) and hamper adherence to medical regimens (Meichenbaum & Turk, 1987; Taylor, 1995). For example, it has been found that patients are less likely to adhere to treatment recommendations when their physicians fail to give clear explanations, provide positive verbal communications, and answer questions (DiMatteo et al., 1993; Hall, Roter, & Katz, 1988).

In one of the few studies to examine patient-practitioner communication in the context of sport injury rehabilitation, Kahanov and Fairchild (1994) found that intercollegiate athletes with injuries and their athletic trainers had discrepancies in their perceptions of several aspects of communication during the initial evaluation. For example, more than one-third of the athletes indicated that they had summarized their athletic trainers' injury explanations when their athletic trainers indicated that they had not.

In a related investigation, Hokanson (1994) asked a sample of competitive and recreational athletes undergoing rehabilitation following knee surgery to describe the nature of their communication with the physical therapist or athletic trainer who was directing their rehabilitation efforts. Analyses of qualitative data revealed that patient-practitioner communication was predominantly informational, characterized by discussion of rehabilitation-related topics. To a lesser extent, there was empathic (or socioemotional) communication between patients and practitioners, in which common interests and patients' lives in general were discussed. Quantitative analyses in which patients' satisfaction with their communication with the rehabilitation professionals was assessed with the Sports Injury Clinic Athlete Satisfaction Scale (SICASS; Taylor & May, 1995b) indicated a nonsignificant relationship between satisfaction and adherence to the rehabilitation program.

Clearly, despite its importance, little is known about patient-practitioner communication in sport injury rehabilitation. Descriptive and inferential investigations are needed to provide a thorough understanding of the nature and implications of communication between athletes with injuries and the professionals attending to their rehabilitation.

Patient and Practitioner Perceptions

During the course of injury rehabilitation, patients and practitioners are likely to form impressions of rehabilitation-related processes and outcomes. These perceptions are important because they may both reflect and influence interactions between patients and practitioners. In this section of the chapter, research on patient and practitioner perceptions associated with sport injury rehabilitation is examined.

Rehabilitation Regimen

Several studies have investigated the congruence between patients and practitioners with regard to the content of sport injury rehabilitation regimens. Kahanov and Fairchild (1994) found that athletes with injuries and athletic trainers had significant disagreement in terms of whether the athlete understood the rehabilitation program and whether a written protocol was given to the athlete. May and Taylor (1994) found that patients at a university-based sport injury clinic gave estimates of the amount of time required to complete their home rehabilitation exercises that were an average of 42% lower than their physiotherapists' estimates. A study by Webborn, Carbon, and Miller (1997) bolstered the findings of Kahanov and Fairchild (1994) and May and Taylor (1994), demonstrating that 77% of sport injury clinic patients who were prescribed home rehabilitation exercises misunderstood at least some aspect of their rehabilitation program. Thus, it appears that patient and practitioner perceptions of something so vital and seemingly objective as the rehabilitation program itself may differ dramatically.

Recovery Progress

There is probably no aspect of the rehabilitation process more on the minds of patients and practitioners than the extent to which patients are progressing toward recovery. Perceptions of poor rehabilitation progress have been linked to negative emotional responses in athletes with injuries (McDonald & Hardy, 1990; Smith, Young, & Scott, 1988). Given the centrality and potential adverse impact of perceptions of recovery progress in sport injury rehabilitation, patient and practitioner perceptions of injury status have been assessed in a number of studies.

Crossman and Jamieson (1985) found that athletic trainer ratings of injury seriousness and injury disruptiveness were significantly correlated with those made by athletes with injuries (r = .56 and r = .39, respectively), indicating a degree of agreement between patients and practitioners on patients' current injury status. The athletes with injuries in this study, however, tended to overestimate the seriousness and underestimate the disruptiveness of their injuries relative to their athletic trainers. Athletes who overestimated the seriousness or disruptiveness of their injuries tended to experience greater pain and mood disturbance than athletes who did not overestimate the seriousness or disruptiveness of their injuries. In a follow-up study, Crossman, Jamieson, and Hume (1990) again found that athletes underestimated the disruptive impact of their injuries relative to medical professionals.

Subsequent research has substantiated the findings of Crossman and her colleagues (Crossman & Jamieson, 1985; Crossman et al., 1990). Van Raalte, Brewer, and Petitpas (1992) documented significant correlations between patient and practitioner estimates of the number of days that the athletes would be prevented from participating in sport (r = .92) and ratings of the extent to which the athletes were fully rehabilitated (r = .35). Athletes in the Van Raalte et al. study viewed themselves as significantly more recovered than did their athletic trainers. Significant correlations between injury appraisals made by sports medicine clinic patients and their physicians were also obtained in investigations by Brewer, Linder, and Phelps (1995) and Brewer, Van Raalte, Petitpas, Sklar, and Ditmar (1995).

Thus, it appears that although patient and practitioner perceptions of recovery progress are often congruent, discrepancies sometimes occur and may influence the emotional state of patients. It should also be recognized that under certain circumstances, athletes may conceal symptoms and downplay the significance of their injuries to return to sport sooner than medically advisable (Nixon, 1994). In such situations, it may be difficult for patients and practitioners to see "eye to eye" with regard to patients' injury status. Fortunately, there is evidence that sport injury rehabilitation professionals are less susceptible than coaches to situational influences in judging the appropriateness of a given athlete's returning to sport following injury (Flint & Weiss, 1992).

Attributions for Recovery

One goal of sport injury rehabilitation practitioners is to instill a sense of responsibility for rehabilitation in their patients (Gordon et al., 1991). By encouraging their patients to take ownership of their rehabilitation, it is presumed that patients will become more invested in completing therapeutic activities and will achieve a more rapid and complete recovery. Research indicates that the extent to which patients accept responsibility for their rehabilitation progress may depend upon the rate of recovery, with athletes recovering slowly less likely to claim responsibility for their rehabilitation progress than athletes recovering rapidly (Brewer, Cornelius et al., 2000; Grove, Hanrahan, & Stewart, 1990; Laubach, Brewer, Van Raalte, & Petitpas, 1996). Because attributions for recovery have been associated with rehabilitation self-efficacy beliefs (Shaffer, 1992) and adherence to sport injury rehabilitation (Brewer, Cornelius et al., 2000; Laubach et al., 1996), they merit further empirical attention.

Psychological Distress

Due in part to the psychological significance of sport participation to many athletes (Brewer, 1993; Kleiber & Brock, 1992), injury may be a major source of stress (Brewer & Petrie, 1995; Wiese-Bjornstal, Smith, & LaMott, 1995) and emotional disturbance (Brewer & Petrie, 1995; Chan & Grossman, 1988; Leddy, Lambert, & Ogles, 1994; Pearson & Jones, 1992; Smith et al., 1993). Because emotional disturbance is inversely related to rehabilitation adherence (Daly, Brewer, Van Raalte, Petitpas, & Sklar, 1995) and rehabilitation outcome (Wise, Jackson, & Rocchio, 1979), it is important for sport injury rehabilitation practitioners to recognize psychological distress in their patients to facilitate appropriate referral. Unfortunately, research indicates that rehabilitation personnel may have difficulty in identifying psychological distress in their patients. Brewer, Petitpas et al. (1995) found that sports medicine clinic patients' self-reported psychological distress was uncorrelated with their physical therapists' or athletic trainers' ratings of patient behaviors indicative of psychological disturbance. This finding signals a potential need for additional emphasis on the psychological realm in the training of physical therapists and athletic trainers.

Adherence to Rehabilitation

Adherence to a sport injury rehabilitation program is a tangible outcome of patient-practitioner interactions. Encouraging patients to adopt treatment recommendations is an essential task of rehabilitation practitioners. Depending on the nature of the particular sport injury rehabilitation regimen, adherence may involve such behaviors as
- complying with practitioner instructions to restrict physical activity,
- completing home rehabilitation exercises,
- completing home cryotherapy (icing),

- complying with medication prescriptions, and
- participating in clinic-based rehabilitation exercises and therapy (Brewer, 1998).

A review of the literature indicated that, depending on how adherence to sport injury rehabilitation is assessed, adherence rates ranging from 40 to 91% have been documented (Brewer, 1998).

Characteristics of both the patient and the rehabilitation context have been linked to adherence to sport injury rehabilitation. Patient characteristics positively associated with adherence include self-motivation (Brewer, Daly, Van Raalte, Petitpas, & Sklar, 1999; Duda et al., 1989; Fields, Murphey, Horodyski, & Stopka, 1995; Fisher et al., 1988; Noyes, Matthews, Mooar, & Grood, 1983), pain tolerance (Byerly et al., 1994; Fields et al., 1995; Fisher et al., 1988), health locus of control (Murphy, Foreman, Simpson, Molloy, & Molloy, 1999), task involvement (Duda et al., 1989), and tough-mindedness (Wittig & Schurr, 1994). Ego involvement (Lampton, Lambert, & Yost, 1993) and trait anxiety (Eichenhofer, Wittig, Balogh, & Pisano, 1986) are patient characteristics that have been negatively correlated with adherence to sport injury rehabilitation programs. Thus, it appears that patients who are stoic, strong-willed, and self-motivated are more likely than other patients to stick with their rehabilitation.

A number of contextual variables have been linked to sport injury rehabilitation adherence. Factors related to greater adherence include belief in the efficacy of the treatment (Brewer et al., 2003; Duda et al., 1989; Noyes et al., 1983; Taylor & May, 1996), comfort of the rehabilitation setting (Brewer et al., 1994; Fields et al., 1995; Fisher et al., 1988), convenience of rehabilitation scheduling (Fields et al., 1995; Fisher et al., 1988), perceived exertion during rehabilitation exercises (Brewer et al., 1994; Fisher et al., 1988), and rehabilitation practitioner expectancy of patient adherence (Taylor & May, 1995a). These factors highlight the importance of patients' interactions with the providers attending to their care and the sport injury rehabilitation environment as a whole. Adherence may be compromised when athletes with injuries are not confident in and comfortable with their rehabilitation regimens.

Fisher and his colleagues investigated the adherence-enhancing strategies and behaviors identified by previously injured athletes (Fisher & Hoisington, 1993) and athletic trainers (Fisher et al., 1993). The former patients noted that having practitioners who were caring, honest, and encouraging helped them through the rehabilitation process (Fisher & Hoisington, 1993). The practitioners indicated that providing patients with education about their injuries and rehabilitation programs, assisting patients with goal setting, offering encouragement to patients, and monitoring the progress of their patients were successful strategies for procuring patient adherence to rehabilitation (Fisher et al., 1993). Goal setting has received empirical support for its efficacy (Evans & Hardy, 2002; Penpraze & Mutrie, 1999). Patients and practitioners alike expressed disdain for athletic trainer threats and scare tactics in gaining adherence (Fisher & Hoisington, 1993; Fisher et al., 1993).

Although the strategies suggested by patients and practitioners may be effective in achieving increased adherence to sport injury rehabilitation programs, it is important to target the strategies appropriately. In particular, the adherence-enhancing interventions should be applied only to rehabilitation regimens for which there is substantial support for their efficacy. Poor adherence may hamper physical recovery for some rehabilitation regimens (Alzate Saez de Heredia, Ramirez, & Lazaro, 2004; Brewer, Van Raalte, Cornelius et al., 2003; Derscheid & Feiring, 1987), but not others (Noyes et al., 1983; Shelbourne & Wilckens, 1990), especially those that are "experimental" or lacking in formal documentation. Along these lines, practitioners are cautioned not to infer that patients are not adhering to the treatment program when their recovery is slower than expected. Healing rate is inappropriate for use as an index of adherence because it is not behaviorally based and therefore does not provide information on how well patients are complying with their rehabilitation programs (Johnson, 1993). In other words, athletes with slow-healing injuries may truly be doing all that has been asked of them, and to assume otherwise may damage the patient-practitioner relationship.

Referral for Psychological Services

Athletes, in general, exhibit a smaller range and frequency of mental disorders than are found in the population at large (Andersen, Denson, Brewer, & Van Raalte, 1994). Nevertheless, an estimated 5–27% of athletes report clinically meaningful levels of psychological distress, at least in the short term (i.e., one to two months) following injury (Brewer, Linder, & Phelps, 1995; Brewer, Petitpas et al., 1995; Brewer & Petrie, 1995; Leddy, Lambert, & Ogles, 1994; Manuel et al., 2002; Smith, Scott, O'Fallon, & Young, 1990). For athletes with injuries who are having difficulties in relationships, school, or work, referral to mental health professionals can improve their quality of life and enhance their sport involvement (Brewer, Petitpas, & Van Raalte, 1999).

Referral is a delicate process. The structure of the referral can set the stage for the quality and efficacy of the therapeutic relationship that follows (Bobele & Conran, 1988). When working with athletes, referrals can be complicated by the stigma associated with mental problems and the derogation of those who seek help from mental health practitioners (Linder, Brewer, Van Raalte, & DeLange, 1991). Although some athletes with injuries may be skeptical about the utility of psychological interventions in sport injury rehabilitation and express reluctance about receiving a psychological referral, research indicates that athletes have generally positive perceptions of psychological interventions in the context of injury rehabilitation (Brewer, Jeffers, Van Raalte, & Petitpas, 1994; DeFrancesco et al., 1994; Durso-Cupal, 1996; Pearson & Jones, 1992; Potter, 1995).

Referral Networks

Having gathered information about psychological problems that may require referral (e.g., anxiety/stress, depression, eating disorders, adjustment reaction to athletic injury, substance abuse), sports medicine practitioners should develop an appropriate referral network. A referral network is a group of people with expertise in a variety of areas to whom patients can be referred. Ideally, the mental health professionals in the referral network have knowledge of sport and experience working with athletes. At the least, they should be interested in learning about sport and exercise and open to working with an athletic population (Van Raalte & Andersen, 2002).

Establishing a referral network takes time and motivation:

- First, appropriate mental health professionals in the local area should be identified (Heyman, 1993). These might include psychologists, psychiatrists, and social workers. Selecting both male and female mental health professionals of various theoretical orientations, racial/ethnic backgrounds, and professional backgrounds can be useful.

- Second, an effort should be made to develop a relationship with these professionals. The referral process is often smoother and more comfortable if practitioners know the professionals to whom they are referring their patients and have asked the referral sources how they would like athletes to be referred (Bobele & Conran, 1988). Athletes seem to find this "team approach" in which various sport professionals work together to be appealing (Andersen, 1992).

- Third, the referral network should be evaluated and modified on an ongoing basis to provide the best service for athletes. Having a broad group of professionals available for referral allows sports medicine practitioners to have some flexibility in the referral process.

When developing a referral network, it is important to keep in mind some of the specific concerns that athletes may have. Athletes generally have limited time due to the demands of training and work or school. Many athletes have limited funds. Thus, it is useful to select local practitioners, at least some of whom provide services on a sliding scale basis. For student-athletes attending colleges or universities, there are usually "free" on-campus services available. Developing a relationship with these providers increases the likelihood that athletes will follow through on referrals made.

The Referral Process

Each athlete's needs and situation are different. Therefore, each referral is different. The likelihood of making successful referrals can be increased by carefully assessing the psychological needs of athletes who are injured, paying attention to the timing of referrals, and following-up on referrals.

Sports medicine providers often observe athletes' psychological responses to injury as a normal part of treatment. For example, practitioners may ask their patients how they are feeling and how their recovery is progressing. Athletes who report that they are having difficulties may be good candidates for referral.

Before referring athletes, it is useful for sports medicine practitioners to consult with mental health professionals in their referral network to discuss the case. Consultation can help clarify the situation and, if referral is necessary, facilitate the referral process.

Sports medicine practitioners who have good relationships with their patients will probably have the easiest time making referrals. Nevertheless, the referral process is tricky, and there is no "perfect time" to make a referral. As a general rule, the more severe the psychological symptoms athletes are experiencing, the sooner athletes should be referred (Heil, 1993b).

Sports medicine practitioners who decide to refer athletes should explain to athletes the reason for the referral and should describe what is involved in working with the mental health professionals to whom they have been referred (Bobele & Conran,

1988; Heil, 1993). Noting the important connection between mind and body and reassuring athletes that they are not "head cases" can also be useful (Heil, 1993).

After a referral has been made, sports medicine practitioners should follow up with the athletes. They might ask, "How is it going with Dr. Smith?" With the athlete's consent, it can also be helpful for the sports medicine and mental health practitioners to consult regarding the athlete's progress. The mental health professional should not reveal confidential details of the patient's discussions, but limited information about the patient's status can be shared.

In some cases, athletes may decide not to follow through on referrals. In these situations, the sports medicine practitioner and the patient might discuss alternate strategies for dealing with the problem. It is appropriate to reintroduce the idea of referral at a later date (Heil, 1993).

Recommendations for Enhancing Patient-Practitioner Interactions

Although the importance of building effective patient-practitioner relationships has been recognized by both injured athletes and sport injury rehabilitation professionals (e.g., DeFrancesco et al., 1994; Gordon et al., 1991), there is little empirical evidence to suggest the best means for enhancing these interactions. However, extensive research from counseling psychology on the nature of the counselor-client relationship may provide a helpful framework for examining patient-practitioner interactions in the sports medicine setting.

The Working Alliance

It has long been believed that the quality of the counseling relationship is a critical variable in predicting successful therapeutic outcomes (Orlinsky & Howard, 1986). Although there are several definitions of the patient-practitioner relationship available in the literature, most contain the notion of establishing a form of collaborative relationship, in which the patient and practitioner come to an agreement about treatment goals and the tasks necessary to achieve them (Petitpas & Cornelius, 2004). However, this relationship is quite complex, may change at different stages in the counseling process, and can be viewed quite differently by counselors and clients (Sexton & Whiston, 1994). Therefore, any recommendations for enhancing patient-practitioner interactions in the sport injury rehabilitation setting should also allow for individual differences, account for the time phase of the injury rehabilitation process, and consider the perceptions of both patients and practitioners.

Bordin (1979) suggested that the counselor-client relationship was a working alliance composed of three main components:
- agreement on goals
- agreement on tasks
- development of an emotional bond between client and therapist

Clearly, agreement on goals and tasks would seem to be a critical component of most patient-practitioner interactions. However, as described earlier, it is not unusual to find discrepancies between patients' and practitioners' perceptions of patients' recovery progress, rehabilitation regimen, or level of psychological distress. In addition, even though athletic therapists may not perceive themselves as establishing emotional bonds with their patients, they have been identified as second only to parents as sources of social support for athletes with injuries (Izzo, 1994). Therefore, a closer examination of how to develop an effective working alliance may enhance sport injury rehabilitation practitioners' ability to facilitate treatment adherence and to positively influence rehabilitation outcomes.

In order to be effective in building working alliances, practitioners should consider their role within the context of the injury rehabilitation process. For the most part, initial interactions between patients and practitioners are marked by interpersonal complementarity. That is, the two participants in the interaction assume unequal status roles, with the practitioner being in the one-up position (Kiesler & Watkins, 1989). As such, athletes with injuries are likely to be dependent on athletic therapists for informational support and to wait for the therapist to take the lead and to establish norms for the interaction.

Ironically, premature attempts to explore feelings or to offer support and encouragement during initial interactions may have a negative impact on the working alliance by putting the patient in a passive role (Kivlighan & Schmitz, 1992). Instead, it may be better to initiate the interaction by providing clear information about the nature of the injury, treatment goals, possible side effects, and coping strategies for adjusting to the rehabilitation process (Petitpas & Danish, 1995). This type of information is often particularly helpful for athletes who experience anxiety over their injuries because it may provide them with a sense of control and predictability that could reduce the levels of stress they experience (Meichenbaum, 1985). However, practitioners must realize that how they present the information is critical in insuring patient understanding (Henderson & Carroll, 1993), adherence to treatment regimens, and patient-practitioner collaboration (Petitpas & Danish, 1995).

Although practitioners may be in a one-up position in the working alliance, they need to take sufficient time to understand problems from the perspectives of the athletes with injuries and to ensure that the athletes understand clearly and accept the information that is provided to them. In addition, the anxiety or power differential that may be inherent in the initial patient-practitioner relationship may interfere with patients' abilities to listen attentively or to be willing to ask for further clarification. Even though practitioners may ask their patients if they have any questions or if everything is understood, many athletes with injuries may still be reluctant to respond. By adopting a working alliance perspective, patients would be required to demonstrate their understanding of the information provided through activities such as summarizing what they have heard, keeping notes, or explaining what the information meant to them. The main objectives at this point in the relationship are to reach agreement on goals and rehabilitation tasks. However, it is doubtful that these objectives will be accomplished unless patients are treated with respect and sensitivity to their unique situations (Taylor, 1995).

To develop an effective working alliance, practitioners must treat their patients with respect and dignity. All patients bring their own set of beliefs or fears about the injury rehabilitation process, and practitioners should always focus first on the patients and not just their injuries (Danish, 1986). The counseling psychology literature suggests that respect, concreteness, genuineness, immediacy, and positive regard are counselor characteristics that are instrumental to the development of empathy and successful therapeutic relationships (Sexton & Whiston, 1994). Inherent in these characteristics is a belief in the dignity and worth of each individual. Therefore, a person sitting in the waiting room should not be treated as just another patient waiting for rehabilitation, but as a unique individual with beliefs, values, strengths, and fears.

Sport injury rehabilitation practitioners who demonstrate an empathic attitude and are able to understand patients' concerns and beliefs about their injuries are likely to create an emotional bond between themselves and their patients. However, care must be taken to understand the nature of this bond in order to avoid dependency or other issues that could negatively affect adherence or motivation. Used appropriately, a working alliance can empower patients to take responsibility for their own rehabilitation.

In addition, the nature of the working alliance may change as a result of the time frame of the rehabilitation process or the situational variables that may be present (e.g., severity of injury, time in athletic career, level of performance). For example, during the time period immediately following an injury, athletes may need a considerable amount of informational support and encouragement from their athletic therapists. However, once exercise regimens have been established and the athletes believe that they are making progress in their workouts, they may have less need for support. Nonetheless, this need could change markedly for athletes who are approaching their recovery target dates and are uncertain about their abilities to trust in their bodies to perform at preinjury levels (Petitpas & Danish, 1995).

Five practical suggestions for enhancing the working alliance

1. *Check perceptions.* Do not assume that patients understand treatment goals, tasks, or exercise prescriptions. You can model the importance of gaining clarity by paraphrasing and summarizing to ensure that you have accurately heard the communications of patients. Then, you can have patients demonstrate their understanding by having them explain what actions they are going to take.
2. *Get specific.* One of the critical elements in building a working alliance is the use of concreteness. That is, you need to move from vague descriptions about what is happening during rehabilitation to specific, concrete examples. Remember the initial objectives of the working alliance are to get agreement on goals and tasks. Specificity can provide a strong base for patient and practitioner problem-solving (Ivey, Ivey, & Simek-Morgan, 1993).
3. *Listen before you fix.* Try to understand patients' problems from their perspectives before you offer suggestions for solving them. Do not make the mistake of assuming that you know what patients need. Instead, listen carefully to what they say about their circumstances, particularly their concerns and situational variables. Use active listening skills, such as paraphrasing and reflection of feelings, to allow patients to feel understood and accepted.

4. *Listen for the "but."* Because of the power differential inherent in the patient-practitioner dyad, many patients may be hesitant to assert their views or express their noninjury-related needs and concerns. Instead, they may simply go along with your lead and reluctantly allow you to set the agenda for your ongoing interactions. By listening carefully for "yes-but" patient responses, you may be able to identify their most pressing fears or concerns. For example, consider the following statement made by a female basketball player. "I can feel my knee getting stronger, but I hope I'm ready for the tournament." In this situation, the use of the "but" discounts the first part of the sentence and places most importance on her doubts about her ability to get back to playing strength in time to play in the league championships. If these doubts are not addressed, she might push herself too hard, which may cause a setback or an injury to another body part. It is also important to recognize that the "but" can be communicated nonverbally. If you get a sense that patients are simply agreeing with you and not fully expressing their doubts or concerns, you might ask them, "What's the 'but'?"

5. *Value patient input.* One proven method for enhancing patient-practitioner interactions is to actively seek out input from patients in a manner that communicates respect (Meichenbaum & Turk, 1987). For example, it is better to ask patients a question like, "What kinds of things are you doing to cope with your injury?" than to ask them a series of "Have you done this?" questions. In addition, allowing patients to complete their sentences, speaking at the appropriate technical level, and using collaborative problem-solving have been shown to increase adherence to medical directives (Meichenbaum & Turk, 1987).

Summary

Social interaction between athletes with injuries and their sports medicine providers is a critical aspect of sport injury rehabilitation, influencing athlete adjustment, treatment adherence, and rehabilitation outcome. Sport injury rehabilitation personnel are in a key position to provide social support for athletes with injuries. However, the ability of practitioners to provide such support for their patients can be compromised by poor communication and discrepant perceptions of rehabilitation processes and outcomes.

Although personal factors undoubtedly contribute to patient adherence to sport injury rehabilitation regimens, adherence may also be affected by the social context in which rehabilitation occurs. Practitioner behavior can help facilitate adherence to prescribed rehabilitation programs.

In some cases, such as when patients are nonadherent or psychologically distressed, referral for psychological services may be warranted. Careful preparation and follow-through are needed to ensure the success of this most delicate and challenging of patient-practitioner interactions.

Sport injury rehabilitation practitioners can enhance their interactions with patients by adopting an approach to building effective therapeutic relationships derived from the counseling psychology literature. By forging an emotional bond with their patients and fostering patient-practitioner agreement on rehabilitation goals and tasks, sports medicine personnel can develop a working alliance that may contribute to positive physical and psychological outcomes for athletes undergoing injury rehabilitation.

References

Alzate Saez de Heredia, R., Ramirez, A., & Lazaro, I. (2004). The effect of psychological response on recovery of sport injury. *Research in Sports Medicine, 12,* 15-31.

Andersen, M. B. (1992). Sport psychology and procrustean categories: An appeal for synthesis and expansion of service. *Association for the Advancement of Applied Sport Psychology Newsletter, 7*(3), 8-9.

Andersen, M. B., Denson, E. L., Brewer, B. W., & Van Raalte, J. L. (1994). Disorders of personality and mood in athletes: Recognition and referral. *Journal of Applied Sport Psychology, 6,* 168-184.

Bobele, M., & Conran, T. J. (1988). Referrals for family therapy: Pitfalls and guidelines. *Elementary School Guidance, 22,* 192-198.

Bordin, E. S. (1979). The generalizability of the psychanalytic concept of the working alliance. *Psychotherapy: Theory, Research, and Practice, 16,* 252-260.

Brewer, B. W. (1993). Self-identity and specific vulnerability to depressed mood. *Journal of Personality, 61,* 343-364.

Brewer, B. W. (1998). Adherence to sport injury rehabilitation programs. *Journal of Applied Sport Psychology, 10,* 1-4..

Brewer, B. W., Cornelius, A. E., Van Raalte, J. L., Petitpas, A. J., Sklar, J. H., Pohlman, M. H., Krushell, R. J., & Ditmar, T. D. (2000). Attributions for recovery and adherence to rehabilitation following anterior cruciate ligament reconstruction: A prospective analysis. *Psychology & Health, 15,* 283-291.

Brewer, B. W., Cornelius, A. E., Van Raalte, J. L., Petitpas, A. J., Sklar, J. H., Pohlman, M. H., Krushell, R. J., & Ditmar, T. (2003). Protection motivation theory and sport injury rehabilitation adherence revisited. *The Sport Psychologist, 17,* 95-103.

Brewer, B. W., Daly, J. M., Van Raalte, J. L., Petitpas, A. J., & Sklar, J. H. (1999). A psychometric evaluation of the Rehabilitation Adherence Questionnaire. *Journal of Sport & Exercise Psychology, 21,* 167-173

Brewer, B. W., Jeffers, K. E., Petitpas, A. J., & Van Raalte, J. L. (1994). Perceptions of psychological interventions in the context of sport injury rehabilitation. *The Sport Psychologist, 8,* 176-188.

Brewer, B. W., Linder, D. E., & Phelps, C. M. (1995). Situational correlates of emotional adjustment to athletic injury. *Clinical Journal of Sport Medicine, 5,* 241-245.

Brewer, B. W., Petitpas, A. J., & Van Raalte, J. L. (1999). Referral of injured athletes for counseling and psychotherapy. In R. R. Ray & D. M. Wiese-Bjornstal (Eds.), *Counseling in sports medicine* (pp. 127-141). Champaign, IL: Human Kinetics.

Brewer, B. W., Petitpas, A. J., Van Raalte, J. L., Sklar, J. H., & Ditmar, T. D. (1995). Prevalence of psychological distress among patients at a physical therapy clinic specializing in sports medicine. *Sports Medicine, Training and Rehabilitation, 6,* 138-145.

Brewer, B. W., & Petrie, T. A. (1995). A comparison between injured and uninjured football players on selected psychosocial variables. *Academic Athletic Journal, 10,* 11-18.

Brewer, B. W., Van Raalte, J. L., Petitpas, A. J., Sklar, J. H., & Ditmar, T. D. (1995). Predictors of perceived sport injury rehabilitation status. In R. Vanfraechem-Raway, & Y. Vanden Auweele (Eds.), *IXth European Congress on Sport Psychology proceedings: Part II* (pp. 606-610). Brussels: European Federation of Sports Psychology.

Byerly, P. N., Worrell, T., Gahimer, J., & Domholdt, E. (1994). Rehabilitation compliance in an athletic training environment. *Journal of Athletic Training, 29,* 352-355.

Chan, C. S., & Grossman, H. Y. (1988). Psychological effects of running loss on consistent runners. *Perceptual and Motor Skills, 66,* 875-883.

Crossman, J., & Jamieson, J. (1985). Differences in perceptions of seriousness and disrupting effects of athletic injury as viewed by athletes and their trainer. *Perceptual and Motor Skills, 61,* 1131-1134.

Crossman, J., Jamieson, J., & Hume, K. M. (1990). Perceptions of athletic injuries by athletes, coaches, and medical professionals. *Perceptual and Motor Skills, 71,* 848-850.

Daly, J. M., Brewer, B. W., Van Raalte, J. L., Petitpas, A. J., & Sklar, J. H. (1995). Cognitive appraisal, emotional adjustment, and adherence to rehabilitation following knee surgery. *Journal of Sport Rehabilitation, 4,* 23-30.

Danish, S. J. (1986). Psychological aspects in the care and treatment of athletic injuries. In P. E. Vinger & E. F. Hoerner (Eds.), *Sports injuries: The unthwarted epidemic* (pp. 345-353). Littleton, MA: PSG.

DeFrancesco, C., Miller, M., Larson, M., & Robinson, K. (1994, October). *Athletic injury, rehabilitation, and psychological strategies: What do the athletes think?* Paper presented at the annual meeting of the Association for the Advancement of Applied Sport Psychology, Incline Village, NV.

Derscheid, G. L., & Feiring, D. C. (1987). A statistical analysis to characterize treatment adherence of the 18 most common diagnoses seen at a sports medicine clinic. *Journal of Orthopaedic and Sports Physical Therapy, 9,* 40-46.

DiMatteo, M. R., Sherbourne, C. D., Hays, R. D., Ordway, L., Kravitz, R. L., McGlynn, E. A., Kaplan, S., & Rogers, W. H. (1993). Physicians' characteristics influence patients' adherence to medical treatment: Results from the Medical Outcomes Study. *Health Psychology, 12,* 93-102.

Duda, J. L., Smart, A. E., & Tappe, M. K. (1989). Predictors of adherence in rehabilitation of athletic injuries: An application of personal investment theory. *Journal of Sport & Exercise Psychology, 11,* 367-381.

Eichenhofer, R. B., Wittig, A. F., & Balogh, D. W. (1986, May). *Personality indicants of adherence to rehabilitation treatment by injured athletes.* Paper presented at the Annual Meeting of the Midwestern Psychological Association, Chicago, IL.

Fields, J., Murphey, M., Horodyski, M., & Stopka, C. (1995). Factors associated with adherence to sport injury rehabilitation in college-age recreational athletes. *Journal of Sport Rehabilitation, 4,* 172-180.

Fisher, A. C., Domm, M. A., & Wuest, D. A. (1988). Adherence to sports-injury rehabilitation programs. *The Physician and Sports Medicine, 16,* 47-52.

Fisher, A. C., & Hoisington, L. L. (1993). Injured athletes' attitudes and judgments toward rehabilitation adherence. *Journal of Athletic Training, 28,* 48-54.

Fisher, A. C., Mullins, S. A., & Frye, P. A. (1993). Athletic trainers' attitudes and judgments of injured athletes' rehabilitation adherence. *Journal of Athletic Training, 28,* 43-47.

Flint, F. A., & Weiss, M. R. (1992). Returning injured athletes to competition: A role and ethical dilemma. *Canadian Journal of Sport Sciences, 17,* 34-40

Ford, I. W., & Gordon, S. (1993). Social support and athletic injury: The perspective of sport physiotherapists. *The Australian Journal of Science and Medicine in Sport, 25,* 17-25.

Gordon, S., Milios, D., & Grove, J. R. (1991). Psychological aspects of the recovery process from sport injury: The perspective of sport physiotherapists. *Australian Journal of Science and Medicine in Sport, 23,* 53-60.

Grove, J. R., Hanrahan, S. J., Stewart, R. M. L. (1990). Attributions for rapid or slow recovery from sports injuries. *Canadian Journal of Sport Sciences, 15,* 107-114.

Hall, J. A., Roter, D. L., & Katz, N. R. (1988). Meta-analysis of correlates of provider behavior in medical encounters. *Medical Care, 26,* 1-19.

Heil, J. (1993). *Psychology of sport injury.* Champaign, IL: Human Kinetics.

Henderson, J., & Carroll, W. (1993). The athletic trainers' role in preventing sport injury and rehabilitating injured athletes: A psychological perspective. In D. Pargman (Ed.), *Psychological bases of sport injuries* (pp. 15-31). Morgantown, WV: Fitness Information Technology.

Heyman, S. R. (1993). When to refer athletes for counseling of psychotherapy. In J. Williams (Ed.) *Applied sport psychology: Personal growth to peak performance* (2nd ed., pp. 299-308). Palo Alto, CA: Mayfield.

Hokanson, R. G. (1994). *Relationship between sports rehabilitation practitioners' communication style and athletes' adherence to injury rehabilitation.* Unpublished master's thesis, Springfield College, MA.

Ivey, A. E., Ivey, M. B., & Simek-Morgan, L. (1993). *Counseling and psychotherapy: A multicultural perspective* (3rd. ed.). Boston: Allyn and Bacon.

Izzo, C. M. (1994). *The relationship between social support and adherence to sport injury rehabilitation.* Unpublished master's thesis, Springfield College, MA.

Johnson, S. B. (1993). Chronic diseases of childhood: Assessing compliance with complex medical regimens. In N. A. Krasnegor, L. Epstein, S. B. Johnson, & S. J. Yaffe (Eds.), *Developmental aspects of health compliance behavior* (pp. 157-184). Hillsdale, NJ: Erlbaum.

Johnston, L. H., & Carroll, D. (1998). The context of emotional responses to athletic injury: A qualitative analysis. *Journal of Sport Rehabilitation, 7,* 206-220.

Johnston, L.H., & Carroll, D. (2000). Coping, social support, and injury: Changes over time and the effects of level of sports involvement. *Journal of Sport Rehabilitation, 9,* 290-303.

Kahanov, L., & Fairchild, P. C. (1994). Discrepancies in perceptions held by injured athletes and athletic trainers during the initial evaluation. *Journal of Athletic Training, 29,* 70-75.

Kiesler, D. J., & Watkins, L. M. (1989). Interpersonal complementarity and the therapeutic alliance: A study of relationship in psychotherapy. *Psychotherapy, 26,* 183-194.

Kivlighan, D. M., & Schmitz, P. J. (1992). Counselor technical activity in cases with improving working alliances and continuing-poor working alliances. *Journal of Counseling Psychology, 39,* 32-38.

Kleiber, D. A., & Brock, S. C. (1992). The effect of career-ending injuries on the subsequent well-being of elite college athletes. *Sociology of Sport Journal, 9,* 70-75.

Lampton, C. C., Lambert, M. E., & Yost, R. (1993). The effects of psychological factors in sports medicine rehabilitation adherence. *Journal of Sports Medicine and Physical Fitness, 33,* 292-299.

Larson, G. A., Starkey, C. A., & Zaichkowsky, L. D. (1996). Psychological aspects of athletic injuries as perceived by athletic trainers. *The Sport Psychologist, 10,* 37-47.

Laubach, W. J., Brewer, B. W., Van Raalte, J. L., & Petitpas, A. J. (1996). Attributions for recovery and adherence to sport injury rehabilitation. *Australian Journal of Science and Medicine in Sport, 28,* 30-34.

Leddy, M. H., Lambert, M. J., & Ogles, B. M. (1994). Psychological consequences of athletic injury among high-level competitors. *Research Quarterly for Exercise and Sport, 65,* 347-354.

Linder, D. E., Brewer, B. W., Van Raalte, J. L., & DeLange, N. (1991). A negative halo for athletes who consult a sport psychologist: Replication and extension. *Journal of Sport & Exercise Psychology, 13,* 133-148.

Manuel, J. C., Shilt, J. S., Curl, W. W., Smith, J. A., DuRant, R. H., Lester, L., & Sinal, S. H. (2002). Coping with sports injuries: An examination of the adolescent athlete. *Journal of Adolescent Health, 31,* 391-393.

May, S., & Taylor, A. H. (1994). The development and examination of various measures of patient compliance, for specific use with injured athletes. *Journal of Sports Sciences, 12,* 180-181.

McDonald, S. A., & Hardy, C. J. (1990). Affective response patterns of the injured athlete: An exploratory analysis. *The Sport Psychologist, 4,* 261-274.

Meichenbaum, D. (1985). *Stress inoculation training.* Elmford, NY: Pergamon Press.

Meichenbaum, D., & Turk, D. C. (1987). *Facilitating treatment adherence.* New York: Plenum.

Murphy, G. C., Foreman, P. E., Simpson, C. A., Molloy, G. N., & Molloy, E. K. (1999). The development of a locus of control measure predictive of injured athletes' adherence to treatment. *Journal of Science and Medicine in Sport, 2,* 145-152.

Myers, C. A., Peyton, D. D., & Jensen, B. J. (2004). Treatment acceptability in NCAA Division I football athletes: Rehabilitation intervention strategies. *Journal of Sport Behavior, 27,* 165-169.

Nideffer, R. M. (1983). The injured athlete: Psychological factors in treatment. *Orthopedic Clinics of North America, 14,* 373-385.

Nixon, H. L. II. (1994). Social pressure, social support, and help seeking for pain and injuries in college sports networks. *Journal of Sport & Social Issues, 18,* 340-355.

Noyes, F. R., Matthews, D. S., Mooar, P. A., & Grood, E. S. (1983). The symptomatic anterior cruciate-deficient knee. Part II: The results of rehabilitation, activity modification, and counseling on functional disability. *Journal of Bone and Joint Surgery, 65-A,* 163-174.

Orlinsky, D. E., & Howard, K. I. (1986). Process and outcome in psychotherapy. In S. L. Garfield & A. E. Bergin (Eds.), *Handbook of psychotherapy and behavior change* (pp. 311-381). New York: Wiley.

Pearson, L., & Jones, G. (1992). Emotional effects of sports injuries: Implications for physiotherapists. *Physiotherapy, 78,* 762-770.

Petitpas, A. & Cornelius, A. (2004). Practitioner-client relationships: Building working alliances. In G. S. Kolt & M. B. Andersen (Eds.), *Psychology in the physical and manual therapies* (pp.57-70). Edinburgh: Churchill Livingstone.

Petitpas, A., & Danish, S. J. (1995). Caring for injured athletes. In S. M. Murphy (Ed.), *Sport psychology interventions* (pp. 255-282). Champaign, IL: Human Kinetics.

Robbins, J. E., & Rosenfeld, L. B. (2001). Athletes' perceptions of social support provided by their head coach, assistant coach, and athletic trainer, pre-injury and during rehabilitation. *Journal of Sport Behavior, 24(3),* 277-297.

Sexton, T. L., & Whiston, S. C. (1994). The status of the counseling relationship: An empirical review, theoretical implications, and research directions. *The Counseling Psychologist, 22,* 6-78.

Shaffer, S. M. (1992). *Attributions and self-efficacy as predictors of rehabilitative success.* Unpublished master's thesis, University of Illinois at Urbana-Champaign, Urbana-Champaign.

Shelbourne, K. D., & Wilckens, J. H. (1990). Current concepts in anterior cruciate ligament rehabilitation. *Orthopaedic Review, 19,* 957-964.

Smith, A. M., Scott, S. G., O'Fallon, W. M., & Young, M. L. (1990). Emotional responses of athletes to injury. *Mayo Clinic Proceedings, 65,* 38-50.

Smith, A. M., Stuart, M. J., Wiese-Bjornstal, D. M., Milliner, E. K., O'Fallon, W. M., & Crowson, C. S. (1993). Competitive athletes: Preinjury and postinjury mood state and self-esteem. *Mayo Clinic Proceedings, 68,* 939-947.

Smith, A. M., Young, M. L., & Scott, S. G. (1988). The emotional responses of athletes to injury. *Canadian Journal of Sport Sciences, 13,* 84P-85P.

Taylor, A. H., & May, S. (1995a). Physiotherapist's expectations and their influence on compliance to sports injury rehabilitation. In R. Vanfraechem-Raway, & Y. Vanden Auweele (Eds.), *IXth European*

Congress on Sport Psychology proceedings: Part II (pp. 619-625). Brussels: European Federation of Sports Psychology.

Taylor, A. H., & May, S. (1995b). Development of a Sports Injury Clinic Athlete Satisfaction Scale for auditing patient perceptions. *Physiotherapy Theory and Practice, 11,* 231-238.

Taylor, A. H., & May, S. (1996). Threat and coping appraisal as determinants of compliance to sports injury rehabilitation: An application of protection motivation theory. *Journal of Sports Sciences,14,* 471-482.

Taylor, S. E. (1995). *Health psychology* (3rd ed.). New York: McGraw-Hill.

Tuffey, S. (1991). *The use of psychological skills to facilitate recovery from athletic injury.* Unpublished master's thesis, University of North Carolina at Greensboro.

Udry, E. (1996). Social support: Exploring its role in the context of athletic injuries. *Journal of Sport Rehabilitation, 5,* 151-163.

Udry, E., Gould, D., Bridges, D., & Tuffey, S. (1997). People helping people? Examining the social ties of athletes coping with burnout and injury stress. *Journal of Sport & Exercise Psychology, 19,* 368-395.

Van Raalte, J. L. & Andersen, M. B. (2002). Referral processes in sport psychology. In J. L. Van Raalte & B. W. Brewer (Eds). *Exploring sport and exercise psychology* (2nd ed., pp. 325-337). Washington, DC: American Psychological Association.

Van Raalte, J. L., Brewer, B. W., & Petitpas, A. J. (1992). *Correspondence between athlete and trainer appraisals of injury rehabilitation status.* Paper presented at the annual meeting of the Association for the Advancement of Applied Sport Psychology, Colorado Springs, CO.

Webborn, A. D. J., Carbon, R. J., & Miller, B. P. (1997). Injury rehabilitation programs: "What are we talking about?" *Journal of Sport Rehabilitation, 6,* 54-61.

Wiese, D. M., Weiss, M. R., & Yukelson, D. P. (1991). Sport psychology in the training room: Implications for the treatment team. *The Sport Psychologist, 5,* 15-24.

Wiese-Bjornstal, D. M., Smith, A. M., & LaMott, E. E. (1995). A model of psychologic response to athletic injury and rehabilitation. *Athletic Training: Sports Health Care Perspectives, 1,* 17-30.

Wise, A., Jackson, D. W., & Rocchio, P. (1979). Preoperative psychologic testing as a predictor of success in knee surgery. *American Journal of Sports Medicine, 7,* 287-292.

Wittig, A. F., & Schurr, K. T. (1994). Psychological characteristics of women volleyball players: Relationships with injuries, rehabilitation, and team success. *Personality and Social Psychology Bulletin, 20,* 322-330.

Chapter Six | Modeling in Injury Rehabilitation: Seeing Helps Believing

Frances A. Flint
York University

Modeling has been used extensively within sport as an instructional tool for the learning of motor skills and social behavior. The extension of this technique into the realm of sport injury rehabilitation affords motivation, injury-rehabilitation information, and behavioral cues for recovering athletes. For athletes who have never experienced a major injury, a key component of a successful recovery involves learning how to cope with the process of rehabilitation and return to competition. Thus, athletes who have already effected a complete recovery from injury are ideal models. Seeing another person successfully overcome a similar injury can help an injured athlete believe that recovery is possible. In this sense, "seeing helps believing."

Introduction

"I thought I was invincible until this happened." Such were the words of a highly recruited, first-year university basketball player as she recounted her reactions to a season-ending knee injury. Never having experienced a major injury before, she suffered through the loss of the image she held of being a physically active, elite-level athlete. In addition, the daily exercise and competitive pursuits to which she was accustomed were now replaced with dependency and physical disability. Consequently, in the hours and days immediately post-injury, despair and depression dominated the psyche of this injured athlete.

Certainly with the current surgical techniques and rehabilitation programs available, this kind of injury scenario no longer need be considered devastating and potentially career-ending. But what of the psychological trauma sustained by the injured athlete? How can therapists, coaches, and teammates support the injured athlete through the difficult periods of depression and despondency that may result from injury? Therapists often ask how they can aid in the recovery process. It has been suggested that psychological skills such as goal setting, visualization, relaxation training, and negative thought stoppage be used to provide psychological rehabilitation in conjunction with physical recovery protocols (Crossman, 2001; Feltz, 1984; Gordon, 1986; Weiss & Troxel, 1986; Wiese & Weiss, 1987). One technique that has been given minimal attention in the psychological rehabilitation of athletic injuries is the use of modeling or observational learning.

Modeling has been described as an ideal way to communicate skills, attitudes, and behaviors through the observation of behavioral or verbal cues provided by a model (Bandura, 1986a). Modeling has been used extensively in sport, and teachers and coaches have often relied on this teaching tool for the transmission of knowledge in motor skill learning (McCullagh, Weiss, & Ross, 1989; Weiss & Klint, 1987). Thus, athletes are familiar with observing models either in a live or filmed format for the purpose of motor skill learning or the transmission of psychological information (e.g., motivation). In order to understand the potential beneficial effects of modeling in a therapeutic context, it is important to understand common affective reactions to injury and the psychological needs of recovering injured athletes.

Psychological Reactions to Athletic Injury

When a university-level basketball player was asked how she felt after suffering a major knee injury she responded,

> That week between the time of the injury and surgery, . . .it was hell—because I didn't know what to think . . . That was the worst week I can ever comprehend in my life . . . my school suffered and I was trying to get around campus on crutches. My social life suffered with respect to relationships with other people, because I was so confused and I was angry. . . I had so many emotions running through my head. (Flint, 1991, p. 142)

The athlete remarked that she also was contending with an overload of medical information on injury and surgery that she didn't understand, while trying to deal with the reality of the sudden end to her playing season. In addition, because she was only a freshman, doubts about whether she would be able to complete her university athletic career were evident.

When a severe injury occurs the injured athlete must often cope with an excess of medically based information, the loss of physical capability, the emotions of withdrawing from a desired activity, and a dependency on others to fulfill daily needs. At the same time, anxiety about the uncertainty of the future may be exacerbated by the severity of the injury and the limitations imposed by it (Lynch, 1988; Purtilo, 1978). Consider the university athlete who prior to the injury was a mobile, active player, now relying on others to get to classes or manage activities of daily living (i.e., eating, dressing). All of these experiences and emotions may overwhelm the injured athlete and create confusion and feelings of helplessness (McDonald & Hardy, 1990; Yukelson, 1986). Consequently the athlete may downplay or exaggerate the extent of the injury and draw unwarranted conclusions as to the implications of the injury. Catastrophizing (seeing only the worst case scenario) is often an athlete's initial reaction to major injury (Flint, 1998). In addition to irrational thoughts, affective reactions can become influential and may partially determine the actions and behavior of the injured athlete (Rotella, 1988; Yukelson, 1986). Anger, depression, and despair emanating from this sense of loss and confusion may become so burdensome as to interfere with the recovery process (Feltz, 1984; Yukelson, 1986).

Thus, the athlete who becomes injured may experience myriad emotions that can be detrimental to the recovery process. Helping the athlete deal with these emotions is an important component in the psychological rehabilitation program.

Psychological Needs during Recovery

For athletes who are accustomed to seeking control over opponents and game situations, their own helplessness due to injury can be overwhelming. Specific psychological needs of injured athletes must be satisfied and strategies developed to promote a complete healing process. In the same way that the athlete requires technical information from coaches in order to develop skill, so too the injured athlete needs guidance from physicians, therapists, and others so that the recovery process can be as comprehensive as possible. Information from sports medicine professionals on both the process of recovery and the potential outcomes of that recovery are important to injured athletes.

Yukelson (1986) has suggested that athletes can overcome injury by employing the same psychological qualities that helped them to excel in their athletic endeavors (e.g., pride, determination, and hard work). Bev Smith, a former Canadian National Women's Basketball team member and All-American, provides an excellent example of this transfer of athletic excellence determination to injury recovery. Bev had sustained several knee injuries and surgery in her illustrious career and remarked that,

If you keep your perspective on it and look one day at a time, then that'll come, but, I mean, you have to get up every morning and you have to do your leg weights. It's the most unromantic thing in the morning . . . a lot of people think comebacks . . . they see TV documentaries on these athletes who have come back and it's all really spectacular and romantic . . . but it's not—it's drudgery, it's getting up every morning and doing these small little things, doing the leg weights, doing them at night before you go to bed even though you're tired—those things really pay off. (Flint, 1991, p. 151)

Bev's dedication to her injury recovery consisted of the same psychological factors (i.e., goal setting, persistence) as her basketball skill development.

Keeping Bev's comments in mind, an identification of the specific psychological needs and strategies for recovery must be the first step in the rehabilitation process. Athletes who have recovered from injury consistently identify the same emotions, needs, and factors as helpful in overcoming injury. For instance, taking an active role and responsibility for the recovery process is perceived as being vital (Ievleva & Orlick, 1991; McDonald & Hardy, 1990; Vergeer, 2006). Also, having a social support structure either through family, peers, and coaches, other injured athletes, or therapists, provides a valuable foundation on which to tackle the hardships of recovery from injury (Flint, 1991; McDonald & Hardy, 1990; Smith, 1980; Udry, 2001; Wiese & Weiss, 1987).

Fisher (1990) concurred with the importance of psychological factors in injury rehabilitation and has identified self-confidence as a primary component in this process. According to Fisher, three aspects of self-confidence that become important in the recovery process include

- competence,
- control, and
- commitment.

Competence relates to the feeling that a task can be accomplished successfully, and in the instance of an injured athlete, this means a successful return to competition. The control aspect describes the athlete's feeling that he or she has the ability to take command of a certain situation such as the rehabilitation program. The last aspect, commitment, refers to the athlete's willingness and capability to stay with a task. Fisher (1990) suggested, "Any strategy that promotes any of these 3 ends will increase the likelihood of treatment adherence" (p. 154). Thus, pertinent injury and rehabilitation information and strategies for coping become critical components for increasing the athlete's confidence in a successful recovery from injury.

Much of the information needed by the injured athlete to promote the psychological aspects of recovery can be gained through the use of modeling. Listening to someone like Bev Smith talk about setting daily goals for recovery and dedication to the small details of rehabilitation, seeing another athlete struggle through reconditioning, or hearing another athlete with similar injury speak of her frustration as well as joy in returning to play can all be influential for the recently injured athlete. This is especially true if the athlete has never experienced a major injury before and has no experience on which to base behavior or hopes for recovery. Not knowing what to expect, how to behave under injury conditions, or how to tackle the challenges of recovery may present a dilemma for the injured athlete.

Modeling: What Is It?

Modeling has long been regarded as a powerful instructional tool for the learning of motor skills and social behaviors (McCullagh et al., 1989). The theoretical strength and empirical support for the effects of modeling make it a viable intervention strategy, particularly in the area of sport and exercise.

A number of theories have been forwarded to explain the modeling-behavior relationship. The most consistent support has come from Bandura (1969, 1977, 1986a, 1986b), with social-cognitive theories of modeling being the most popular. This theory proposes that modeling or observational learning is one of the primary modes used by individuals to gain socialization information and cognitive skills. Behaviors, attitudes, and skills can be learned through modeling via behavioral and verbal cues provided by the model (Bandura, 1986a). As the observer views a model, symbolic representation or verbal coding takes place and these cues are placed in memory. Through this vicariously gained information, judgment criteria are established and new behavioral patterns can be learned. Judgments about capabilities are often comparative in nature; therefore, seeing someone similar to oneself perform a novel task or particular behavior can enhance the perception about the observer's capacity to recreate the action (Bandura, 1986a). This is very evident in sport injury situations as athletes watch others who have overcome a particular roadblock during injury recovery.

A number of significant factors help to determine the effectiveness of a modeling experience and whether the observer will have incentive to copy the modeled behavior. These factors may include

- physical characteristics of the model (e.g., physique, age, sex),
- model type (e.g., mastery vs coping), and
- the number of models.

By presenting multiple, diversified models, it is hoped that at least one of the models will demonstrate characteristics similar to the observer and will capture the attention of the observer creating a common bond.

The importance of model/observer characteristics has been stressed by Bandura (1977) and McCullagh et al. (1989). It is proposed that the observer will form a bond with the model through the identification of similarities and, thus, the observer will be more motivated to pay attention to the message the model is conveying (McCullagh et al., 1989). In sport these similarities may relate to playing position, level of competition, or style of play. Therefore, the selection of specific characteristics of the model, creating a "similar other," is critical for effecting behavioral change in observers.

Model similarity is a particularly salient aspect of the observer/model relationship because it may determine if the observer will pay attention to the model. A perfect example of the effect of model/observer similarity was provided by an injured female basketball player who had just undergone anterior cruciate ligament surgery. While watching a videotape of other female basketball players who had experienced the same surgery, she described one of the models who had caught her attention and why she had noticed the model. "One of the girls who talked about the pain after coming out of surgery, I had it too. Because I could relate completely to what she was talking about, I understood it" (Flint, 1991, p. 246). Obviously, this model had an impact on the observer through the shared experience of pain. This common bond, which had been formed between the two, may have been influential in encouraging the observer to pay attention to the verbal and behavioral cues provided by the model.

Another important aspect of the model/observer relationship is the type of model presented. Model similarity is established through the level of expertise displayed by the model such as a mastery or expert model as compared to a coping model. Mastery or exemplary models demonstrate errorless task execution and show tasks as they are to be performed perfectly (Schunk, Hanson, & Cox, 1987). On the other hand, coping models initially demonstrate negative cognitions and affects and an imperfect performance. Gradually, the coping model demonstrates positive thoughts, high self-efficacy, and strategies needed to overcome problems and improve performance. The use of coping models is particularly pertinent to injury rehabilitation because the injured observer can relate to the stages of recovery demonstrated by the model who is overcoming an injury. If we constantly point to previously injured, elite-level athletes as mastery models, the recovery may appear too easy or too far out of reach for the ordinary injured athlete.

The last factor, the use of multiple, diversified models has also been demonstrated as effective in the learning of new behaviors and motor skills (Thelen, Fry, Fehrenbach, & Frautschi, 1979). This modeling strategy entails the use of at least two, but possibly more, persons who demonstrate the target behavior. The models should be diverse, however, in terms of personal characteristics (e.g., sex, age), and physical attributes (e.g., size, physical abilities) to increase the likelihood that the observer will be able to identify with at least one of the models. The visible characteristics of the model may result in a psychological bonding effect by the observer because a similarity with the model is recognized. This aspect of bonding may have a motivational effect on the observer and may prompt the observer to expend more effort to "be like" the model. The use of multiple models also provides the observer with more than one exposure to the target behavior, which enhances the opportunity for learning.

When modeling is used as a psychological intervention in therapeutic situations, it is felt that the model/observer relationship will act as a catalyst to effect a positive approach to the rehabilitation process. By watching the model, the injured athlete gains knowledge about rehabilitation, strategies for handling setbacks, and the confidence that, if others can recover from injury, so can he or she (Flint, 1998). Feltz (1988) suggests that the effect of modeling resides in experience with the task or behavior: "The less experience one has had with a task or situation, the more one will rely on others to judge one's own capabilities" (p. 427). Thus, athletes injured severely for the first time would be considered extremely naive in terms of what is required to accomplish a complete recovery.

In summary, strong empirical evidence exists for the powerful effects of modeling on performance, cognitions, and emotional responses in observers. In particular, the use of specific strategies such as similar, diversified, and coping modeling has been shown to have enduring beneficial effects in anxiety-producing, clinical, and therapeutic settings. The provision of coping models via videotape presentation may be particularly salient to athletes as they pursue physical rehabilitation post injury. The psychological benefits of watching a similar other recover from injury could have far-reaching effects on effort and persistence in adherence to rehabilitation programs.

Informal and Formal Modeling in the Medical Context

Both informal and formal modeling techniques have been used within a medical context to bolster the observer's sense that recovery from a serious health threat is possible. In many cases, these observer/model situations occur informally and naturally within a rehabilitation setting as a therapist points out another athlete with the same injury who is progressing with the rehabilitation process. Often, an athlete who has returned to competition after recovering from a serious injury is identified by coaches or therapists as an example for the injured athlete. This is a form of informal modeling where the main benefit to the observer is a motivational boost and very little hard data on psychological strategies or ways of overcoming obstacles to recovery is conveyed.

An excellent example of informal modeling was provided by Kerrin Lee-Gartner at the 1992 Winter Olympics and Jennifer Heil in the 2006 Winter Olympics when both recovered from serious injuries to win Olympic gold. The head coach of the Canadian women's ski team remarked, "It'll make us believe again. It'll make injured skiers like Kate Pace and Lucie LaRoche say, 'I can win again'" (Byers, 1992, p. E18). Kerrin became a model for injured downhill skiers because, despite five knee surgeries and a broken ankle, she was able to recover and win Olympic gold. Jennifer Heil had experienced chronic back injuries and became a model for freestyle skiers as she overcame this roadblock to excellence. These are instances of informal modeling because strategies for recovery were not provided by Kerrin or Jennifer, but rather, motivational examples were set for others to follow. Even though these are elite-level models, they both demonstrate the use of their athletic excellence psychological determination to overcoming injuries.

In order to ensure that pertinent, useful information and strategies for a complete rehabilitation process are being displayed by the model, the modeling process should be formalized. In formal modeling, a situation is created whereby one or more models present specific verbal or visual cues that expose the observer to

- vicarious experiences,
- verbal persuasions, and
- emotional exhortations.

Depending on how the modeling experience is structured, all three of these sources of self-confidence information can be presented or one specific source can be isolated and highlighted. In formal modeling, the model/observer situation is created to gain the maximum benefit from the exposure.

For instance, in order to reduce preoperative anxiety, increase postoperative ambulation, and decrease the number of days in the hospital after surgery, newly hospitalized patients can be exposed to post-surgery roommates who demonstrate various coping behaviors (Kulik & Mahler, 1987). The exposure to postoperative sensations and events through a coping model better prepares the observer by providing accurate information on which cognitive appraisal of the situation can be made (Kulik & Mahler, 1987). According to Lazarus (1966) the observer will experience less stress in these situations because the events are now interpreted as less threatening due, in large part, to the newly acquired cognitive and behavioral responses. In other words, because of the modeling experience, the preoperative patient now knows what to expect and this may help alleviate fear.

In order to provide the observer with a maximal amount of pertinent information regarding medical procedures and outcomes, videotape or film modeling may be used to augment therapy in clinical settings (Thelen et al., 1979; Melamed & Siegel, 1975). Videotape modeling has also been used as a psychological intervention within an athletic population (Flint, 1991) dealing with recovery from knee injury. Female athletes who had just undergone a surgical repair of the anterior cruciate ligament (ACL) in the knee watched a videotape of several coping models. The videotape consisted of interviews with seven basketball players who had all recovered from knee ligament surgery. Six of the players in the videotape were interviewed at various stages of recovery from anterior cruciate ligament surgery extending from 2 weeks to 7 years post surgery. The seventh player was an example of complete progress of a full recovery from a few weeks post surgery to 16 months post surgery. These players were interviewed in a question-and-answer format describing the playing situation in which they were injured, the problems and fears they experienced during their recovery from surgery, and various aspects of their rehabilitation. Heavy emphasis was placed on how they had overcome the problems they faced during recovery and on a positive outlook with respect to their return to a basketball career. At the end of each interview were scenes of the recovered player during practice and game sessions demonstrating a total capability to participate.

The modeling videotape was seen by the injured athletes on three separate occasions: immediately post surgery, at 2 months post surgery, and at 4 months post surgery. These time frames coincide approximately to the phases of healing: acute, inflammatory phase, fibroblastic or tissue regeneration phase, and maturation phase (Flint, 1998). Pertinent insights into the needs of the recovering athletes were provided and this information affords us a guideline for the designing of modeling interventions for athletic injury rehabilitation.

In general, immediately post surgery, the injured athletes tended to notice things that related to the emotions associated with the injury and the surgery. For example, one subject picked out a specific model in the videotape as similar to herself "... because when she injured it she said 'F—' and I knew exactly what she was going through because the same thing was going through my mind too!" (Flint, 1991, p. 243). Another recovering athlete commented that she felt comforted knowing that "other basketball players had some of the same feelings about the injury. Even though I feel a lot of support from parents and teammates it is good to know that other injured athletes have similar feelings and that I'm not going crazy" (Flint, 1991, p. 246). Most of the comments initially noticed by the injured athletes who watched the videotape were in some way connected to affective responses to the injury and surgery that were verbalized by the models.

Later, at 2 and 4 months post surgery, the verbal statements and actions of the models that attracted more notice tended to change as the rehabilitation process continued. One injured athlete summed this up perfectly when she said, "Everybody in the tape said something that I could relate to, but it has changed as my rehab progressed" (Flint, 1991, p. 246). Several of the injured athletes remarked about their recovery and said that some of the statements made by the models meant more to them now that they were experiencing the struggles of rehabilitation. One injured athlete commented that the model who was cycling with one leg and then both legs caught her attention because, "I remember how frustrated I was when I couldn't do a single rotation and finally being able to cycle without any pain and actually sweating!" (Flint, 1991, p. 241). In general, there was an overwhelmingly positive response to the verbalizations and actions of the models and it appears that a bonding effect did occur between models and observers.

Injured athletes who watched the videotape also provided insight and qualitative information on their perceptions relative to their rehabilitation progress. They were asked to outline what factors had helped them adhere to the rehabilitation program or why they had not persisted in their physical rehabilitation. They were also asked to reflect on their experience and discuss what assistance would have been helpful to them in their recovery (i.e., more social support, more advice).

It was interesting to note that the injured athletes who watched the videotape

- appeared to be motivated to adhere to their rehabilitation programs,
- had knowledge about what had helped them throughout rehabilitation, and
- were definitive about their needs during the recovery period (e.g., goal setting).

The videotaped modeling experience appeared to have a positive effect on the perceptions of the injured athletes in terms of their ability to handle a physical rehabilitation program.

When combined with the use of the videotape medium, coping models can be effective in reducing fears and anxiety in therapeutic settings. Thelen et al. (1979) supported the efficacy of videotape or film modeling over live modeling because the opportunity to present naturalistic modeling sequences would be difficult or unrealistic to create in a clinical setting. The videotape format also allows for the reconstruction of the most desirable scenes and the multiple viewing of specific situations or conditions (Anderson, DeVellis, & DeVellis, 1987). This format is versatile in that it affords self-administration by the injured athlete at times when the need is greatest, such as when setbacks occur in the recovery process. In terms of costs, after an initial relatively high expenditure, the videotape becomes an inexpensive tool for augmenting the rehabilitation process. Much support exists in the literature for the use of videotape modeling in therapeutic settings (Anderson, L.A. et al., 1987; Kendall & Watson, 1981; Thelen et al., 1979).

Information Provided Through Modeling: The Specifics

What information should be provided through formalized modeling experiences? Is there information that would be of prime benefit to the observer and other information that could be harmful? These questions and others related to the modeling experience have been posed in the medical psychology literature (Weinman & Johnston, 1988). Within the dimensions of sport psychology and sports medicine, however, the use of multiple coping models to demonstrate behavior and attitudes conducive to the rehabilitation of athletic injuries is a relatively new strategy. Thus, it is important that direction be sought from allied medical and health fields in order to discern valid content and composition guidelines for modeling interventions in rehabilitation.

In addition to injury and rehabilitation information, common questions asked by injured athletes, parents, and coaches relate to

- the procedures of surgery,
- its potentially disfiguring effects, and
- the prospects for complete recovery.

Often, the shock of a major injury and fear of possible surgery create a mental obstruction, and the injured athlete is unable to be receptive to injury information. In some cases, too much information or too many medical technicalities create an overload situation, and details of the injury are forgotten or misunderstood (Flint, 1991; Samples, 1987). If a videotaped presentation by a former injured athlete outlining pertinent injury information was available through either the physician or therapist's office, then the injured athlete could refer to it as needed. Information about surgery or rehabilitation that the athlete had missed because of the stress of the injury or the announcement that surgery was needed could then be gained at a time when the athlete was more receptive.

Van der Ploeg (1988) provides us with useful information on the perceptions of hospital patients relative to stressful medical situations, and this furnishes guidance on the development of modeling experiences. He found that hospital patients described the most stressful medical situations and events to include

- pain,
- not being able to discuss their problems, and
- the lack of sufficient information on medical conditions.

Thus, information provided to medical patients should be designed to ameliorate these stressful situations. In terms of athletes, there are few concrete guidelines concerning patient information (Flint, 1998; Heil, cited in Samples, 1987, p. 174). Basically, information to athletes should include

- the exact nature of the injury,
- the procedures and rationale for rehabilitation,
- potential obstacles that lie ahead and how to overcome them, and
- feelings the athletes may experience through the recovery period.

Obviously, this information must be specific to the athlete's sport and position and the competitive schedule. Thus, the recommendations from Flint and Heil concerning injured athletes are in concert with Van der Ploeg's (1988) research.

Kulik and Mahler (1987) suggest that, in general, the more information a patient has preoperatively about what to expect, the better are the chances of recovery being facilitated. One concern with this approach of full injury and surgery disclosure are the aspects of fear and the impression of control. If the information provided to the injured athlete is too detailed and graphic, then the fear experienced may be overwhelming and the athlete will suffer from a feeling of loss of control over the situation. In this case, the stress and fear created by explicit details of the injury and surgery may be greater than the perception that the athlete has of his or her ability to overcome the injury. It is vital that any information provided or psychological interventions applied help injured athletes gain more confidence that they are capable of performing activities that may benefit overall recovery. Gaining insight from a similar other who has successfully rehabilitated an athletic injury could help reduce fear and increase confidence for a complete recovery.

The concept of fear reduction and perceptions of control are two important aspects of information provided to the injured athlete. Few guidelines exist for the composition or content of information designed to reduce stress in medical settings (Johnson, 1984; Wilson, 1981). According to Anderson and Masur (1983), the best kind of information is a combination of sensory and procedural details that can help foster accurate expectations and allow for correct cognitive interpretations of sensations to be experienced. Through this information, both procedural stress (immediate aspects) and outcome stress (long- term factors) can be alleviated (Weinman & Johnston, 1988). The procedural stress relates to details of the surgery (pain, disfigurement), and outcome stress is associated with the prognosis for a complete recovery. Perhaps in this situation, a previously injured athlete who has recovered from a similar injury can provide valuable information on the immediate effects of injury and surgery, obstacles to be expected, strategies to encourage adherence to rehabilitation, and realistic expectations for future recovery. Care must be ensured, however, that negative modeling situations, in which either the model or the viewer is not progressing as appropriate, are anticipated and open lines of communications maintained.

Athletes sustaining injury for the first time have no experience on which to base their expectations for a full recovery. Fear of the unknown may result in dysfunctional attitudes on the part of the injured athlete and may delay the recovery process (Rotella & Heyman, 1986). This situation creates the perfect opportunity for vicarious learning from a similar other who can provide an accurate account of the road ahead (Kulik & Mahler, 1987; Weiss & Troxel, 1986; Wiese & Weiss, 1987). Models who provide cues to coping behavior and effective strategies for dealing with challenging or threatening situations are an untapped resource in the rehabilitation of athletic injuries. The use of models may also be of benefit to athletes who are close to resuming their competitive careers (Podlog and Eklund, 2006).

Summary

The old adage "Treat the person, not the injury" has specific implications in the rehabilitation of athletic injuries. Injured athletes will experience a psychophysiological response to trauma that dictates a need to consider their physical and psychological requirements when designing a rehabilitation protocol (Brewer et al., 2002; Flint, 1998; Lynch, 1988; Weiss & Troxel, 1986; Wiese & Weiss, 1987). It is inappropriate to treat tissue damage, but not trauma to the psyche. As Chesterfield remarked, "I find by experience that the mind and the body are more than married, for they are most intimately united; and when one suffers, the other sympathizes" (cited in Frost, 1971, p. 191).

Recovery from major injury, both physically and psychologically, is a long and arduous process requiring adherence to a comprehensive rehabilitation program. As we know, "Compliance may currently be one of the greatest challenges facing the health professions" (Cerkoney & Hart, 1980 cited in Turk, Meichenbaum, & Genest, 1983, p. 177). Any strategies that are effective in encouraging persistence in the face of obstacles to recovery are vital components of any rehabilitation protocol. One of the most effective means of conveying information and psychological strategies for injury rehabilitation that may be helpful to the recovering athlete is modeling and, after all, "Now that I have seen that others can recover from serious injury, then so can I!"

References

Anderson, K. O., & Masur, F. T. (1983). Psychological preparation for invasive medical and dental procedures. *Journal of Behavioral Medicine, 6*, 1-40.

Anderson, L. A., DeVellis, B. M., & DeVellis, R. F. (1987). Effects of modeling on patient communication, satisfaction, and knowledge. *Medical Care, 25*, 1044-1056.

Bandura, A. (1969). *Principles of behavior modification.* New York: Holt, Rinehart & Winston.

Bandura, A. (1977). Self-efficacy: Toward a unifying theory of behavioral change. *Psychological Review, 84*, 191-215.

Bandura, A. (1986a). *Self-efficacy mechanism in psychological activation and health-promoting behavior.* Stanford University, Department of Psychology, Stanford, CA.

Bandura, A. (1986b). *Social foundations of thought and action: A social cognitive theory.* Englewood Cliffs, NJ: Prentice-Hall.

Brewer, B. W., Anderson, M. B., & Van Raalte, J. L. (2002). Psychological aspects of sport injury rehabilitation: toward a biopsychosocial approach. In D. L. Mostofsky and D. Zaichkowsky (Eds.) *Medical aspects of sport and exercise.* Morgantown, WV: Fitness Information Technology.

Byers, J. (1992, February 16). Canadian ski gold an inspiration to others. *The Toronto Star,* p. E18.

Crossman, J. (2001). Managing thoughts, stress, and pain. In J. Crossman (Ed.), *Coping with sports injuries: Psychological strategies for rehabilitation* (pp. 128-144). New York: Oxford University Press.

Dishman, R. (1986). Exercise compliance: A new view for public health. *The Physician and Sportsmedicine, 14*(5), 127-145.

Feltz, D. L. (1984). The psychology of sports injuries. In P. F. Vinger & E. F. Hoerner (Eds.), *Sports injuries: The unthwarted epidemic* (2nd ed., pp. 336-344). Littleton, MA: PSG.

Feltz, D. L. (1988). Self-confidence and sports performance. In K. B. Pandolf (Ed.), *Exercise and sport sciences reviews* (Vol. 16, pp. 423-457). New York: Macmillan.

Fisher, C. A. (1990). Adherence to sports injury rehabilitation programmes. *Sports Medicine, 9,* 151-158.

Flint, F. A. (1991). The psychological effects of modeling in athletic injury rehabilitation. (Doctoral dissertation, University of Oregon, 1991). *(Microform Publications No. BF 357).*

Flint, F. A. (1998). *Psychology of sport injury.* Champaign, IL: Human Kinetics.

Frost, R. B. (Ed.). (1971). *Psychological concepts applied to physical education and coaching.* (pp. 191-210). Reading, MA: Addison-Wesley.

Gordon, S. (1986, March). Sport psychology and the injured athlete: A cognitive-behavioral approach to injury response and injury rehabilitation. *Science Periodical on Research and Technology in Sport, BU-1,* pp. 1-10.

Gordon, S., Potter, M., & Hamer, P. (2001). The role of physiotherapist and sport therapist. (pp. 66-82). In J. Crossman (Ed.), *Coping with sports injuries: Psychological strategies for rehabilitation.* New York: Oxford University Press.

Iveleva, L., & Orlick, T. (1991). Mental links to enhanced healing: an exploratory analysis. *The Sport Psychologist, 4,* 25-40.

Johnson, M. (1984). Dimensions of recovery from surgery. *International Review of Applied Psychology, 33,* 505-520.

Kendall, P. C., & Watson, D. (1981). Psychological preparation for stressful medical procedures. In C. K. Prokop & L. A. Bradley (Eds.), *Medical psychology: Contributions to behavioral medicine* (pp. 198-218). New York: Academic Press.

Kulik, J. A., & Mahler, H. I. (1987). Effects of preoperative roommate assignment on postoperative anxiety and recovery from coronary-bypass surgery. *Health Psychology, 6,* 525-543.

Lazarus, R. S. (1966). *Psychological stress and the coping process.* New York: McGraw-Hill.

Lynch, G. P. (1988). Athletic injuries and the practicing sport psychologist: practical guidelines for assisting athletes. *The Sport Psychologist, 2,* 161-167.

MacDonald, S. A., & Hardy, C. J. (1990). Affective response patterns of the injured athlete: an exploratory analysis. *The Sport Psychologist, 4,* 261-274.

McCullagh, P., Weiss, M. R., & Ross, D. (1989). Modeling considerations in motor skill acquisition and performance: An integrated approach. In K. B. Pandolf (Ed.), *Exercise and sport sciences reviews* (Vol. 17, pp. 475-513). Baltimore: Williams & Wilkins.

Melamed, B. G., & Siegel, L. J. (1975). Reduction of anxiety in children facing hospitalization and surgery by use of filmed modeling. *Journal of Consulting and Clinical Psychology, 43,* 511-521.

Podlog, L., & Eklund, R. C. (2006). A longitudinal investigation of competitive athletes' return to sport following serious injury. *Journal of applied sport psychology, 18*(1), 44-68.

Purtilo, D. T. (1978). *Health professional/patient interaction* (2nd ed.). Philadelphia: Saunders.

Rotella, R. J. (1988). Psychological care of the injured athlete. In D. N. Kulund (Ed.), *The injured athlete* (2nd ed., pp. 151-164). Philadelphia: Lippincott.

Rotella, R. J., & Heyman, S. R. (1986). Stress, injury and the psychological rehabilitation of athletes. In J. M. Williams (Ed.), *Applied sport psychology: Personal growth to peak performance* (pp. 343-364). Palo Alto, CA: Mayfield.

Samples, P. (1987). Mind over muscle: Returning the injured athlete to play. *The Physician and Sportsmedicine, 15*(10), 172-180.

Schunk, D. H., Hanson, A. R., & Cox, P. D. (1987). Peer-model attributes and children's achievement behaviors. *Journal of Educational Psychology, 79,* 54-61.

Smith, R. (1980). Development of an integrated coping response through cognitive-affective stress management training. In C. H. Nadeau, W. R. Halliwell, K. M. Newell, & G. C. Roberts (Eds.), *Psychology of motor behavior and sport: 1979* (pp. 54-72). Champaign: Human Kinetics.

Thelen, M. H., Fry, R. A., Fehrenbach, P. A., & Frautschi, N. M. (1979). Therapeutic videotape and film modeling: A review. *Psychological Bulletin, 86*, 701-720.

Turk, D. C., Meichenbaum, D., & Genest, M. (1983). *Pain and behavioral medicine.* New York: Guilford Press.

Udry, E. (2001). The role of significant others: Social support during injuries. (pp. 148-161). In J. Crossman (Ed.). *Coping with sport injuries: Psychological strategies for rehabilitation.* New York: Oxford University Press.

Van der Ploeg, H. M. (1988). Stressful medical events: A survey of patients' perceptions. In S. Maes, C. D. Spielberger, P. B. Defares, & I. G. Sarason (Eds.), *Topics in health psychology* (pp. 193-203). New York: Wiley.

Vergeer, I. (2006). Exploring the mental representation of athletic injury: A longitudinal case study. *Psychology of Sport and Exercise, 7*, 99-114.

Weinman, J., & Johnston, M. (1988). Stressful medical procedures: An analysis of the effects of psychological interventions and of the stressfulness of the procedures. In S. Maes, C. D. Spielberger, P. B. Defares, & I. G. Sarason (Eds.), *Topics in health psychology* (pp. 205-217). New York: Wiley.

Weiss, M. R., & Klint, K. A. (1987). "Show and tell" in the gymnasium: An investigation of developmental differences in modeling and verbal rehearsal of motor skills. *Research Quarterly for Exercise and Sport, 58*, 234-241.

Weiss, M. R., & Troxel, R. K. (1986). Psychology of the injured athlete. *Athletic Training, 21*, 104-109, 154.

Wiese, D. M., & Weiss, M. R. (1987). Psychological rehabilitation and physical injury: The role of the sports medicine team. *The Sport Psychologist, 1*, 318-330.

Wilson, J. F. (1981). Behavioural preparation for surgery: Benefit or harm. *Journal of Behavioural Medicine, 4*, 79-102.

Yukelson, D. (1986). Psychology of sport and the injured athlete. In D. B. Bernhardt (Ed.), *Clinics in physical therapy* (pp. 175-195). New York: Churchill Livingstone.

Chapter Seven

Psychosocial Considerations of the Return to Sport Following Injury

Leslie Podlog
Charles Sturt University

Robert C. Eklund
Florida State University

"I had lost a lot of confidence during the long layoff. And for a long time after I returned, I still held back. All I could think about was protecting my knee from another injury."
    Earvin "Magic" Johnson (cited in Taylor & Taylor, 1997, p. 273)

As Magic Johnson's quote suggests, returning to sport following a serious injury may be a difficult transition for athletes. Too often, however, coaches, practitioners, and athletes equate psychological readiness to resume sport participation with physical readiness. Research over the past ten years indicates that this assumption may be inaccurate (e.g., Bianco, 2001). Athletes' psychological reactions to their return to sport may have important implications for their subjective well-being and their return-to-sport outcomes (e.g., confidence levels, quality of performances). Consequently, the purpose of this chapter is to examine the psychosocial issues associated with the return-to-sport transition following serious injury. We begin by examining two conceptual models—the biopsychosocial model and the stages of Return to Sport Model—that have been used to describe the return to sport following serious injury. We then discuss some of the empirical literature that has examined the psychosocial stressors associated with the return to sport, drawing from our recent qualitative research involving high performance athletes (Podlog & Eklund, in press) and coaches (Podlog & Eklund, under review). Finally, we discuss the implications of these findings and offer strategies for clinicians, coaches, and practitioners aiming to prevent and/or reduce athlete stressors during the return-to-sport transition.

Conceptual Models and the Return to Sport Following Injury

Researchers have employed conceptual models to better understand the return-to-sport transition following injury. Conceptual models enable the systematic study of potential variables of interest and provide practitioners with a framework for guiding and targeting treatment interventions. Two conceptual models have been used to describe the return to sport transition: A Biopsychosocial Model (Andersen, 2001, Brewer, 2001, Brewer, Andersen & Van Raalte, 2002) and the Stages of Return to Sport Model (Taylor & Taylor, 1997).

A Biopsychosocial Model

An athlete's return to full activity is a complex process influenced by numerous factors, including the characteristics of the injury along with biological, psychological, and social variables (Andersen, 2001). Andersen (2001) suggests that a biopsychosocial model is particularly germane when preparing an athlete for a return to sport as it reminds coaches and practitioners of the myriad factors influencing return-to-sport outcomes (e.g., re-injury concerns, performance levels, confidence). As shown in Figure 1, the model has seven key components:
- characteristics of the injury
- sociodemographic factors
- biological factors
- psychological factors
- social/contextual factors
- intermediate biopsychological outcomes
- sport injury rehabilitation outcomes

According to Brewer (2001), the rehabilitation process is best initiated immediately following sport injury. It is proposed that the characteristics of the injury (e.g., severity, location, history) as well as sociodemographic factors (e.g., age, gender, socioeconomic status), influence biological (e.g., circulation, tissue repair, neurochemistry), psychological (personality, cognition, affect, and behavior), and social/contextual factors (e.g., social support, life stress, rehabilitation environment). Psychological factors are posited to have a reciprocal relationship with biological and social/contextual factors, all of which influence intermediate biopsychological rehabilitation outcomes (e.g., range of motion, strength, rate of recovery). Psychological factors and intermediate rehabilitation outcomes are also suggested to influence sport injury rehabilitation outcomes (e.g., functional performance, quality of life, readiness to return to sport).

The model has heuristic utility as a framework for giving coaches and practitioners clues as to how athletes will respond to a return to sport following injury (Andersen, 2001). Exploring the characteristics of the injury (e.g., severity, location, or history) may provide useful information about the ways in which athletes may respond to the prospect of returning to sport. If, for example, a soccer player tears her anterior cruciate ligament (ACL), this injury may produce greater re-injury fears than an injury to the athlete's forearm or shoulder. Given the importance of the injured limb to the sport performance, it seems more likely that the athlete will have concerns about re-injury and regaining pre-

Figure 1.

A biopsychosocial model of sport injury rehabilitation.

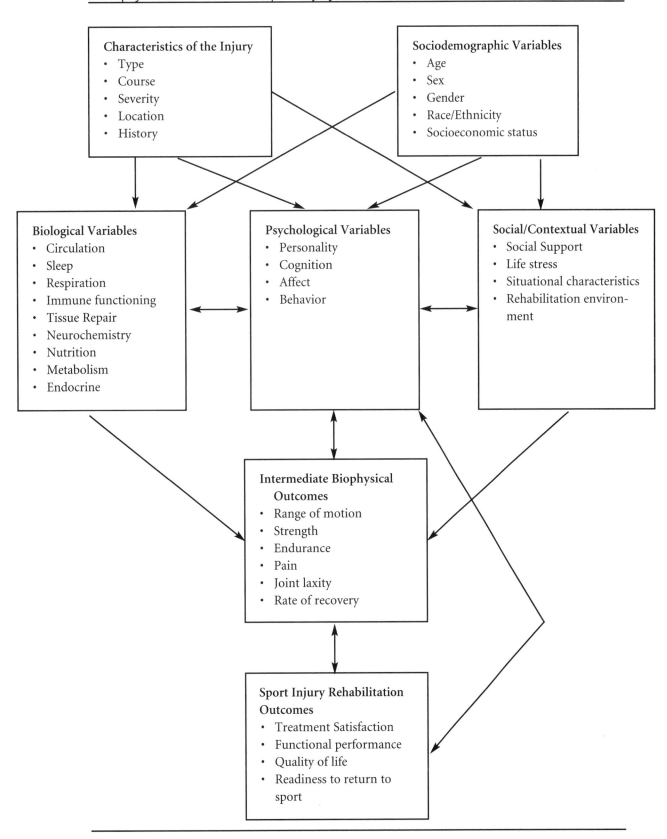

Note:
Brewer, B. W., Andersen, M. B., & Van Raalte, J. L. (2002). Psychological aspects of injury rehabilitation: Toward a biopsychosocial approach. In D. I. Mostofsky & L. Zaichkowsky (Eds.), *Medical and psychological aspects of sport and exercise* (pp. 41-54). Morgantown, WV: Fitness Information Technology.

injury form. The athlete with the ACL injury may also experience psychosocial disruptions due to the severity of the injury, the associated period of rehabilitation, and the perceived likelihood of full recovery. Finally, if the athlete has not had any previous injury experience she may have a more difficult time adapting to the demands of the return to sport since she has never had the experience of successfully returning.

Other factors such as sociodemographic, biological, psychological, and social/contextual variables may play an equally important role in an athlete's course of recovery and ability to return to full activity (Brewer et al., 2002). If for instance, the athlete has received effective social support from the coach and teammates, has stayed involved with the team and has not been pressured to come back too early (i.e., social/contextual factors), then the athlete may feel more confident and supported in returning to play. Conversely, if the athlete has been isolated from the team and has had his or her position taken by another, then the athlete may feel pressured and anxious about returning to play. These and many other factors listed in the model may directly and indirectly influence sport injury rehabilitation outcomes and ultimately return-to-sport outcomes.

The biopsychosocial model provides a general framework for investigating the numerous factors affecting sport injury rehabilitation outcomes. Specifically, the model includes an extensive list of variables and identifies general relationships among variable categories that may influence injury rehabilitation outcomes. Even while identifying relevant variables and general relationships, however, it is not a theory, and as a consequence does not (and cannot) provide a coherent explanation of how variables within and across categories might interact to produce different return-to-sport outcomes. Moreover, no indication is provided in the model of which factors may be most salient in producing various return-to-sport outcomes or why such factors are significant. Finally, the biopsychosocial model was not specifically designed to examine the return-to-sport transition. Although Andersen (2001) has extended the model to examine return-to-sport outcomes, the model was not created with the a priori intent of examining the issues and concerns relevant to athletes in this phase of injury recovery. In order to appreciate the psychosocial sequelae of events moving from readiness to return to sport (i.e., sport injury rehabilitation outcomes) to training and competition, it is informative to examine psychological models detailing this transition. Taylor and Taylor's (1997) "Stages of Return to Sport" is one model that has been proposed in the literature.

Stages of the Return to Sport Model

Taylor and Taylor's (1997) stage model of the return to sport is composed of five physical and psychological stages:
- the initial return
- recovery confirmation
- return of physical and technical abilities
- high-intensity training
- return to competition

Taylor and Taylor contended that athletes' ability to pass successfully from one stage to the next in their return to sport may be strongly contingent upon the injury healing, physical conditioning, and the psychological rehabilitation that has proceeded the return-to-sport phase of recovery. The model is presented in Figure 2.

The first stage, the initial return, provides athletes with their first opportunity to test the rehabilitated area. Taylor and Taylor (1997) suggested that the entire stage is dedicated to giving athletes a number of tests of the healed area that will lead to the second stage of the return to sport. This stage is one of the most difficult from a psychological standpoint, as it provides the athlete with feedback regarding the effectiveness of the rehabilitated area. The success of the initial phase dictates subsequent attitudes and feelings that athletes carry with them and that influence the ultimate outcome of rehabilitation and return to sport. Taylor and Taylor address a number of concerns that should be considered as athletes enter the initial return. These include unrealistic expectations about the ability of the rehabilitated area to withstand new levels of exertion, a desire to return too quickly, and progressing through this stage in an overly aggressive or overzealous manner.

The second stage is entitled recovery confirmation (Taylor & Taylor, 1997). It involves athletes obtaining feedback from the initial return that their injury is, in fact, healed and that they are ready to face the demands of training and competition. Again, this stage is more psychological than physical in nature as it involves athletes' emotional and cognitive responses to their initial return. It is also of psychological importance

Figure 2.

Stages of return to sport.

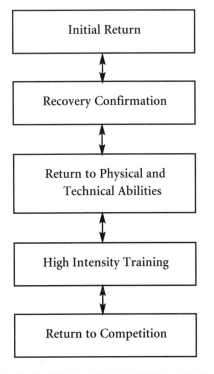

From Taylor, J., & Taylor, S. (1997). *Psychological approaches to sports injury rehabilitation.* Gaithersburg, MD: Aspen Publication

because how athletes feel about their initial return will affect their attitudes and approaches to subsequent stages. According to Taylor and Taylor, the primary goal of this phase is for athletes to have a strong belief that the rehabilitation was successful and that they are completely ready to move on to more intensive stages of the return to sport. While a successful initial return will provide athletes with a clear confirmation that the rehabilitation was effective, an unsuccessful initial return can produce physical and psychological problems that negatively impact further integration to sport.

As its name implies, the third stage—return of physical and technical abilities— focuses on restoring athletes' levels of physical conditioning and technical proficiency in preparation for the later stages. According to Taylor and Taylor (1997), this stage is significant, as it marks the end of rehabilitation and healing. It does so by marking the point at which athletes no longer see themselves as rehabilitating but rather as fully functioning athletes who are returning to training and competition.

The fourth stage is entitled high-intensity training (Taylor & Taylor, 1997). This stage is the final step in the return to full sport participation prior to a return to competition; it marks the complete conclusion of athletes' identification as injured or rehabilitating. At this point, athletes should perceive themselves as completely healed and capable of functioning at their pre-injury level. During this stage, athletes' physical conditioning and technical base are built upon in order to prime them for a return to a high level of competitive performance equal to or surpassing their pre-injury level. The aim at this stage is for the athlete to feel little anxiety about the health of the rehabilitated area or ability to perform at the desired level. The athlete should also be able to maintain a narrow focus on the final aspects of preparation before returning to competition and should have no awareness of, or preoccupation with, the former injured area.

The final phase and ultimate goal of rehabilitation is the return to competition. Entering the competitive arena may be both a source of excitement and anticipation as well as concern. After what might have been a lengthy rehabilitation, the athlete once again is able to demonstrate his or her skills and abilities in a public setting. At the same time, athletes may have some trepidation and anxiety over the fact that they cannot be certain that their return is truly successful until they demonstrate their skills in competition. As well, athletes may be putting themselves in the same situation in which the initial injury occurred. This may also be a cause of worry or concern. Taylor and Taylor (1997) suggested that a discussion with athletes at this time is beneficial in allowing them to express any concerns or fears and to redirect their focus onto the positive aspects of the competition.

A number of criticisms can be leveled against Taylor and Taylor's (1997) model:

- First, it is unclear where the first stage, the initial return, begins and ends or what the stage actually consists of. Taylor and Taylor do not specify what type of tests they are referring to in suggesting that the initial return provides athletes with a "series of tests" that the injured area is healed.
- Second, the model fails to account for individual differences with regard to athletes' ability to move from one stage to the next. That is, the model gives no

indication why some athletes progress through the stages at varying speeds and with varying degrees of success.

- Third, no empirical research exists to support the contention that the return-to-sport transition is best conceptualized in terms of the five-stage approach outlined by Taylor and Taylor. Although the model is prescriptive of the level of physical and psychological functioning that athletes should be at in particular points of their return to sport, it remains unclear if in fact they are. That is, the model seems to present the ideal return to sport versus the reality of what athletes may or may not experience.

- Fourth, the model assumes that athletes move in a linear fashion from the initial return to a return to competition. It may be, however, that various feedback mechanisms prevent an athlete from progressing in a sequential manner from Stage 1 to 5. For example, the athlete who does not receive recovery confirmation feedback (i.e., Stage 2) from the first stage may not progress onto the third stage. Unfortunately, no such contingencies are considered in the model.

Despite these criticisms, the return-to-sport model proposed by Taylor and Taylor (1997) is helpful insofar as it reminds practitioners, clinicians, and coaches that it may take athletes some time before they are able to compete to their full capabilities. Taylor and Taylor suggested that knowing the various stages of a return to sport will help make the arduous journey from rehabilitation to training and competition seem more achievable for athletes. It will also give athletes a greater sense of predictability and control over their return-to-sport transition.

An important implication of the biopsychosocial and the stages of return-to-sport models is that there may be myriad difficult "tests" facing athletes returning to sport following injury. Empirical research and clinically based evidence support this contention (e.g., Bianco, 2001; Gould, Udry, Bridges, & Beck, 1997; Kvist, Ek, Sporrstedt, & Good, 2005; Williams & Roepke, 1993). As Taylor, Stone, Mullin, Ellenbecker & Walgenbach (2003) suggest, for many athletes these tests may be inherently stressful. The nature of athlete stressors in returning to sport from injury can have an important impact on their psychological well-being and the quality of their return to sport. It is therefore important to understand the types of stressors that athletes experience in returning to sport as well as the most effective ways to assist them in dealing with these stressors. The next section of the chapter examines the psychosocial stressors associated with returning to sport from injury. The perspectives of athletes and coaches are considered. We then discuss the implications of these findings as well as some strategies for addressing athletes' return-to-sport stress sources.

Psychological Stressors Associated with Returning to Sport from Injury

Athlete Perceptions of the Stressors of Returning to Sport from Injury

According to Taylor et al. (2003) athletes returning to sport following injury can interpret their return in one of two ways—as a threat or as a challenge. Athletes who appraise their return to sport as threatening tend to avoid difficult aspects of the return to sport to avoid being considered a failure. Taylor et al. (2003) suggested that comments about not being ready to return, complaints of instability, unsubstantiated pain, and reduced adherence to rehabilitation typify this response. These individuals may exhibit low confidence, reluctance or resistance to return, stress, and a negative-outcome focus. Conversely, athletes who perceive their return to sport as a challenge look forward to their return with excitement and anticipation, exhibit high motivation to return, and display a process-oriented focus. Elite-level athletes in a recent longitudinal qualitative investigation also described their return to competition with a mixture of positive and negative appraisals and emotions (Podlog & Eklund, in press). Feelings of excitement and anticipation about being able to compete and experience the benefits of sport participation were described. Making a return to competition, however, was also perceived as threatening because there were so many "unknowns" about how things would unfold following the return to competition. These unknowns created a sense of anxiety and insecurity. The following comments typified the mixed emotions about returning to competition: "I'm excited because I haven't played for ages but I'm also a bit nervous because I'm going to be expected to perform" or:

Figure 3.

Athlete Perceptions of the Stressors of Returning to Sport from Injury.

Athlete Perceptions of the Stressors of Returning to Sport from Injury

Stress Sources Prior to a Return to Competition

- Return-to-Sport Appraisals
  - threat vs. challenge
- Pre-competition stressors:
  - anxiety about "unknowns" i.e.,
    - fear of re-injury
    - reaching pre-injury levels and achieving goals
    - self-presentational concerns
      - performance expectations
      - letting down teammates/coach
      - upholding one's reputation

From Podlog & Eklund (in press) A longitudinal investigation of competitive athletes' return to sport following serious injury, *Journal of Applied Sport Psychology*.

Stresss Sources Following a Return to Competition

- Adapting to increased intensity of competition:
  - increased fatigue from competition
  - physical abuse from competition
  - regaining match fitness
  - increased performance anxiety
  - difficulties with competition focus
- Injury flareups/injury to another body part:
  - frustration over:
    - uncertainty/
    - lack of control over one's body
    - training/competing with pain
- Not making/getting dropped from teams:
  - frustration over "falling behind others"
- Reduced confidence:
  - doubts the ability to achieve one's goals

> I'm excited that it's finally here, that I can start playing again. It's just all the
> things that I miss I get to do once again so I can't wait for it. But I know that
> it's not going to be the same as if I didn't have the injury because I might
> be….I won't be scared but I've got to wait and see. I can't wait for it.

Researchers have found that feelings of threat or trepidation regarding an upcoming
return to competitive sport are often based on several prominent concerns. The next
section of the paper discusses athlete stressors at the end of rehabilitation, prior to a
return to competition.

Stress sources prior to a return to competition. One of the most common sources of
stress identified in the literature among returning athletes is a fear of re-injury (Bianco,
Malo, & Orlick, 1999; Cox, 2002; Kvist et al. 2005). Podlog and Eklund (in press) also
found that re-injury concerns were conspicuous in their interviews with high-performance athletes. Discussing her fear of re-injury, a high-jumper commented:

> I'm a little bit nervous actually. I've been out a year and I don't think the
> nerves are about other people. I think my nerves are more about making sure
> the knee doesn't blow up now that I've gotten this far. Competition puts a lot
> more stress on the knee than training does. I think most of the nerves come
> from not knowing whether the knee's going to hold together.

Athletes with re-injury fears indicated that overcoming this fear would be important
in order for them to achieve their goals. Thus, re-injury was a concern for many of the
participants because they wanted to avoid any setbacks in pursuit of their aspirations.
Re-injury concerns were also prominent because athletes felt they had invested so
much time, energy, and effort into their recovery and did not want their efforts "all to
be for nothing." Athletes without any previous injury experience appeared to have
heightened re-injury fears. These athletes commented that they had no way of knowing how their bodies would respond to the return because they had never had the experience of successfully returning to competition.

Fears of re-injury also appeared more predominant for participants whose injuries
had a chronic component (e.g., knee "flare-ups") (Podlog & Eklund, in press). For
participants who had experienced recurring problems, their fears were understandably
greater than those who were confident that their acute injury had sufficiently healed to
warrant a return. As one rower stated:

> I [have a fear of re-injury] mainly because I had a few recurrences and I hurt
> it a few times. So when I'm training now I'm always thinking about it and if it
> feels uncomfortable I think maybe something is going to happen. I've spoken
> to the physio and he said you just need to relax and be confident that if you're
> doing the rehabilitation then it will be all right. I'm a bit hesitant when I do
> some exercises now, especially if we have do high-intensity stuff, which I
> haven't done much of since I've been injured.

Concerns over reaching pre-injury levels have also been identified as a salient concern
among athletes returning to sport from injury (Bianco, 2001; Rotella, 1985; Williams
& Roepke, 1993). Similarly, athletes in Podlog and Eklund's (in press) investigation
indicated that the ability to achieve short- and long-term goals was a prominent concern. This concern was suggested to be "only natural" after being out of sport for such

a long time. For some athletes, apprehensions about achieving personal goals were related more to the time away from sport than to the injury itself. Having a long break created a sense of uncertainty about achieving one's goals given that others had improved during the time away. A field hockey player's comment was typical:

> If I don't perform that would be a fear because there are always selectors and national coaches watching and I want to make the next team. I don't want to be dropped out of the system. With the time that I've had off, everyone else has improved and I've missed out on a whole lot of training and stuff.

Concerns about accomplishing goals were also common because in some cases, athletes were worried about the effect the injury would have on their ability to train properly or to continue their sport participation (Podlog & Eklund, under review). One rower, for example, described how his chronic back pain might prevent him from continuing to row:

> I went through a period of about a month just after I did the injury where I had no improvement and I couldn't sit down. Everywhere I went I had to lie down or stand up. I had a lot of trouble driving a car and even walking and lifting my knee up was hurting. At that point, I was contemplating whether it was worth continuing. I've still got a fear that if I keep pushing and pushing for years, it might affect me later on. I'll do everything I can to row this year but if my back's a big problem then I might think about not rowing again after the Olympics.

An issue that has not received a lot of attention in the literature is that of self-presentational fears regarding the outcome of the return to competition. Athletes in Podlog and Eklund's (in press) investigation indicated that a fear of not meeting others' performance expectations, letting down teammates or the coach, and concerns over upholding one's reputation were conspicuous. Self-presentational concerns appeared more pronounced for athletes cognizant of coaches', fans', and teammates' interest in their upcoming performances. Prolonged absences from sport participation (often for the first time) typically led to uncertainty about how one would perform and whether such performances would meet the expectations of others. A swimmer commented:

> Obviously, I'm going to be worried whether I'm going to make a fool of myself but I'm pretty sure that will be all right... The other people have been training while you've had time off so you could make a fool of yourself if you're not going as fast as them. Not make a fool of myself, maybe I phrased that a bit wrong. It's more of a concern about making your reputation go down a bit if you're not swimming as fast. It's not for other people, it's for yourself because you want to keep your reputation up and keep positive thoughts.

Stress sources following a return to competition. Another issue that has not received a lot of empirical attention is that of athlete stressors following a return to competition after injury. Bianco (2001) reported that skiers who had unrealistically high performance expectations for their return, and who failed to achieve these goals, experienced drops in confidence. Unrealistic expectations were more common among those who "naively" believed that because they had worked so hard to recover and were disciplined in rehabilitation they would immediately perform well. Athletes in

Podlog and Eklund's (in press) investigation also discussed a number of stressors following their return to competition:

- adapting to the increased intensity of competition
- difficulties with injury flare-ups or injury to another body part
- missing out on team selection
- reduced confidence

It was suggested that moving from training to competition placed increased physical and psychological demands on participants that were believed to be greater than normal due to their competitive absence. For some athletes, the increased level of physical fatigue brought on by competition was difficult, particularly the first few competitions. As a rower described it:

> It's difficult going from just doing a lot of steady training, not pushing really hard, and just being cautious to going back into a full program where 90% of it is pretty intense, a lot of racing. It was harder the first few weeks but it's slowly getting back to normal. I'm getting used to being tired again all the time, which is good. It's something you have to deal with.

Difficulties associated with the physical abuse and punishment of returning to competition after a significant lay-off were reported among a few contact sport athletes. An Australian Rules football player, for example, suggested that after 12 months away from the game, his body was simply not used to the "rough and tumble" that took place on the football field. Regaining "match fitness" was also a concern for some participants, especially within the first couple of months of the return. A field hockey player indicated that the fitness aspect of his game was never his forte. His lack of fitness was even more apparent upon his initial return to competition:

> At the start it was really difficult because as much as I was on the bikes and in the gym and running, getting back into it was the hardest part. You can never get that match fitness until you actually start playing. After being out for about 5 months it's really difficult, especially because there was a lot of wind down when I was in hospital. I had five operations and I was lying down a lot and I put on quite a bit of weight. It was really difficult physically for me when I initially came back. Slowly I got better but again I was never at the point where I was before the injury. I guess it's only now that I'm really getting my body into good physical shape.

A lack of game fitness had a detrimental effect on athletes' ability to exert themselves over the course of the entire game, their reaction time, and their ability to "read the play." According to the field hockey player, these difficulties were much more apparent after returning from injury because he had never been away from training and competition for such an extended period (i.e., 5 months).

Athletes also reported psychological obstacles associated with the increased intensity of competition and/or game situations (Podlog & Eklund, in press). In particular, increased performance anxiety and difficulties remaining focused were articulated. Just over 2 months into the competitive season, a netball player commented, "I'm a lot more nervous before games because I still feel like I haven't played for ages….I think it's more the mental side of netball that I've got to get used to playing again, not so much the physical." Staying focused during the games was difficult for the netballer because of the increased pace and tenacity of the players on the floor.

The occurrence of injury flare-ups or injury to another body part was another salient form of adversity mentioned by participants. A rower, for example, expressed disappointment and frustration over a new back injury he acquired before he even had a chance to compete. Not knowing if (or when) the bulging disc in his back would settle down was disconcerting and frustrating. Moreover, having the doctor tell him to take three weeks off on three separate occasions meant that his hopes of returning were continually raised and dashed. For this particular athlete, not having control over his situation was difficult:

> I'm the kind of person that likes to be in control of my surroundings and be able to see into the future. But with this injury, I haven't been able to do that....I like to plan ahead and set goals to achieve things and I can't do that. Even if I say okay I'll go down and row 4 kilometers this morning and then I'll start rowing 8 kilometers each morning, I can't do that. If I go down and row 4 kilometers and my back feels so sore I can hardly straighten it, then all the goals that I'd just set become useless and get thrown away.

Not making or being dropped from particular teams was another stressor described by athletes. A soccer player commented on his frustrations in seeing others progress into the first division team while he remained on the reserve squad. Before his injury the athlete felt he was "moving up in the ranks"; however, after being out for so long, he felt had fallen behind others:

> It's just hard seeing people that I know that I'm better than being able to play there. You look at others and you think you should be there but you can't do anything because you're still coming back. Even still, you want to be there because you know you're good enough. It's just a matter of putting in a few good performances and the coaching staff will see that.

Stressors such as fitness concerns, increased performance anxiety, injury flare-ups, not making or being dropped from teams, and performance declines were often reported to have a negative effect on athletes' confidence (Podlog & Eklund, in press). Evans, Hardy, and Flemming (2000) and Johnston and Carroll (1998) also found that difficulties such as performance declines resulted in a diminished sense of confidence for athletes following their return to sport from injury. While several participants in Podlog and Eklund's investigation were surprised at how quickly they were able to compete at a high level, the majority struggled with various physical and/or psychological obstacles. A field hockey player, for example, related some of his self-doubt and lack of confidence during the first few months following his return from injury:

> Mentally, at the beginning, it was pretty difficult. I always felt that having gone through this, I could do anything else, like why can't I play for Australia? But as much as you can think that, you start to have these doubts. Can I play as well as I played before my injury and how long will that take? Can I take the next step? Can I get to the next level? As much as you say to yourself you've been through a [hand] injury, you're going to be mentally tough and push

yourself more, you always seem to question yourself and wonder is it holding you back? And could you have been better if it hadn't happened?

Coach Perceptions of the Stressors of Returning to Sport from Injury

A second qualitative investigation by Podlog & Eklund (under review) has revealed that coaches' perceptions of the stressors of returning to sport largely parallel those discussed by athletes. In this qualitative investigation professional coaches articulated a variety of physical, social, and performance-related stressors among returning athletes (See Figure 4). Although coaches suggested that individual differences were apparent to the extent to which athletes' experienced these stressors, it was noted that athletes often experienced stressors in at least one of these areas.

Common physical stressors included

- a fear of re-injury,
- fitness concerns, and
- the effect of physical limitations on the athlete's ability to perform (Podlog & Eklund, under review).

These findings replicate those in the extant literature on athlete fears of re-injury (Andersen, 2001; Kvist et al. 2005), concerns over physical fitness (Taylor & Taylor, 1997; Tracey, 2003), and difficulties making technical adjustments as a result of the injury (Gould et al., 1997). Coaches reported believing that the fear of re-injury was

Figure 4.

Coach perceptions of the stressors of returning to sport from injury.

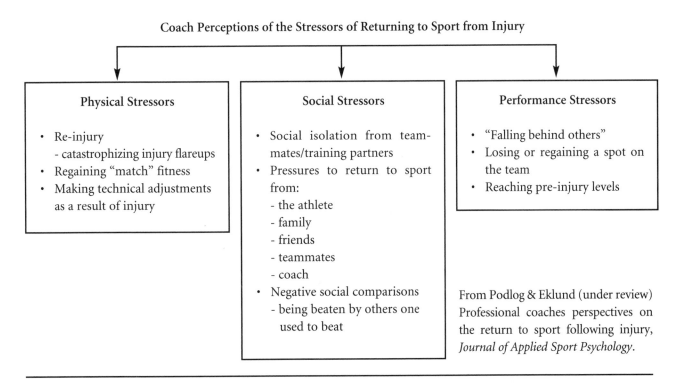

Coach Perceptions of the Stressors of Returning to Sport from Injury

Physical Stressors

- Re-injury
  - catastrophizing injury flareups
- Regaining "match" fitness
- Making technical adjustments as a result of injury

Social Stressors

- Social isolation from teammates/training partners
- Pressures to return to sport from:
  - the athlete
  - family
  - friends
  - teammates
  - coach
- Negative social comparisons
  - being beaten by others one used to beat

Performance Stressors

- "Falling behind others"
- Losing or regaining a spot on the team
- Reaching pre-injury levels

From Podlog & Eklund (under review) Professional coaches perspectives on the return to sport following injury, *Journal of Applied Sport Psychology.*

one of the most salient issues for returning athletes. As one of the rowing coaches commented:

> They may not be 100% sure their [rehabilitated body part] is going to hold up. Competition pressure is very different from training pressure so if they get to competition sometimes they doubt that their body can actually make it through this without breaking down.

In contrast to these findings, athletes in Tracey's (2003) investigation did not report experiencing fears of re-injury. According to Tracey (2003), these fears may not yet have become salient because some participants were still a long way from their return to sport at the time of their final interview. It is also possible that athletes in Tracey's investigation did not report fears of re-injury since some of the participants experienced only moderately severe injuries (e.g., a sprained ankle, a strained back). Regardless, it seems likely that different types of stressors may be more or less significant depending upon the stage of injury recovery and/or return to sport. This assumption, however, requires greater attention in future research.

Coaches suggested that it was not uncommon for athletes to catastrophize minor injury "flare-ups" once they resumed training and competition given their preoccupation with re-injury (Podlog & Eklund, under review). As one coach remarked:

> It's not always a smooth transition from rehab into the program and sometimes it's a couple of steps forward and a couple back and that is probably the hardest time for them. They think that it's all okay. They come back in and a little niggle comes up and they wonder, "Is it just what I've had before, do I have to stop, what's happening?" The hardest time for them is if something doesn't go right, how bad is it and what can I do now? Can I do normal training? The transition back into training and competition is very emotionally tough for them.

Difficulties associated with regaining competitive (i.e., "match") fitness was also raised as a salient stressor among returning athletes (Podlog & Eklund, under review). Coaches reported feeling that athletes were often worried about their fitness levels because the fitness requirements for effective competitive play were higher than in training, a finding echoed in Tracey's (2003) investigation with injured athletes.

Finally, adjusting technical aspects of one's play because of injury restrictions and/or limitations was perceived to be another potential stressor for returning athletes (Podlog & Eklund, under review). A squash coach described how one of his players had to alter the mechanics of his swing because of his injury. Not being able to swing the same way that he had done for years previously was believed to be difficult and frustrating for the athlete under discussion. Similarly, US national team skiers commented on the stress they experienced in adjusting to the physical changes brought about as a result of their surgeries (Gould et al., 1997). One skier discussed her frustrations over not having the same amount of feeling or proprioception in her leg upon first returning to skiing after knee surgery. Another skier commented that after returning to skiing, she had to adjust the alignment of her legs to accommodate her post-injury knee brace. The skier suggested that because this type of adjustment was not normal for her, seeing videos of her post-injury performances "was hard, it was really hard" (Gould et al., 1997, p. 371).

Coaches' discussions of the social stressors associated with returning to sport were also generally consistent with previous research examining return to sport issues following injury (Bianco, 2001; Curry, 1993; Gould et al., 1997; Nixon, 1992; Young, White, & Mcteer, 1994). In particular, discussion about

- social isolation from teammates and training partners,
- pressures to return quickly, and
- negative comparisons

emerged from coach interviews. Feelings of social isolation were believed to be common both during injury rehabilitation and upon the return to sport, a finding also reported in several investigations examining athlete stressors during the rehabilitation period (Bianco, 2001; Gould et al., 1997; Johnston & Carroll, 1998). Because athletes (especially those in interactive team sports) were often working on an individual basis with coaches during the return to sport, coaches reported believing that feelings of isolation and separation from the team lingered during this time (Podlog & Eklund, under review). Several interactive team sport coaches commented that athletes often did not seem to feel like full team members unless they were training with the team and helping them achieve their goals.

Pressure to return quickly was another social stressor discussed by coaches (Podlog & Eklund, under review). It was felt that these pressures emanated from a variety of sources including the athletes themselves, family and friends, teammates, and the coach. Several coaches recognized that they could inadvertently place pressures on the athlete to return because they were "only human" and wanted to see the athlete compete once again. Although a conscious effort was made not to rush athletes into returning, coaches indicated that ultimately they too wanted to see the athlete accomplish particular goals.

Ensuring that the athlete was not coming back because they were made to feel guilty or because they felt pressured to return was considered important by the coaches. According to a gymnastics coach:

> We try not to bully them into feeling they should be doing it to please the coach because there can be an aspect of that if you're not careful. You can bully an athlete into doing things going: "Oh, my foot's really sore." "Is it? Okay. Well, I suppose we won't be ready for nationals, but okay don't do anything then."—as opposed to: "My foot's really sore." "Okay. Well, what do you feel you can handle? Do you feel you can do a few of these?" "No, not really." "Well, leave that for today. We'll try it tomorrow." That's a very different approach to making the athlete feel guilty if they've come to you and said, "I can't do it," and you go, "That's fine," or you make some snide or underhand remark, and that's very easy to do.

The gymnastics coach emphasized the importance of keeping the "locus of control with athletes" by teaching them to make good judgments about what they were capable of doing. It was recognized that pressuring an athlete to return was only doing a disservice to the athlete because performances were likely to suffer, the chances of re-injury were increased, and the athlete was likely to suffer reduced confidence. Coaches also indicated that pressuring an athlete to return could be counterproductive, as athletes might question whether the coach had their best interests in mind. These results support previous research examining the negative consequences regarding pressures to return to sport following injury (Bianco, 2001; Curry, 1993; Frey, 1991; Messner, 1992; Nixon, 1992; Young, White, & Mcteer, 1994). For example, Canadian national team skiers reported returning to competition because they felt pressure to prove themselves to the coaches and they wanted to avoid losing a spot on the team (Bianco, 2001). All of the rookie team members in Bianco's purposive sample suffered further injuries that they attributed to their premature returns. The skiers commented that much of the pressure they experienced to return could be alleviated if there were no performance expectations placed on them by the coach or specific return deadlines.

Negative social comparisons were perceived to be another stressor for returning athletes (Podlog & Eklund, under review). Coaches suggested that athletes were often either unprepared or had difficulties accepting the fact that their skills may have diminished while others had improved during their competitive absence. It was reported that for many athletes, this reality did not completely set in until they resumed their training and competing and were beaten by others they used to beat. This experience was believed to be very frustrating for returning athletes. One of the rowing coaches remarked:

> Most of them think they're going to be back at the level they stopped pre-injury. It's a big shock to them that they come back and other people who've had 6 to 12 months more training have moved forward one or two steps and the injured athlete is probably one or two steps below where they were. So the gap has increased and someone they were beating easily before is now beating them easily. Sometimes that's a bit of a shock to them.

Gould et al. (1997) also found that injured athletes identified social comparisons as a source of stress upon returning to competitive skiing. One returning athlete indicated that it was hard to "lose to people I used to beat," and another stated frustration over "being beat by people I used to beat" (Gould et al., 1997, p.368).

Finally, coaches articulated performance concerns and difficulties among returning athletes (Podlog & Eklund, under review). In particular, concerns about "falling behind others," losing or regaining a spot on the team, and reaching pre-injury levels were suggested to be common performance stressors among returning athletes. Coaches also indicated that athletes often had unrealistic expectations regarding their ability to remain competitive with former opponents and to return to pre-injury levels. It was reported that unrealistic expectations could result in a "vicious circle" of frustration, poorer performances, and reduced confidence. Their comments on this account are consistent with athlete descriptions of stressors encountered in returning to sport in the extant literature (e.g., Bianco, 2001; Evans et al., Johnston & Carroll, 1998; Rotella, 1985; Tracey, 2003; Williams & Roepke, 1993).

Implications of Athlete Stressors in Returning to Sport

Coach and athlete discussions of the stressors of returning to sport have important implications for the management of this transition phase. Examination of the afore-mentioned findings indicates that returning athletes may commonly experience stressors relating to three psychosocial areas:

- competence
- autonomy
- relatedness

The finding that returning athletes have re-injury fears and concerns about how their body will adapt to the increased demands and intensity of competition (Bianco, et al., 1999; Gould et al., 1997) suggests that issues of physical competency may be significant. Athletes may also experience competency-related concerns about reaching pre-injury levels, achieving future goals and the ability to fulfill personal or external expectations (e.g., Bianco, 2001; Feltz, 1986; Gould et al., 1997; Johnston & Carroll, 1998; Taylor & Taylor, 1997; Williams & Roepke, 1993). Athletes discussed concerns such as a fear of not meeting other's performance expectations, letting down team-mates or the coach, and concerns over upholding their reputation. Although such concerns were self-presentational in nature they were implicitly related to participants' need to appear competent. That is, all of the self-presentational concerns mentioned above were in some capacity related to participants' need to create a desired impression of "athletic competency" in the minds of others. Finally, recognition that athletes may suffer decreases in confidence and performance following injury indicates that competency concerns may be significant when athletes resume their sport participation (Evans et al., 2000; Johnston & Carroll, 1998).

Knowledge that athletes may receive (and often internalize) external pressures to return to sport from injury (e.g., Curry, 1993; Frey, 1991; Messner, 1992; Nixon, 1992) suggests that one's level of autonomy in returning to sport may play an important role in the outcome of that return. Support for this contention was received in studies by Bianco (2001) and Gould et al. (1997). In both investigations, athletes who reported pressures to return to sport (i.e., those less autonomous) also indicated less favorable return-to-sport outcomes (i.e., re-injury, performance decrements, reduced confidence). Similarly, Podlog and Eklund (under review) revealed that coaches were aware of the importance of not putting pressure on athletes to return to sport before they were physically and psychologically ready. It was indicated that doing so could result in negative psychological consequences and return-to-sport outcomes.

Finally, recognition that injured athletes may often feel a sense of alienation and social isolation from their friends, teammates, and fellow competitors suggests that the need for relatedness (i.e. connectedness) may be significant among returning athletes (e.g., Ermler & Thomas, 1990; Gould et al., 1997a; Thomas & Rintala, 1989). A good deal of research indicates that social support and assistance from a variety of sources (e.g., coaches and rehabilitation specialists) may act as prophylaxis against the isolation and alienation commonly associated with injury recovery and rehabilitation (e.g, Bianco & Eklund, 2001; Andersen, 2001).

Self-Determination Theory

As we have argued previously (Podlog & Eklund, 2004; 2005), self-determination theory (SDT) may be valuable for understanding injury recovery and return to sport processes as the theory deals explicitly with notions of competence, autonomy, and relatedness. Ryan and Deci (2000) propose that environments that satisfy people's basic needs for competence, autonomy, and relatedness are likely to result in enhanced psychological and social well-being. Conversely, in environments that fail to meet these needs or that thwart their satisfaction, individuals may display non-optimal functioning, for example, apathy, alienation, and lethargy. Self-determination-grounded research indicates that environments supportive of individuals' psychological needs yield beneficial consequences for social development, health, well-being, and human performance (e.g., Frederick & Ryan, 1993; Grolnick, Deci & Ryan, 1997; Miserando, 1996). In education, for example, researchers have found that autonomy-supportive (as opposed to controlling) teachers foster greater intrinsic motivation, curiosity, and desire for challenge in their students (e.g., Flink, Boggiano, & Barrett, 1990). Similarly, supports for autonomy and competence by parents and sport mentors have been found to stimulate intrinsic motivation in kids and sport participants (e.g., Grolnick, Deci & Ryan, 1997; Frederick & Ryan, 1995). More research is needed to validate these findings in a sport injury context; nonetheless, the notion that environments supportive of injured athletes' needs for competence, autonomy, and relatedness may yield enhanced physical and psychological recovery and return-to-sport outcomes holds strong intuitive appeal.

Strategies for Addressing Athletes' Return-to-Sport Stress Sources

Given that: (a) athletes may commonly experience competence, autonomy, and relatedness type stressors, and that (b) self-determination research supports the benefits of enhanced competence, autonomy, and relatedness, it may be useful to structure programs in ways that meet these three basic needs. Based on this assumption, the following suggestions are offered to coaches and practitioners as a guideline for meeting both the physical and psychological needs of returning athletes.

Address Issues of Competence

Help establish realistic expectations. Having discussions with athletes about what they hope to achieve and how they expect to perform following their return may be useful for revealing unrealistic goals and expectations. Recognizing that making a return to sport is a gradual process may help athletes avoid creating overly high expectations that in turn lead to frustration, decreased confidence, and negative social comparisons. Expecting "too much too soon" (which is not uncommon among elite athletes) may often lead to a sense of frustration, reduced confidence, and ultimately poorer performances (Bianco, 2001; Podlog & Eklund, under review). Encouraging athletes to create realistic expectations upon returning to sport is important.

Develop short-term process goals. Encouraging athletes to focus on short-term process (i.e., task-oriented) goals upon their initial resumption of sport-related training may be a useful way to help them build competence in their physical and mental capabilities. Providing them with as many opportunities as possible to experience success may assist them in avoiding a sense of frustration and decreased confidence should they struggle to immediately return to pre-injury form (Gilbourne & Taylor, 1998).

Assist athletes in overcoming return-to-sport fears and building confidence. The two most common fears associated with a return to sport appear to be a fear of re-injury and concern over not performing to pre-injury levels. Providing athletes with progressive physical challenges that they can successfully meet without physical pain can enhance their sense of competency regarding their capabilities and their bodies' ability to remain uninjured (Cox, 2002). Reassuring athletes that they have met all the physical requirements necessary for their return may help alleviate concerns about re-injury and performance issues. Finally, discussion of return-to-sport fears or concerns can provide an opportunity to dispel irrational beliefs and to "get out in the open" any issues the athlete might have (Cox, 2002; Taylor et al., 2003).

Provide athlete role models. Putting returning athletes in contact with other athletes who have experienced and overcome similar injuries may be highly beneficial for the returning athletes' level of confidence. Having models who have come back from a similar injury may give athletes returning from injury a sense that if others can do it, so can they (i.e., "seeing helps believing") (Flint, 1993).

Address Issues of Autonomy

Discuss motivations to return to sport. Having a discussion with athletes prior to their return to training and competition about why they are returning may help the practitioner establish which athletes are returning for the "wrong" reasons (e.g., pressure from a coach or teammate; guilt about missing an important competition the athlete does not feel prepared to compete in). Previous research by Podlog and Eklund (2005) revealed that an athlete whose motivation to return to sport was more self-determined (e.g., the love of the sport) appeared to have ameliorated psychological outcomes in returning (i.e., a renewed perspective on sport) than an athlete whose motivations were less self-determined (e.g., returning in order to demonstrate one's skills to others).

Help ensure the autonomy of the returning athlete. Given that athletes may be susceptible to receiving pressure to return to sport (and that they typically want "freedom from pressure"), coaches and medical practitioners need to ensure that athletes have the freedom to return at a time and manner of their own choosing (Bianco, 2001). Thus coaches need to be aware of any personal tendencies toward pressuring the athlete or creating feelings of guilt during his or her return. Additionally, physiotherapists, athletic trainers, or medical practitioners may be ideally positioned to act as mediators between athletes and those encouraging them to return possibly before they are physically or psychologically prepared to do so. Having the time to recover from their injury and slowly progress will not only meet the autonomy needs of returning athletes, but will provide them with a sense of confidence that they are healed and ready to perform at a high level. Taylor and Taylor's (1997) Stages of Return to Sport model may serve as a useful reminder of the various stages in which athletes *should* progress en route to a successful, healthy, and satisfying return to sport from injury.

Address Issues of Relatedness

Keep athletes involved in sport. Staying involved with the team during the injury rehabilitation may help team sport athletes as they make the transition from injury to training and competition. Injured athletes often miss the social aspect of their sport participation. Staying in contact with the team can provide athletes with a sense of connectedness and provide them with the opportunity to observe, learn, and analyze their sport from the sidelines (Ermler & Thomas, 1990). Research by Tracey (2003) as well as our recent research with coaches, however, indicates that coaches and others may need to be cautious about attempts to keep athletes involved in sport. Injured athletes have suggested that attending practice may provoke concerns about fitness loss, remind athletes of their participation restrictions, and reinforce beliefs about letting down their team simply by watching (Tracey, 2003). Ensuring that athletes are given meaningful interaction opportunities (e.g., participating in team activities where they can be physically active, such as weight training) may help mitigate feelings of frustration over not being able to participate, not contributing to the team, or not having a particular team role/function. Additionally, recognizing that individual differences may be apparent in terms of the extent to which athletes want to be involved with their teammates (specifically in terms of practice attendance) and the degree to which such involvement is psychologically beneficial may be important.

Hold individual training sessions with athletes. Taking the extra time to work on a one-to-one basis with athletes making the transition back into sport can help to remind athletes that coaches are concerned about their well-being. Not only can this have the potential to meet athletes' needs for connectedness, but it can provide coaches with opportunities to monitor athlete activities, introduce skills gradually, assess athletes' physical conditioning, and give athletes skill-related feedback.

Provide athletes with social support. Providing athletes with various types of social support can also be highly beneficial in meeting their relatedness needs. A good deal of empirical research has found support for the notion that social support among athletes recovering from injury may lead to enhanced psychological functioning and ameliorated recovery outcomes (e.g., see Bianco & Eklund, 2001 for a review). Canadian national team skiers reported that support from coaches was important in holding them back, helping them set realistic performance expectations, building confidence, and recognizing improvements (Bianco, 2001). Providing athletes with emotional support by taking a personal interest in them and providing positive encouragement can go a long way to meeting their needs for connectedness. Similarly, providing athletes with tangible (e.g., assistance with goal setting) and informational support (e.g., video analysis) can send the implicit message that coaches are willing to facilitate athletes' return to sport from injury.

Summary

In this chapter we have addressed some of the key psychosocial considerations among athletes returning to sport from injury. After considering two models that have been used to describe the return to sport transition, we examined some of the psychosocial stressors associated with the return to sport, taking into account the perspectives of athletes and coaches. That elite-level, full-time coaches reported similar stressors as athletes suggests that the former appear to possess a good understanding of the stressors associated with the return-to-sport transition. Examination of athlete and coach perceptions of the stressors of returning to sport revealed that issues of competence, autonomy, and relatedness were prominent. Targeting strategies in ways that address these three general psychological areas may be of great utility in maximizing the quality and nature of athletes' return to sport following injury. Given their understanding of return-to-sport stressors as well as their close contact with athletes, coaches may be ideally positioned to assist the latter in making a complete physical and psychological recovery and return from injury.

References

Andersen. M. B. (2001). Returning to action and the prevention of future injury. In J. Crossman (Ed.), *Coping with Sports Injuries: Psychological Strategies for Rehabilitation* (pp.162-173). Melbourne: Oxford University Press.

Bianco, T. (2001). Social support and recovery from sport injury: Elite skiers share their experiences. *Research Quarterly for Exercise and Sport, 72,* 376-388.

Bianco, T., & Eklund, R. C. (2001). Conceptual considerations for social support research in sport and exercise settings: The instance of sport injury. *Journal of Sport & Exercise Psychology, 2,* 85-107.

Bianco, T., Malo, S., & Orlick., T. (1999). Sport injury and illness: Elite skiers describe their experiences. *Research Quarterly for Exercise and Sport, 70,* 157-169.

Brewer, B.W. (2001). Emotional adjustment to sport injury. In J. Crossman (Ed.), *Coping with Sport Injuries: Psychological Strategies for Rehabilitation* (pp.1-19). Melbourne: Oxford University Press.

Brewer, B. W., Andersen, M. B., & Van Raalte, J. L., (2002). Psychological aspects of sport injury rehabilitation: Toward a biopsychosocial approach. In D. Mostofsky & L. Zaichkowsky (Eds.), *Medical Aspects of Sport and Exercise* (pp. 41-54). Morgantown, WV: Fitness Information Technology.

Cox, R. (2002). The psychological rehabilitation of a severely injured rugby player. In. I Cockerill (Ed.), *Solutions in Sport Psychology* (pp. 159-172). London: Thomson.

Curry, T. (1993). A little pain never hurt anyone: Athletic career socialization and the normalization of sports injury. *Symbolic Interaction, 16,* 273-290.

Ermler, K. L., & Thomas, C. E. (1990). Interventions for the alienating effect of injury. *Athletic Training, 25,* 269-271.

Evans, L., Hardy, L., & Fleming, S. (2000). Intervention strategies with injured athletes: An action research study. *The Sport Psychologist, 14,* 186-206.

Feltz, D. L. (1986). The psychology of sports injuries. In P. E. Vinger, & E. F. Hoerner (Eds.), *Sports Injuries: The Unthwarted Epidemic* (2nd ed., pp.336-344). Boston, Massachusetts: John Wright.

Flink, C., Boggiano, A. K., & Barrett, M. (1990). Controlling teaching strategies: Undermining children's self-determination and performance. *Journal of Personality and Social Psychology, 59,* 916-924.

Flint, F (1993). Seeing helps believing: Modeling in injury rehabilitation. In D. Pargman (Ed). *Psychological Bases of Sport Injuries* (pp. 183-198). Morgantown, WV: Fitness Information Technology.

Frederick, C. M., & Ryan, R. M. (1993). Differences in motivation for sport and exercise and their relations with participation and mental health. *Journal of Sport Behavior, 16,* 124-146.

Frederick, C. M., & Ryan, R. M. (1995). Self-determination in sport: A review using cognitive evaluation theory. *International Journal of Sport Psychology, 26,* 5-23.

Frey, J. H. (1991). Social risk and the meaning of sport. *Sociology of Sport Journal, 8,* 136-145.

Gilbourne, D., & Taylor, A. H. (1998). From theory to practice: The integration of goal perspective theory and life development approaches within an injury-specific goal-setting program. *Journal of Applied Sport Psychology, 10,* 124-139.

Gould, D., Udry, E., Bridges, D., Beck, L. (1997). Stress sources encountered when rehabilitating from season-ending ski injuries. *The Sport Psychologist, 11,* 361-378.

Grolnick, W. A., Deci, E. L., & Ryan, R. M. (1997). Internalization within the family. In J.E. Grusec & L. Kuczynski (Eds.), *Parenting and children's internatlization of values: A handbook of contemporary theory* (pp. 135-161). New York: Wiley.

Johnston, L. H., & Carroll, D. (1998). The provision of social support to injured athletes: A qualitative analysis. *Journal of Sport Rehabilitation, 7,* 267-284.

Kvist, J., Ek, A., Sporrstedt, K., & Good, L. (2005). Fear of re-injury: a hindrance for returning to sports after anterior cruciate ligament reconstruction. *Knee Surgery, Sports Traumatology, Arthroscopy, 13,* 393-397.

Messner, M. (1992). *Power at Play: Sports and the Problem of Masculinity.* Boston: Beach Press.

Miserando, M. (1996). Children who do well in school: Individual differences in perceived competence and autonomy in above-average children. *Journal of Educational Psychology, 88,* 203-214.

Nixon, H. L. (1992). A social network analysis of influences on athletes to play with pain and injuries. *Journal of Sport and Social Issues, 16,* 127-135.

Podlog, L., & Eklund, R. C. (2004). Assisting injured athletes with the return to sport transition. *Clinical Journal of Sport Medicine, 14,* 257-259.

Podlog, L., & Eklund, R. C. (2005). Return to sport after serious injury: A retrospective examination of motivation and outcomes. *Journal of Sport Rehabilitation, 14,* 20-34.

Podlog, L., & Eklund, R. C. (in press). A longitudinal investigation of competitive athletes' return to sport following serious injury. *Journal of Applied Sport Psychology.*

Podlog, L., & Eklund, R. C. (under review). Professional coaches' perspectives on the return to sport following serious injury. *Journal of Applied Sport Psychology.*

Rotella, R. J. (1985). The psychological care of the injured athlete. In L. Bunker, R. J. Rotella, & A. S. Reilly (Eds.), *Sport psychology: Psychological Considerations in Maximizing Sport Performance* (pp. 273-287). Ithaca, N.Y.: Mouvement.

Ryan, R., & Deci, E. L. (2000). Self-Determination Theory and the facilitation of Intrinsic motivation, social development and well-being. *American Psychologist, 55,* 68-78.

Taylor, J., Stone, K. R., Mullin, M. J., Ellenbecker, T., & Walgenbach, A. (2003). *Comprehensive Sports Injury Management: From Examination of Injury to Return to Sport.* Austin, Texas: Pro-ed.

Taylor, J., & Taylor, S. (1997). *Psychological Approaches to Sports Injury Rehabilitation.* Gaithersburg, MD: Aspen.

Thomas, C., & Rintala, J. (1989). Injury as alienation in sport. *Journal of the Philosophy of Sport, 16,* 44-58.

Tracey, J. (2003). The emotional response to the injury and rehabilitation process. *Journal of Applied Sport Psychology, 15,* 279-293.

Williams, J. M., & Roepke, N. (1993). Psychology of injury and injury rehabilitation. In R. N. Singer, M. Murphy, & K. Tennant (Eds.), *Handbook of Research on Sport Psychology (pp.815-839).* New York: MacMillan.

Young, K., White, P., & McTeer, W. (1994). Body talk: Male athletes reflect on sport, injury, and pain. *Sociology of Sport Journal, 11,* 175-194.

Chapter Eight

The Use of Imagery in the Rehabilitation of Injured Athletes

Lance B. Green
Tulane University

Kimberlee Bethany Bonura
Florida State University

The purpose of this chapter is to provide an educational text that
(a) cites existing literature supporting a mind-body paradigm for rehabilitation from psychophysiological and psychomotor perspectives,
(b) demonstrates the application of imagery techniques within the chronology of an athletic injury, and
(c) describes the performance-related criteria to which an athlete can compare his or her progress during rehabilitation.

The chronology includes the period of time preceding the injury, the attention given to the athlete immediately following the injury, and the subsequent rehabilitation program leading to the return of the athlete to practice and competition. Examples of imagery experientials are used to illustrate application of imagery throughout the chronology.

Introducion

A study conducted by Wiese, Weiss, and Yukelson (1991) reported that athletic trainers support the use of psychological strategies when dealing with injury rehabilitation of athletes. Listening to coaches and trainers, intrinsic motivation on the part of the athlete, and social support were identified as key strategies and skills in the recovery process. It was also reported that the use of imagery was not perceived as important relative to the other techniques. When Francis, Andersen, and Maley (2000) replicated the Wiese, Weiss, and Yukelson study with Australian physiotherapists and professional basketball players, they again found support for the use of psychological skills in injury recovery, specifically those skills designed to enhance, such as communication and motivation. A lack of belief in the use of imagery and relaxation techniques for rehabilitation was also identified, mirroring Wiese, Weiss, and

Yukelson's previous findings. In contrast, a study of Division I collegiate athletes revealed that, of all psychological interventions, student athletes were most likely to use goal-setting and imagery—but they were more comfortable seeking help from a coach than from a sport-titled professional (for instance, sport psychologist; Maniar, Curry, Sommers-Flanagan, & Walsh, 2001). Therefore, it may be important for coaches and athletic trainers to become proficient in providing services such as imagery, so that athletes can receive the guidance and assistance that they seek.

Wiese et al. (1991) indicated that the reluctance on the part of trainers to advocate the use of imagery techniques may have resulted from their not feeling qualified to use them and/or not believing in their efficacy. Health professionals involved in the rehabilitation of injured athletes should therefore be educated about the "why and how to" of imagery techniques because imagery has been depicted as a multifaceted process that is not easily understood (Hall, 2001).

Perspectives on Mind-Body Integration

In most cases, athletes are assigned to rehabilitation programs based upon traditional medical models that do not include a mind-body orientation. That athletes may have the capacity to expedite their own recovery with the use of cognitive strategies such as imagery does not seem to be recognized to the degree that it should. Sordoni, Hall, and Forwell (2000) reported that injured athletes are more likely to use motivational imagery than cognitive imagery during the rehabilitation process, but that athletes report less use of imagery during injury than in other aspects of sport (for instance, training and competition). Athletes may require guidance in understanding the potential applications of imagery in sport injury rehabilitation. Academic preparation in the area of psychophysiology will facilitate the understanding and application of imagery to the rehabilitation process (Collins and Hale, 1997).

Psychophysiological Perspectives

Substantial evidence exists that speaks to the credibility of using a mind-body approach in explaining human existence and the intricacies of the healing process. Viewing the human being as a package that contains a constant interchange between mental and physiological functions helps in recognizing the interdependence of their interaction. Historically, patients' beliefs about the efficacy of the treatment they received and their own input into the process have been at the forefront of both Chinese and Navajo practices (Porkert, 1979; Sandner, 1979). Indeed, Gardner (1985) speaks of multiple intelligences that an individual possesses to varying degrees. One of these is the "body-kinesthetic intelligence . . . the ability to use one's body in highly differentiated and skilled ways." These skilled ways include "the body being trained to respond to the expressive powers of the mind" (p. 206).

At the cornerstone of this position, however, lies the principle of homeostasis advanced by Cannon (1932, cited in Ievleva & Orlick, 1991), which establishes "a process of interaction between the brain and the body toward maintaining internal stability."

Green, Green, and Walters (1979) adhere to what they call the psychophysiological principle, which suggests that for every physiological change that occurs in the body, there is an appropriate change in the mental-emotional state. They also suggest that the converse of this phenomenon is equally true. Others have established that imagery triggers similar neurophysiological functions as does actual experience (Leuba, 1940; Perky, 1910; Richardson, 1969). In recent research with patients with complete spinal cord injury (SCI), when the patients practiced mental imagery of motor activity, "the primary motor cortex was consistently activated, even to the same degree as during movement execution in the controls" (Alkadhi, Brugger, Boendermaker, Crelier, Curt, & Hepp-Reymond et al., 2005). The extent of activation in the primary motor cortex was significantly correlated with the vividness of movement imagery.

Surgent (1991) suggests that there is a mind-body connection which facilitates the healing process. He indicates that:

> Your immune system doesn't work alone. . .your mind also has a voice in what goes on. There is a communication network between your brain and your immune system, like telephone lines between a general and his field commanders. . . . Feelings, attitudes, and beliefs are organized in your brain and communicated to your immune system by chemical messengers. These can have an effect on the healing process which can be either positive or negative. (pp. 4-5)

This claim has been substantiated by findings reported by Hall (1983), who revealed an increased immune response when he tested the effects of hypnosis and imagery on lymphocyte function. The most recent support for the interplay between the use of imagery and immune system responses has been reported by Achterberg (1991), AuBuchon (1991), and Post-White (1991). They have provided evidence that describes the positive effects the immune system experiences when triggered by imagery.

Literature pertaining to psychoneuroimmunology further establishes the plausibility of the mind-body paradigm during rehabilitation. Achterberg, Mathews-Simonton, and Simonton (1977), as well as Fiore (1988), have reported that certain psychological characteristics of patients influenced recovery from cancer. Simonton, Matthews-Simonton, and Creighton (1978) provide evidence that supports the use of imagery in the treatment for cancer. Others have reported positive effects of the use of imagery during the rehabilitation of various illnesses and injuries such as psoriasis (Gaston, Crombez, & Dupuis, 1989); stress management (Hanley & Chinn, 1989); ulcers, paraplegia, fractures, hip disarticulations, and intra-abdominal lesions (Korn, 1983).

In addition, a large number of studies have indicated that the use of imagery produces altered autonomic activity (Lutze, Scheler, Tan, Braun, & Birbaumer, 2003), physiological responses such as salivation (Barber, Chauncey, & Winer, 1964), increase in pupillary size (Simpson & Paivio, 1966), increased heart rate (May & Johnson, 1973), changes in electromyograms (Sheikh & Jordan, l983; Tremblay, Tremblay, & Colcer, 2001; Lutz & Lindner, 2001), increases in blood-glucose, inhibition of gastrointestinal activity, and changes in skin temperature (Barber, 1978).

When these findings are taken to their logical end, it may be worth considering that when one takes physiologic measurements, he or she is in fact taking corresponding psychological indicators simultaneously. The results reported may depend entirely on what category of measurement is being taken and the perspective from which the investigator originates, e.g., psychology, physiology, psychophysiology.

The possibility exists that the specialization in professional orientation prevalent in today's scientific community is merely part of the lasting ripple effect created by Cartesian's medical model and does nothing but perpetuate an all-too-narrow perspective from which to draw conclusions concerning the human condition. As a consequence, the thoughts of Diderot from the middle 19th century may be applicable today. He spoke of the intention at that time of scholars to reinstate holism as an appropriate perspective for medicine so that it "may be advanced to the point of where it was two thousand years ago" (McMahon & Sheikh, 1986, p. 12).

Psychomotor Perspectives

From a sport psychology perspective, it appears that there is, at the very least, a logical leap from the relationship between imagery and sport performance to the impact of imagery on the healing process of injuries. The premise that the use of mental rehearsal facilitates EEG activity (Romero, Lacourse, Lawrence, Schandler & Cohen, 2000), activity in some of the higher brain centers (Malouin, Richard, Jacksons, Dumas, & Doyon, 2003), the activation of motor pathways (Stinear & Byblow, 2004), as well as the execution of certain motor skills under certain conditions is well documented (for reviews see Corbin, 1972; Feltz & Landers, 1983; Hall, 2001).

In addition, Hecker and Kaczor (1988) have summarized existing theoretical models that have been advanced to explain the processes involved with mental imagery and its influence on athletic performance, e.g. motor skill development. These include

(a) the symbolic learning theory, which posits that symbolic rehearsal advances the development of skills requiring cognitive processes (Sackett, 1935);

(b) the psychoneuromuscular theory associated with Jacobsen's work (1938), which identified muscular innervations during imagery that are similar to those occurring during actual performance;

(c) the attention-arousal set, which integrates cognitive and physiological aspects of rehearsal in order to distinguish between relevant and irrelevant cues (Vealey, 1987; Feltz & Landers, 1983); and

(d) the bioinformational theory of Lang (1979), in which imagery processes the stimulus characteristics of an imagined scenario and the physiological/behavioral responses that accompany them.

Other models such as Greene's (1972) multi-level hierarchical control of motor programs and Pribram's (1971) two-process model of imagery have been applied to the development of motor programs and further describe the interdependence of mind and body. Greene maintains that movement is the result of a mind-body system composed of a number of levels. The higher levels initiate a "ballpark" motor response to environmental input that is then refined by lower levels of neuromuscular processing. The end result is the appropriate movement that meets the requirements of the task.

Pribram's two-process model of imagery includes neuropsychological processes identified as TOTE and TOTEM systems. The TOTE system refers to the exchange of feedback and feed-forward mechanisms between the environment and the organism in order to produce movement. The TOTEM system is an application of these processes in which images conduct TOTE operations on each other exclusively within the mental environment.

It seems viable to suggest, therefore, that the same models that attempt to explain psychophysiological and psychomotor processes used in athletic performance can be applied when describing the place of imagery during the rehabilitation associated with the healing of athletic injuries, e.g., the re-establishing of fine and gross motor movements, the re-establishing of psychoneurological pathways. However, as Hecker and Kaczor (1988) have indicated, when these theories are taken alone, they prove to be inadequate in explaining the complex mind-body process of imagery. What is needed is a more integrated approach to any attempt at explanation (Lavallee, Kremer, Moran, & Williams, 2004), such as a "systems theory" as suggested by Schwartz (1984).

Schwartz maintained that systems theory "has the potential to provide a metatheoretical framework for integrating the biological, psychological, and social consequences of imagery on health and illness" (Schwartz, 1984, p. 35). In describing the synthesis attained by systems theory, he elaborated on its metaprinciples:

> A system is an entity (a whole) which is composed of a set of parts (which are subsystems). These parts interact. Out of the parts interaction emerge unique properties that characterize the new entity or system as a whole. These emergent properties represent more than the simple, independent sum of the properties of the parts studied in isolation. It is hypothesized that the emergent properties appear only when the parts are allowed to interact. (p. 39)

Thus, independent theories that appear to be in competition can be integrated into a comprehensive perspective that appears to be both logical and substantiated by scientific evidence. It is proposed that this may provide the necessary body of knowledge from which the education of health professionals (i.e., athletic trainers) may be enhanced. The use of psychophysiological techniques such as imagery may increase when the educational barriers are weakened. Hopefully, this will lead to the use of psychological techniques that go beyond the traditional skills of communication and motivation.

What follows is an example of how the mind-body perspective might be applied in the development of a rehabilitation program for injured athletes. It is offered with the understanding that it is not all-encompassing. However, it should provide a starting point from which sport medicine teams can develop programs of rehabilitation from a mind-body perspective.

The Chronology of an Injury

The following is a chronology of athletic injuries adapted from Nideffer's scheme (1987). Although his scheme included factors related to the onset of the injury as well as the athlete's coping and recovery, this chronology addresses three periods of time associated with injuries:

- pre-injury
- attention to the athlete immediately following the injury

- the rehabilitation program leading to the recovery and re-integration of the athlete into the competitive situation

Each will be described with the intended purpose of demonstrating the application of imagery techniques within the context of an integrated mind-body approach to rehabilitation.

Figure 1.

The Uses of Imagery during Rehabilitation.

The Chronology of an Injury	The Potential Use of Imagery
Pre-injury	**Preventive Medicine** * enhances relaxation * facilitates self-regulation * enhances perspective toward stressors
Immediately Subsequent to Injury	**Developing Awareness** * knowledge base of the injury * what is to be expected during rehabilitation (instant pre-play of rehab program) * maintenance of positive attitudes * reinforce efficacy of treatment * knowledge of potential emotions associated with rehabilitation
During Rehabilitation	**Creating the Mindset for Recovery** * eliminating counterproductive thoughts * developing "possible selves" * facilitate goal setting * affirmation imagery * performance-related mental rehearsals * rehabilitative imagery * coping with pain * bringing closure to the injury

Pre-injury

All athletes experience periods in their lives during which the probability of injury is high. As noted in Selye's (1974) classic work, such periods are characterized by an abundance of stressors. These stressors may be categorized as either general life stressors or athletic stressors. General life stressors may include

- the transition to college life for incoming freshmen,
- the homesickness experienced by athletes of all levels, and
- the feelings of sorrow and anguish that accompany the death of someone close.

Athletic stressors might include

- trouble with a coach, teammate, or fans;
- loss of playing status; and
- the athletic event itself

(Bramwell, Holmes, Masuda, & Wagner, 1975; Kerr & Minden, 1988; Lynch, 1988; Rotella & Heyman, 1986).

The resultant injury may be the function of the fatigue associated with having to deal with these situations or the divisive effect on concentration the athlete may experience (Kerr & Minden, 1988). Inasmuch as an athlete may experience any of these, or other circumstances that have an adverse effect on his or her "normal" life pattern, injury is often the result.

As a form of preventive medicine that would serve to lessen the impact of stressors and thus reduce the potential for injury, imagery techniques that enhance relaxation and perspective toward specific situations of stress may be developed and implemented throughout the season as circumstances mandate. For example, an athlete may experience stress as the result of homesickness. An imagery experiential can be developed that puts the immediate needs of the athlete in a long-term perspective while enhancing a relaxed state of mind. It could be implemented by introducing a relaxed state, possibly with some form of Jacobsen's (1938) progressive relaxation. This may then be followed by guided imagery intended to gain perspective on the situation. This has also been described by Samuels and Samuels (1975) as developing the ability "to see . . . to look at an object from different mental points of view, as well as from different vantage points" (p. 115), for example:

> Imagine yourself as a freshman entering college. As soon as the Thanksgiving break arrives, you can't wait to get on the first plane home. Same for the December/January break. Same for the summer break.
>
> Now, you are a sophomore. When Thanksgiving comes, you definitely want to go home, but now you'll miss some of your college friends. Same for the December/January break. Same for the summer break.
>
> Now, you're a junior. You've established your "place" on campus. You have developed close relationships with both male and female friends. As Thanksgiving break approaches, you weigh the pros and cons of going home or staying on campus. You decide to go home as usual. The same thoughts occur, but not as strongly when December rolls around. But with summer, you make plans to travel with your friends and tell your parents you'll see them when you finish your trip.
>
> Now, you're a senior. Your apartment or room seems more like home to you than your parents' home. Since Thanksgiving and the December break are family occasions, it's your parents who want you home more than it's you wanting to go. But, still, you go. Then it's summertime and your parents are calling you to come home instead of you calling them. What does it feel like to be self-reliant, self-sufficient?

Immediately Subsequent to the Injury

When the injury occurs, standard first aid procedures should be followed so that further complications are not created unnecessarily. The athlete should be accompanied to the physician by someone associated with the program (e.g., trainer, coach, sport psychologist, parent) and should be given at least "the illusion of hope" at the outset (Nideffer, 1987).

After the athlete has seen a physician, there should be an exchange of information concerning the injury between the attending medical personnel, the athlete, the team trainer/physician, and coaches. This should include specifics about the anatomy and physiology of the injured area. By using anatomical models and photographs, the abstraction of the injury is translated into more tangible and recognizable terms. In addition, the injury might be explained in lay terms that facilitate an image, e.g., "the rubber bands (ligaments) need to grow back onto the bone." This knowledge is critical as it may be applied to the use of rehabilitative imagery that would be employed later (Surgent, 1991).

During Rehabilitation of the Injury

The structure of the rehabilitation program (e.g., an instant pre-play of the program) should be discussed by all parties directly involved as the sports medicine team, e.g., trainers, coaches, athletes. This may include the expected time frame associated with recovery, as well as the general parameters of the physical as well as mental program to be used during rehabilitation. Expectations of the athlete such as appointments with trainers, coaches, and sport psychologists, attendance at practice and games, and the criteria to be used to determine when the athlete is ready to return to practice and competition should also be identified. In addition, *who* will make the final decision (e.g., the athlete, the coach, the physician) as to the athlete's readiness may also be discussed as part of the criteria used for return (Thomas, 1990). Of considerable importance are the factors relating to the athlete's adherence to the rehabilitation. These should be identified and discussed with the athlete. It should be pointed out that successful rehabilitation is characterized by specific behaviors associated with adherence to the rehabilitation process. Wiese et al. (1991) have identified the following:

(a) the willingness on the part of the athlete to listen to the trainer

(b) the athlete maintaining a positive attitude

(c) intrinsic motivation on the part of the athlete

In addition, characteristics described by Duda, Smart, and Tappe (1989) include

- the athlete's belief in the efficacy of the treatment,
- the presence of a social support system, and
- the athlete's orientation toward task-related goals in his or her sport.

Imagery experientials in which the athlete envisions the overt behaviors associated with these factors may become an integral part of daily treatments in the training room. An example of such an application of imagery may be created by adapting the work of Lazarus (1984), who has developed procedures that depict an individual taking psychological risks. After the behaviors associated with

- carrying out specific instructions from the trainer,
- personifying positive attitudes,
- demonstrating intrinsic motivation, and
- task-related goal setting

have been imagined, the athlete is then encouraged to go out and perform them.

Finally, Rotella and Heyman (1986) and Lynch (1988) have discussed the application of Kubler-Ross' (1969) work concerning the emotional recovery from the death of a loved one to the athletic setting and the recovering athlete. It is suggested that athletes may experience similar patterns of emotional reaction during their rehabilitation. This might include

- denial,
- anger,
- bargaining,
- depression, and
- acceptance.

Were an athlete given insight into the process of recovery with imagery depicting each stage, he or she may be able to facilitate the transition from one stage to the next.

For example, an experiential entitled "Time Projection or Time Tripping" (Lazarus, 1984, pp. 131-137) may facilitate the development of an athlete's awareness concerning potential emotional reactions throughout rehabilitation. By projecting himself or herself back or forward in time and describing the emotions associated with different stages of rehabilitation from retrospective or futuristic perspectives, the athlete is encouraged to recognize various stages of recovery. For example, the athlete may recognize that he or she may become depressed during the rehabilitation. But, he or she may also recognize that depression may be part of the process that eventually leads to recovery.

In summary, the following four examples have been described to demonstrate how imagery might be applied to the first two phases of the chronology of an injury:
- for the pre-injury phase—
  (a) relaxation and perspective imagery as preventative medicine
- for the time immediate following the injury—
  (b) an instant pre-play of the rehabilitation program
  (c) attitude and belief imagery
  (d) imagery depicting emotional stages of transition during recovery

The Mind-Body Rehabilitation Process

The rehabilitation program for athletes should be devised by a sports medicine team composed of the attending physician, the athlete, trainers, coach, and sport psychologist. The resulting program should reflect a mind-body approach to the process of recovery (Gordon, Jaffe, & Bresler, 1984; Peper, Ancoli, & Quinn, 1979) that includes the use of imagery in the recovery from and coping with pain associated with the injury (Morris, Spittle, & Watt, 2005). It should address the creation of the appropriate mindset for the recovering athlete as well as the physical dimensions of rehabilitation.

Creating the Mindset for Recovery

A character named Socrates from Dan Millman's (1984) book *The Way of the Peaceful Warrior* describes the part one's mind plays in creating his or her way of being. He suggests that

"Mind" is one of those slippery terms like "love." The proper definition depends on your state of consciousness. . . . We refer to the brain's abstract processes as "the intellect.". . . The brain and the mind are not the same. The brain is real; the mind isn't. The brain can be a tool. It can recall phone numbers, solve math puzzles, or create poetry. In this way, it works for the rest of the body, like a tractor. But when you can't stop thinking of that math problem or phone number, or when troubling thoughts and memories arise without your intent, it's not your brain working, but your mind wandering. Then the mind controls you; then the tractor has run wild, (p. 62).

In essence, an athlete in rehabilitation must accomplish the same task of getting rid of a mind full of negative and counterproductive wanderings. Only then might the brain be able to do its work. These counterproductive wanderings might include certain fears associated with being injured:

- the fear of re-injury
- the fear of the pain associated with the original injury and/or of that experienced during rehabilitation
- the fear of not returning to previous level of ability
- the fear of the loss of status

In addition, Ievleva and Orlick (1991) reported that recovery time for injured athletes was faster for those who did not engage in injury-replay imagery. Thus, athletes must use their intellect to guide the neuropsychological processes of the brain in such a manner as to facilitate recovery.

Developing "Possible Selves"

Upon injury, athletes are faced with what Cantor and Kihlstrom (1987) refer to as a life task. They are immediately confronted with a problem that must be resolved before normal existence can continue. In truth, the athletes must make a conscious effort to redirect their attention from playing the game to playing a new game called rehab. The game in which they must now perform becomes that associated with recovery. They must adopt a mindset that focuses all of their energies toward that end. The immediate life task then becomes one of rehabilitation. It's a brand new game that requires a conscious shift of attention that has as its ultimate goal their return to competition.

In addressing the task of goal setting associated with the rehabilitation process, sport psychologists might consider applying the theoretical framework of Markus and Ruvolo (1989). This framework depicts the development of "possible selves." Their notion of developing possible selves addresses the potential for "personalized representations of goals" (p. 211). They discuss goal setting in terms of "constructing a possible self in which one is different from the now self and in which one realizes the goal" (p. 211). Thus, a progression of possible selves "becomes a part of the working self-concept" (Markus & Kunda, 1986; Markus & Nurius, 1986).

What is critical is the ability of the athletes to formulate and maintain the possible selves that lead toward the desired goal. They must be able to repress possible selves that are inconsistent with the task of recovery, e.g., a possible self depicting injury-replay or negative attitudes. The desired possible selves might depict the athlete as an individual having

- a positive outlook,
- descriptive self-talk, and
- performance-related goals.

As a number of authors have suggested, the athlete should engage in affirmation imagery that portrays him or her fulfilling short-term goals (Korn & Johnson, 1983; Ievleva and Orlick, 1991). To the extent that they are able to accomplish these tasks, their behavior will be "focused, energized, and organized by this possible self" (Markus & Ruvolo, 1989, p. 214).

For example, imagery scenarios could be patterned after the work of Maxwell Maltz concerning the self-image. Ishii (1986, pp. 313-323) describes a number of provocative experientials that focus on developing positive, assertive, and successful self-images as well as attitudes pertaining to happiness and willpower. One in particular places the client in an empty theater. From this setting, the client is asked to imagine a movie unfolding in which he or she handles a problem successfully. Another technique requires that the client visualize an unerasable chalkboard on which he or she lists past successes.

The task of the sport psychologist then becomes the creation of a series of "programmed visualizations" (Samuels & Samuels, 1975, p. 229) that reflect the rehabilitative tasks and outcomes established by the sports medicine team. That possible selves may depict performance goals as well as outcome goals presents the sport psychologist with the task of identifying specific scenarios depicting each. In fact, Bandura (1986, 1988) maintains that performance and outcome selves should be separated.

Korn (1983) agrees that there should be a progression from product to process goals. That is, as an initial step, athletes should imagine themselves as completely recovered and able to do all the things they were capable of doing prior to the injury. After they have have become reasonably proficient at this form of product-oriented image, they may then progress to more specific, process-oriented images.

These process-oriented possible selves should reflect instrumental selves. That is, they should represent a sequence of possible selves that depicts the athlete in the process of performing specific motor skills, each leading to a self that is one step closer to total recovery. In essence, the instrumental possible selves are intended to result in a summation effect, with the eventual result matching or surpassing the initial product-oriented image.

For example, a female basketball player undergoing rehabilitation for a knee injury consisting of a torn interior cruciate ligament with cartilage strains used the following series of possible selves over nine months of rehabilitation.

Possible Self #1 "Knee at 90 Degrees: "I Want to Be a Success Story,"
    e.g., following surgery, getting out of bed and out of the hospital, establishing image of desired outcome.

Possible Self #2 "Strut Your Stuff,"
    e.g., getting off crutches, watching other people walk, establishing own gait.

Possible Self #3 "Hurt to Get Better,"
    e.g., progression of physical therapy that included, in part, weight training, electric stimulation, stationary bike, stair master.

Possible Self #4 "Spring Forward,"
    e.g., running at 75 %, jumping exercises, increasing work load.

Possible Self #5 "Let's Play,"
e.g., pick-up games.

Possible Self #6 "Dribble, Drive, and Dive!"
e.g., playing with no fear of failure.

Possible Self #7 "No Brace,"
e.g., the final stage due to school policy of mandatory use of brace following such an injury.

Other Uses of Imagery

The processes of guided and non-directed imagery can also be utilized by the athlete in the form of

- relaxation techniques,
- motor skill rehearsals, and
- rehabilitative experientials.

(Surgent, 1991). Rehabilitative imagery has been shown to have significant effects on recovery time (Ievleva & Orlick, 1991). Imagery training during rehabilitation can improve outcomes. In a controlled study with random assignment, Cupal and Brewer (2001) assigned 30 patients who were in rehabilitation for anterior cruciate ligament (ACL) reconstruction to one of three groups:

- treatment group (guided relaxation and imagery)
- placebo group (social support and attention)
- control group (no intervention)

Imagery group participants had significantly greater knee strength and significantly less re-injury anxiety and pain at 24 weeks post-surgery than did participants in the other two groups.

As described earlier during the chronology of an injury, information gathered from the physician concerning the anatomy and physiology of the injury facilitates the use of rehabilitative imagery. In addition, Day (1991) has developed an educational discourse on the immune system through the use of cartoon imagery that uses immune cell caricatures to explain the function of each cell involved in the rehabilitation process. Korn (1983) described a technique of rehabilitation imagery that consists of envisioning the wounds as filling from the inside out rather than just being covered over at the surface. The filling material was cement and the repair process was analogous to the method of repair of a hole in a concrete walkway (p. 28). Computer technology can also be used to facilitate the use of imagery for rehabilitation (Gaggioli, Morganti, Walker, Meneghini, Alcaniz, & Lozano, et al., 2004). Gaggioli et al. have developed a protocol that provides in-home computer-based imagery support for rehabilitation for patients after they have moved from in-patient to out-patient status. Gaggioli indicated that the use of the technological support of imagery practice—after imagery training with a medical professional—will reduce the need for expensive skilled support during practice of the skills.

Specific mindsets that might be addressed through the use of imagery include the following:

- maintaining a positive outlook
- stress control
- the use of positive and descriptive self-talk
- sustaining belief in the rehabilitation process

Performance-related imagery may take the form of mental rehearsal while attending practices and competitions in which the athletes imagine themselves as if they were playing. Mental rehearsal of the sport activity may also increase an athlete's self-efficacy for his or her sport after injury. Chase, Magyar, and Drake (2005) reported that previously injured gymnasts may fear re-injury. Lack of practice during rehabilitation may cause a gymnast's self-efficacy for his or her sport to diminish. However, mental practice of skills and techniques can help maintain self-efficacy for the sport and therefore diminish fear re-injury. In addition, imagery has been shown to be effective in coping with pain (Achterberg, Kenner, & Lawlis, 1988; Korn, 1983; Samuels & Samuels, 1975; Simonton, Mathews-Simonton, & Creighton, 1978; Spanos & O'Hara, 1990).

Rotella and Heyman (1986) recommended the use of videotapes of past performances. This technique may serve to reinforce the symbolic learning and psychoneuromuscular processes. Imagery may also be used to facilitate closure of the rehabilitation process when the athlete has returned to competition.

Physical Rehabilitation

The use of targeted performance criteria facilitates the athlete's return to pre-injury performance levels on specific tasks associated with his or her sport. They may also serve as the impetus for creating specific instrumental and performance-related possible selves. The groundwork for this, however, must be laid at the onset of training prior to the season and, most certainly, prior to injury.

At the beginning of the season's training, baseline data should be gathered for the athletes on specific tasks associated with their training, e.g., maximum weight, sets, and repetitions for a variety of weightlifting routines; range of motion measurements for flexibility; physiologic parameters such as heart rate, time of recovery, max VO2 for endurance; and recorded times on specific distances for indication of speed, etc. These data provide the target criteria to which an athlete can compare his or her progress during rehabilitation.

In addition, a functional progression of specific sport skills should be identified that represent "being back" to the athlete. For example, baseball pitchers who have been out with elbow injuries may wish to use a particular pitch (e.g., breaking off a hard slider) to gauge effectiveness upon return. Tennis players may engage in the side shuffle used on the base line as an indicator that they have recovered from the pain associated with shin splints.

Each of these tasks, in addition to other methods of progressive resistance exercises and cross training, forms the foundation for physical rehabilitation with tangible indicators of recovery. Of course, these are undertaken in proper sequence relative to the initial training room duties prescribed by the trainers and physician (e.g., whirlpool, electrical stimulation, iced therapy).

Summary

Wiese et al. (1991) have reported that many athletic trainers agree with the need for further education in the area of psychology and, in particular, for methods that can be applied in the athletic setting. To that end, Morris, Spittle and Watt (2005) maintained that sport medicine personnel should be trained in the use of video modeling, biofeedback, and flotation devices.

The purpose of this chapter has been to provide an educational text that
* supports a mind-body paradigm for rehabilitation from psychophysiological and psychomotor perspectives,
* demonstrates the application of imagery within the chronology of an injury, and
* describes performance-related criteria used in physical rehabilitation.

The chronology includes that period of time preceding the injury, the attention given to the athlete immediately following the injury, and the subsequent rehabilitation program leading to the return of the athlete to practice and competition. It is suggested that imagery techniques may be applied during the pre-injury stage as a tool for preventive maintenance. During the actual rehabilitation program, its purpose is

(a) to facilitate the healing process,

(b) to promote the development of a positive and relaxed outlook toward recovery,

(c) to create the mindset required for optimum performance, and

(d) to bring closure to the injury experience.

References

Achterberg, J., (1991, May). *Enhancing the immune function through imagery.* Paper presented at the Fourth World Conference on Imagery, Minneapolis, MN.

Achterberg, J., Kenner, C., & Lawlis, G. F. (1988). Severe burn injury: A comparison of relaxation, imagery and biofeedback for pain management. *Journal of Mental Imagery, 12*(1), 71-88.

Achterberg, J., Matthews-Simonton, S., & Simonton, O. C. (1977). Psychology of the exceptional cancer patient: A description of patients who outlive predicted life expectancies. *Psychotherapy: Theory, research, and practice, 14,* 416-422.

Alkadhi, H., Brugger, P., Boendermaker, S. H., Crelier, G., Curt, A., & Hepp-Reymond, M. et al. (2005). What disconnection tells about motor imagery: Evidence from paraplegic patients. *Cerebral Cortex, 15*(2), 131-140.

AuBuchon, B. (1991, May). *The effects of positive mental imagery on hope, coping, anxiety, dypsnea, and pulmonary function in persons with chronic obstructive pulmonary disease: Tests of a nursing intervention and a theoretical model.* Paper presented at the Fourth World Conference on Imagery, Minneapolis, MN.

Bandura, A. (1986). *Social foundations of thought and action: A social cognitive theory.* Englewood Cliffs, NJ: Prentice-Hall.

Bandura, A. (1988). Self-regulation of motivation and action through goal systems. In V. Hamilton, G. H. Bower, & N. H. Frijda (Eds.), *Cognitive perspectives on emotion and motivation* (pp. 37-61). Dordrecht, Netherlands: Kluwer Academic Publishers.

Barber, T. X. (1978). Hypnosis, suggestions and psychosomatic phenomena, a new look from the standpoint of recent experimental studies. *The American Journal of Clinical Hypnosis, 21,* 13-27.

Barber, T. X., Chauncey, H. M., & Winer, R. A. (1964). The effect of hypnotic and nonhypnotic suggestions on parotid gland response to gustatory stimuli. *Psychosomatic Medicine, 26,* 374-380.

Bramwell, S. T., Holmes, T. H., Masuda, M., & Wagner, N. N. (1975). Psychosocial factors in athletic injuries: Development and application of the social and athletic readjustment rating scale (SARRS). *Journal of Human Stress, 1*(2), 6-20.

Cannon, W. B. (1932). *The wisdom of the body.* New York: Norton.

Cantor, N., & Kihlstrom, J. (1987). *Personality and social intelligence.* Englewood Cliffs, NJ: Prentice-Hall.

Chase, M. A., Magyar, T. M., & Drake, B. M. (2005). Fear of injury in gymnastics: Self-efficacy and psychological strategies to keep on tumbling. *Journal of Sports Sciences, 23*(5), 465-475.

Collins, D., and B. D. Hale. (1997). Getting closer . . . but still no cigar! Comments on Bakker, Boschker, and Chung (1996). *Journal of Sport and Exercise Psychology* 19: 207-212.

Corbin, C. (1972). Mental practice. In W. Morgan (Ed.), *Ergogenic aids and muscular performance* (pp. 93-118). New York: Academic Press.

Cupal, D. D., & Brewer, B. W. (2001). Effects of relaxation and guided imagery on knee strength, reinjury anxiety, and pain following anterior cruciate ligament reconstruction. *Rehabilitation Psychology, 46*(1), 28-43.

Day, C. H. (1991). *The immune system handbook.* North York, Ontario: Potentials Within.

Duda, J. L., Smart, A. E., & Tappe, M. K. (1989). Predictors of adherence in the rehabilitation of athletic injuries: An application of personal investment theory. *Journal of Sport and Exercise Psychology, 11,* 367-381.

Feltz, D. L., & Landers, D. M. (1983). The effects of mental practice on motor skill learning and performance: A meta-analysis. *Journal of Sport Psychology, 5,* 25-27.

Fiore, N. A. (1988). The inner healer: Imagery for coping with cancer and its therapy. *Journal of Mental Imagery, 12*(2), 79-82.

Francis, S. R., Andersen, M. B., & Maley, P. (2000). Physiotherapists' and male professional athletes' views on psychological skills for rehabilitation. *Journal of Sports Science and Medicine in Sport, 3*(1), 17-29.

Gaggioli, A., Morganti, F., Walker, R., Meneghini, A., Alcaniz, M., & Lozano, J. A. et al. (2004). Training with computer-supported motor imagery in post-stroke rehabilitation. *CyberPsychology & Behavior, 7*(3), 327-332.

Gardner, H. (1985). *Frames of mind: The theory of multiple intelligences.* New York: Basic Books, Inc.

Gaston, L., Crombez, J. & Dupuis, G. (1989). An imagery and meditation technique in the treatment of psoriasis: A case study using an A-B-A design. *Journal of Mental Imagery, 13*(1), 31-38.

Gordon, J. S., Jaffe, D. T., & Bresler, D. E. (1984). *Mind, body, and health: Toward an integral medicine.* New York: Human Sciences Press.

Green, E. E., Green, A. M., & Walters, E. D. (1979). Biofeedback for mind/body self-regulation: Healing and Creativity. In E. Peper, S. Ancoli, & M. Quinn (Eds.), *Mind/body integration: Essential readings in biofeedback.* New York: Plenum Press.

Greene, P. H. (1972). Problems of organization of motor systems. In R. Rosen & F. M. Snell (Eds.), *Progress in theoretical biology* (Vol.2, pp. 304-333). New York: Academic Press.

Hall, C. R. (2001). Imagery in sport and exercise. In R. N. Singer, H. A. Hausenblas, & C. M. Janelle (Eds.), *Handbook of research on sport psychology* (2nd ed., pp. 529-549). New York: Wiley.

Hall, H. R. (1983) Hypnosis and the immune system: A review with implications for cancer and the psychology of healing. *American Journal of Clinical Hypnosis, 25*(3), 92-103.

Hanley, G. L., & Chinn, D. (1989). Stress management: An integration of multidimensional arousal and imagery theories with case study. *Journal of Mental Imagery, 13*(2), 107-118.

Hecker, J. E., & Kaczor, L. M. (1988). Application of imagery theory to sport psychology: Some preliminary findings. *Journal of Sport and Exercise Psychology, 10,* 363-373.

Ievleva, L., & Orlick, T. (1991). Mental links to enhanced healing: An exploratory study. *The Sport Psychologist, 5,* 25-40.

Ishii, M. M. (1986). Imagery techniques in the works of Maxwell Maltz. In A. A. Sheikh (Ed.), *Anthology of imagery techniques* (pp. 313-323). Milwaukee, WI: American Imagery Institute.

Jacobsen, E. (1938). *Progressive relaxation.* Chicago: University of Chicago Press.

Kerr, G., & Minden, H. (1988). Psychological factors related to the occurrence of athletic injuries. *Journal of Sport and Exercise Psychology, 10,* 167-173.

Korn, E. R. (1983). The use of altered states of consciousness and imagery in physical and pain rehabilitation. *Journal of Mental Imagery, 7*(1), 25-34.

Korn, E. R., & Johnson, K. (1983). *Visualization: The uses of imagery in the health professions.* Homewood, IL: Dow Jones-Irwin.

Kübler-Ross, E. (1969). *On death and dying.* New York: Macmillan.

Lang, P. J. (1979). A bio-informational theory of emotional imagery. *Psychophysiology, 16,* 495-512.

Lavallee, D., Kremer, J., Moran, A. P., & Williams, M. (2004). *Sport psychology: Contemporary themes.* Basingstoke, Hampshire, England: Palgrave MacMillan.

Lazarus, A. (1984). *In the mind's eye: The power of imagery for personal enrichment.* New York: The Guilford Press.

Leuba, C. (1940). Images as conditioned sensation. *Journal of Experimental Psychology, 26,* 345-351.

Lotze, M., Scheler, G., Tan, H. R .M., Braun, C., & Birbaumer, N. (2003). The musician's brain: Functional imaging of amateurs and professionals during imagery and performance. *NeuroImage* 20: 1817-1830.

Lutz, R., and Lindner, D. E. (2001). Does electromyographic activity during motor imagery predict performance? A test of bioinformational theory and functional equivalence. *Journal of Sport and Exercise Psychology* 23, S63.

Lynch, G. P. (1988). Athletic injuries and the practicing sport psychologist: Practical guidelines for assisting athletes. *The Sport Psychologist, 2*, 161-167.

Malouin, F., Richards, C. L., Jackson, P. L., Dumas, F., & Doyon, J. (2003). Brain activations during motor imagery of locomotor-related tasks: A PET study. *Human Brain Mapping 19*, 47-62.

Maniar, S. D., Curry, L. A., Sommers-Flanagan, J., & Walsh, J. A. (2001). Student-athlete preferences in seeking help when confronted with sport performance problems. *Sport Psychologist, 15*(2), 205-223.

Markus, H., & Kunda, Z. (1986). Stability and malleability of the self-concept. *Journal of Personality and Social Psychology, 51*, 858-866.

Markus, H., & Nurius, P. (1986). Possible selves. *American Psychologist, 41*, 954-969.

Markus, H., & Ruvolo, A. (1989). Possible selves: Personalized representations of goals. In L.A. Pervin (Ed.), *Goal concepts in personality and social psychology* (pp. 211-241). Hillsdale, NJ: Erlbaum.

May, J., & Johnson, H. (1973). Psychological activity to internally elicited arousal and inhibitory thoughts. *Journal of Abnormal Psychology, 82*, 239-245.

McMahon, C. E., & Sheikh, A. (l986). Imagination in disease and healing processes: A historical perspective. In A. A. Sheikh (Ed.), *Anthology of imagery techniques* (pp. 1-36). Milwaukee, WI: American Imagery Institute.

Millman, D. (1984). *The way of the peaceful warrior.* Tiburon, CA: H.J. Kramer, Inc.

Morris, T., Spittle, M., and Watt, A. P. (2005). *Imagery in sport.* Champaign, Il.: Human Kinetics.

Nideffer, R. (1987, October). *Psychological aspects of injury.* Paper presented at the National Conference on Sport Psychology, Arlington, VA.

Peper, E., Ancoli, S., & Quinn, M. (1979). *Mind/body integration: Essential readings in biofeedback.* New York: Plenum Press.

Perky, C. W. (l910). An experimental study of imagination. *American Journal of Psychology, 21*, 422-452.

Porkert, M. (1979). Chinese medicine: A tradition healing science. In D. S. Sobel (Ed.), *Ways of health: Holistic approaches to ancient and contemporary medicine* (pp. 117-146). New York: Harcourt Brace Jovanovich.

Post-White, J. (199l, May). *The effects of mental imagery on emotions, immune function and cancer outcome.* Paper presented at the Fourth World Conference on Imagery, Minneapolis, MN.

Pribram, K. (1971). *Languages of the brain.* Englewood Cliffs, NJ: Prentice-Hall.

Richardson, A. (1969). *Mental imagery.* London: Routledge and Kegan Paul, Ltd.

Romero, D. H., Lacourse, M. G., Lawrence, K. E., Schandler, S., and Cohen,, M. J. (2000). Event-related potentials as a function of movement parameter variations during motor 47-62.imagery and isometric contraction. *Behavioral Brain Research 117*, 83-96.

Rotella, R. J., & Heyman, S. R. (1986). Stress, injury, and the psychological rehabilitation of athletes. In J. M. Williams (Ed.), *Applied sport psychology: Personal growth to peak performance* (pp. 343-364). Palo Alto, CA: Mayfield.

Sackett, R. S. (1935). The relationship between the amount of symbolic rehearsal and retention of a maze habit. *Journal of General Psychology, 13*, 113-128.

Samuels, S., & Samuels, N. (1975). *Seeing with the mind's eye.* New York: Random House.

Sandner, D. F. (1979). Navaho Indian medicine and medicine men. In D.S. Sobel (Ed.), *Ways of health: Holistic approaches to ancient and contemporary medicine* (pp. 117-146). New York: Harcourt Brace Jovanovich.

Schwartz, G. E. (1984). Psychophysiology of imagery and healing: A systems perspective. In A. A. Sheikh (Ed.), *Imagination and healing* (pp. 38-50). Farmingdale, NY: Baywood Publishing Company, Inc.

Selye, H. (1974). *Stress without distress.* Philadelphia: J.B. Lipincott.

Sheikh, A. A., & Jordan, C. S. (1983). Clinical uses of mental imagery. In A. A. Sheikh (Ed.), *Imagery: Current theory, research, and applications* (pp. 391-435). New York: Wiley.

Simonton, O. C., Matthews-Simonton, S., & Creighton, J. (1978). *Getting well again.* New York: St. Martin's Press.

Simpson, H. M., & Pavio, A. (l966). Changes in pupil size during an imagery task without motor involvement. *Psychonomic Science, 5*, 405-406.

Sordoni, C., Hall, C., & Forwell, L. (2000). The use of imagery by athletes during injury rehabilitation. *Journal of Sport Rehabilitation, 9*(4), 329-338.

Spanos, N. P., & O'Hara, P. A. (1990). Imaginal dispositions and situation-specific expectations in strategy-induced pain reductions. *Imagination, Cognition and Personality, 9*(2), 147-156.

Stinear, C. M., and Byblow, W. B. (2004). Modulation of corticospinal excitability and intracortical inhibition during motor imagery is task-dependent. *Experimental Brain Research, 157,* 351-358.

Surgent, F. S. (1991, January). Using your mind to beat injuries. *Running and Fit News, 9*(l), 4-5.

Thomas, C. (1990, October). *Locus of authority, coercion, and critical distance in the decision to play an injured player.* Paper presented at the Philosophic Society for the Study of Sport, Ft. Wayne, IN.

Tremblay, F., Tremblay, L. E., and Colcer, D. E. (2001). Modulaton of corticospinal excitability during imagined knee movements. *Journal of Rehabilitation Medicine, 33,* 230-234.

Vealey, R. S. (1987, June). *Imagery training for performance enhancement.* Paper presented at the Sports Psychology Institute, Portland, ME.

Wiese, D. M., Weiss, M. R., & Yukelson, D. P. (1991). Sport psychology in the training room: A survey of athletic trainers. *The Sport Psychologist, 5,* 15-24.

Section Three | Counseling the Injured Athlete

Section 3 comprises four chapters, all of which focus upon counseling issues as they pertain to rehabilitation from sport injury. The first two (9 and 10), address the matter of psychological assistance rendered to injured and disabled college student athletes. Chapter 9 is written by Edward Etzel, Sam Zizzi, A.P. Ferante, Frank Perna, and Renee Newcomer, and chapter 10 by Michael L. Sachs, Michael R. Sitler and Gerry Schwille. Although there is some overlap in content, the chapters contribute different perspectives and complement one another

The section's third chapter, chapter 11, presented by Keith Henschen and Gregory A. Shelly, is concerned exclusively with counseling needs of athletes with permanent disabilities. In chapter 12, Trent Petrie advocates an approach, namely support group therapy, which he believes to be very effective when working with injured athletes. He describes two such formats: the psychoeducational strategy and the counseling group strategy.

Chapter Nine

Providing Psychological Assistance to College Student-Athletes with Injuries and Disabilities

Edward F. Etzel and Sam Zizzi
West Virginia University

R. Renee Newcomer-Appeneal
University of North Carolina at Greensboro

A.P. Ferrante
Private Practice, Hilliard, OH

Frank M. Perna
Boston University

Numerous college student-athletes regularly incur athletic injuries and disabilities. In this chapter the authors discuss challenges that may be faced by professionals working with members of this population, the unique consequences associated with their losses in functioning, their need to cope with associated lifestyle changes, and ways of providing psychological assistance. Two cases are offered illustrating the nature and course of work with injured and disabled student-athletes.

> "The misfortunes of good people are not only a problem to the people who suffer and to their families. They are a problem to everyone who wants to believe in a just, fair and livable world." (Kushner, 1981, pp. 6-7)

Introduction

Nearly two decades ago, The National Collegiate Athletic Association's (NCAA) President's Commission hired The American Institutes for Research (AIR) to conduct a comprehensive survey of college student-athletes. The end product, **The National Study of Intercollegiate Athletes** (NSIA) (AIR, 1988), provided an unprecedented view of the reported experiences of both female and male NCAA

Division I sport participants from 42 institutions throughout the country. This study remains a landmark for researchers in the field of student-athlete services today. Among many findings, slightly more than half of the respondents said that they had incurred an injury during their college days. As the NSIA summary results indicate, this figure would not be too shocking, given the frequency and intensity of physical activity associated with sport, if it were not also learned that 70% of football and basketball players and 50% of those who participated in other sports also said that **they had experienced "intense" or "extremely intense" pressure to disregard their injuries** (AIR, 1988, p.52). Other authors have also noted high rates of injury across intercollegiate sports, in particular during pre-season training and competition (Klossner, 2005; Lanese, Strauss, Leizman, & Rotondi, 1990; National Collegiate Athletics Association, 2006; Zemper, 1989).

Before proceeding any further, it would seem useful to clarify for the reader what "student-athletes" are for the purposes of this chapter. A "student-athlete" will mean an undergraduate and a limited number of graduate level students enrolled in universities and colleges in the United States who participate in competitive sports sponsored by their university or college, not including intramural or club level sports. There are a substantial number of student-athletes today. In 2006, approximately 360,000 women (150,000) and men (210,000) participated in NCAA intercollegiate sports on roughly 1,250 campuses across the country (NCAA, 2006a). It should be further noted that the NCAA is not the only organization in which student-athletes participate. Smaller organizations such as The National Association of Intercollegiate Athletics (NAIA), National Christian College Athletic Association (NCCAA), and the National Junior College Athletics Association (NJCAA) also sponsor intercollegiate athletics programs across the U.S.

Injury is a very common phenomenon in sport. At one time, it was estimated that the annual rate of sport injury in the United States was roughly 17 million (Booth, 1987). It is likely greater than that now. For readers interested in keeping up with current college injury prevalence information across sports, the NCAA's Committee on Competitive Safeguards and Medical Aspects of Sports has operated an Injury Surveillance System (ISS) since 1982 for the purpose of annually collecting and making available data on student-athlete injury rates and trends over time by sports. (See www.ncaa.org/health-safety) (NCAA, 2006b.) A so-called "reportable injury" is defined as meeting three essential criteria:

(1) The injury is the consequence of involvement in an "organized intercollegiate practice or contest,"

(2) it necessitates medical attention or treatment by a team athletics trainers or team physician, and

(3) it leads to "restriction of the student-athlete's participation for one or more days beyond the day of injury" (NCAA, 2006c).

Recent data suggest that injury risk in intercollegiate athletics is significant and variable across sports and times of the year. "Participation in intercollegiate athletics involves unavoidable exposure to an inherent risk of injury" (NCAA Sports Medicine Handbook, 2006d, p. 4). **It is widely understood that athletic injury, especially severe or chronic injury, often involves emotional adjustment as well as physical recovery.** Taken together, NCAA ISS data reveal the pervasiveness of injury experienced by female and male college student-athletes and point to the need for mental health professionals (e.g., psychologists, counselors) to help members of this challenged on-campus population cope with losses in functioning that they sometimes are discouraged from addressing.

Challenges Associated with Providing Psychological Services to Student-Athletes

Rehabilitative support to injured student-athletes is typically provided by well-trained and caring sports medicine staff including athletic trainers, student athletics trainers, and physical therapists, as well as various sport medicine physicians (Kolt, 2000; Ray, Terrell, & Hough, 1999; Silva & Hardy, 1991). Their rehabilitative efforts traditionally focus on the current physical trauma associated with injury and with treatment(s) directed toward returning the student-athlete to the field, court, track, or pool as soon as possible, unless the injury is disabling (i.e., it is a condition that is characterized by long-term or permanent losses in functioning). Current thinking in this area supports a broader "biopsychosocial" view of injury response and rehabilitation beyond the medical model (Wiese-Bjornstal, Smith, Shaffer, & Morrey, 1998).

In light of the potentially serious short- and long-term impact and complexity of injury and disability, affected **athletes often are not prepared to return to participation.** This may be the case because, given the efficiency of modern rehabilitative interventions, they

- may have had little time to adjust to loss,
- may have a limited experience with injury or loss, or
- may have limited coping skills,

and therefore are vulnerable to experience a wide range of concomitant psychological responses (e.g., anxiety, fear, depression) (Rotella & Heyman, 1986). Although it is difficult to pinpoint the prevalence of post-injury psychological disturbance, it appears that the number of athletes who do struggle psychologically seems considerable (Brewer, Linder, & Phelps, 1995). Unfortunately, these psychological responses appear to be infrequently attended to by coaches and inconsistently addressed by collegiate sports medicine professionals, even in the case of distressing, disabling conditions. Today, however, incorporating psychological support into the overall rehabilitation process seems to be a "natural extension" of the physical rehabilitation process (Taylor & Taylor, 1997, pp. 35-55). For example, counseling of injured athletes has been noted as a universal competency for athletic trainers (Roh & Perna, 2000). Other authors argue that all sports medicine staff members have a legal and ethical obligation to provide at least basic counseling to injured athletes (Ray & Wiese-Bjornstal, 1999).

Several problems emerge, however, when attempting to expand the medical approach to recovery and return to play:

- First, sports medicine professionals are usually not extensively trained to consider various psychological aspects of assisting the injured and disabled. They may not understand or consider tapping the potential usefulness of psychological consultation or intervention for the impaired student-athlete who is attempting to cope with loss of functioning. Although occasionally there are on-campus helping professionals (e.g., psychologists, counselors, or psychiatrists), formally affiliated with the university sports medicine team, who could be helpful to the psychological rehabilitation of injured or disabled student-athletes, this does not seem to be the norm. Even though universities appear to be increasing their use of the services of mental health professionals, more commonly, athletic department staffs are not aware of either the availability of mental health professionals or the ways in which this expertise can be relevant to the rehabilitative process. Lack of awareness, in turn, may lead to problems in knowing when or how to refer an injured student-athlete. Even in the case of those sports medicine professionals who are sensitive to emotional consequences of injury, given the other extensive demands of their jobs, they may have very little time to devote to this complementary aspect of rehabilitation.

- Another noticeable obstacle is the pervasiveness and probable influence of the so-called "medical model," which does not incorporate psychosocial aspects and approaches to the treatment of injury. Accordingly, helping professionals seem to see fewer referrals of injured and disabled student-athletes from sports medicine professionals to on-campus psychological services than might be warranted given the frequency and severity of athletic injury. Although it can be argued that many sports medicine staff (in particular, athletic trainers) know the student-athletes they serve very well, adhering too closely to the medical model of care may unduly limit the range of complimentary care that facilitates athletic injury rehabilitation. It has been shown that psychological and social support can be a very useful adjunct to medical interventions because the effects of injury are not limited to the afflicted body part(s) alone (Eldridge, 1983; Hardy, Burke, & Crace, 1999; Heil, 1993; Lynch, 1988). For example, psychological skill training has been shown in randomized controlled trials both to lessen the incidence of athletic injury and to speed recovery following injury (Perna et al 2004).

- Reluctance to involve mental health professionals in rehabilitation is somewhat understandable. Even in the New Millennium among educated people, psychological treatment (i.e., counseling, psychotherapy, "sport psychology") remains a mystery and taboo. Stereotypic images of the analyst's couch and the bearded "shrink" persist; misconceptions about who seeks help from such people (i.e., only those who are weak, mentally ill, or crazy) may contribute to the avoidance of on-campus mental health professionals and their services, even if they are affiliated with the athletic department staff. In fact, college students in general, and student-athletes in particular, tend to underutilize psychological services for a variety of practical and age-appropriate, development-related reasons (Pinkerton, Hinz, & Barrow, 1987). This is normal and understandable and appears to be linked to some extent to college student developmental issues of struggling to become independent and dealing with perceived authority figures (Astin, 1977; Chickering, 1969; Farnsworth, 1966).

Even if student-athletes recognize the usefulness of psychological services, have an interest in obtaining counseling, and/or are referred for help, several obstacles may make such assistance difficult to tap or completely inaccessible to them. Barriers include

(a) the "high visibility" of student-athletes on campus,

(b) the limited amount of time available to seek psychological consultation,

(c) misconceptions about the makeup and personalities of student-athletes,

(d) the restrictive and controlled nature of the athletic environment, and

(e) certain personal characteristics of student-athletes (Ferrante, Etzel, & Lantz, 2002).

High visibility. Willingly or unwillingly, student-athletes are often high-profile members of their school's community. One athletic director described their experience as "living in a fishbowl." The names and faces of many of them appear regularly in the media. They can also stand out in a crowd because of their physical size and the gear they often wear: a well-known personality in a team jersey on crutches is quite recognizable hopping down the sidewalk. To avoid being seen and being seen as weak or in need, student-athletes often avoid places like counseling and psychological service centers because they cannot easily seek assistance as privately as others can. "I didn't feel comfortable sitting in the waiting room with everyone looking at me," one injured client complained. There is also often reluctance to seek help that is manifested as anxiety, shame, and procrastination that makes it difficult for students in general to seek help. Their notoriety can further compound the problem and prolong student-athletes overall recovery.

Time demands. Whether in or out of season, student-athletes typically lead hectic, stressful lifestyles (AIR, 1988; Etzel, 1989). Time, especially "free time," is a precious commodity. Although NCAA legislation puts a cap on the number of hours that college athletes may be involved in sport-related activities (i.e., 20 hours per week), historically many student-athletes have spent much more than 20 hours conditioning, practicing, and competing. The National Study of Intercollegiate Athletes (AIR, 1988) revealed that in 1987-88 student-athletes reported participating in excess of 30 hours per week in their chosen sport(s). The more-is-better approach to training appears prevalent. Participants in that same study reported that they spent more time participating in athletics-related activities than they did preparing for and attending classes. It appears that this has not changed much, if at all, in The New Millennium, especially in big-time, high-profile sports like football and basketball. The so-called "off season" too seems to have vanished as "individual workouts" and "voluntary" year-round training and "captain's practices" become more of the norm. (One recent client described his out-of-season training as the "fake" off-season.)

Clearly, there are individual differences in the amount of time devoted to participation across schools and programs of various competitive levels. Nevertheless, when combined with the amount of time that must be devoted to academics, daily individual responsibilities, and a limited personal life, usually little time is left during a highly structured day to seek professional help at mental health services that are typically open from 8 a.m. to 5 p.m. Not surprisingly, student-athlete frustration with this situation is common. We cannot recall the number of times a student-athlete has said to us: "Doc, I just can't seem to make it in to meet with you. Got any time after 7 tonight or this weekend?" Involvement in rehabilitation can be very time-consuming and exhausting as well. Indeed, a seriously injured person can spend many hours each day, sometimes visiting the training room twice a day, rehabilitating an injury. Coach pressure to return to play can put considerable pressure on athletes to "get it done."

Misconceptions about student-athletes. Student-athletes, in particular football and men's basketball players, and members of other athletic teams on certain campuses, are often seen by the community as a spoiled, "over-privileged" group (Remer, Tongate, & Watson, 1978). Some may assume that the athletic department is taking care of all of their needs. Therefore, on-campus mental health professionals who could be of assistance to the injured or disabled may not see a need to reach out to a group perceived as "spoiled" and treated quite differently than non-athletes by the university. Some providers do not have competency with the issues athletes bring to the counseling services. They may also be reluctant to provide student-athletes services as they do not see it as their role. Although some student-athletes may well be pampered, some are challenged young people who truly have a need for personal assistance in the wake of an injury. Services should be as available to them as they are to any other student.

Restrictive environments. Over the years, many athletic departments have come to be seen by others, and often by themselves, as autonomous organizations and entities on campus. Sperber (1990) goes so far as to say that many athletic departments are merely entertainment businesses that have essentially no bona fide connection to the mission of their respective academic institutions. They are now sometimes referred to as "auxiliaries" of the university, acting as agents of the NCAA described by Zimbalist (1999) as a "cartel . . . [whose purpose is] to maintain a player reserve system and contain its costs for profit" (p. 18). Independent-minded, controlling athletic department staff also may not trust mental health professionals or other "outsiders" with the care of their student-athletes. Somehow, it is erroneously assumed by some that all student-athlete needs can be met by athletic department staff alone (except in times of true crisis). Indeed, the "We can take care of our own in-house" attitude appears to be held by many athletic department staff, particularly coaches. Those departments or teams who have healthy budgets also may hire external consultants to provide help to injured athletes instead of using free on-campus professionals. Indeed, a colleague recently commented: "The higher the athlete's profile, the further from the counseling service they are treated."

Student-athlete attributes and developmental tasks. Other perceived barriers to injured college student-athletes seeking psychological assistance are linked to a mixture of personal characteristics (e.g., behaviors and attitudes), as well as certain so-called "developmental tasks" that all college students face (Astin, 1977; Chickering, 1969; Farnsworth, 1966; Pascarella & Terenzini, 2005). As a group, student-athletes tend to be rather independent. This is understandable in view of some of the messages they may learn from influential others in the athletic world. Also, individualism is characteristic of college students in general. Indeed, one of the major developmental tasks of college students involves struggling to become an independent adult (Chickering, 1969). Over time, many student-athletes seem to acquire a sense that they can solve most (if not all) of their difficulties. They also learn through sport to be strong and to minimize or deny physical and emotional pain. If one is not tough or "macho," one is somehow an inferior or weak person. These messages may be heard from coaches, peers, and our culture.

This is particularly applicable to young males who are reluctant in general to adopt heath-promoting behavior and tend to hide illness and injury (Courtenay, 1998). Therefore, injured or disabled student-athletes, especially young men, may not be inclined to ask for or seek help even though they may be experiencing considerable distress and suffering. Some suggest that the tendency to avoid discussion of the physical and emotional impact of injury is present in adolescence prior to entering college (Newcomer & Perna, 2003). "When rugged individualism . . . leads to, or heightens, an unwillingness to seek or accept assistance, athletes will find themselves separated from existing and potential sources of social support" (Pearson & Petitpas, 1990, p. 9). Consequently, persistent encouragement to seek outside psychological assistance on the part of referral sources (e.g., athletic trainers) is often necessary to get assistance from helping professionals for an independent-minded, injured or disabled student-athlete.

Another developmental task that this group must work through involves learning to deal effectively with authority (Farnsworth, 1966). Those who have problems relating to powerful others often will not respond to their guidance or direction or do so grudgingly (e.g., in the case of forced referrals). Consequently, referral for psychological assistance may be met with considerable resistance, even though it is a suggestion that is likely in the best interest of the injured person. If people with such difficulties who do come to obtain help are forced to do so by others (e.g., coaches or trainers), they must be handled with sensitivity so as not to alienate them.

It is not uncommon for those who do ultimately make contact with a helping professional to expect that they can obtain relief in a very brief amount of time and/or without much personal effort. Upon becoming aware of this agenda (the "quick fix"), the astute clinician must carefully educate the injured person about the nature of psychological treatment (e.g., roles of client and therapist, goal setting, responsibility for change and ways in which it may occur) so as to create realistic expectations for their work together. Solution-based approaches and motivational interviewing can be very useful to such referrals (Friedman & Fanger, 1993; Miller & Rollnick, 2002). Additionally, efforts can be made to train sports medicine staff properly to educate clients prior to making referrals regarding the nature, scope, and pace of psychological services.

Finally, for those who can have an impact on assisting injured or disabled student-athletes, it will be helpful to assume a broader view of the individuals who are both college students and participants in athletics. Student-athletes are not students or athletes first and foremost. Rather, they are at their core developing young *people* in transition who are in the process of becoming adults. They are continuously working through the many developmental tasks of their stage in life such as

(a) becoming independent;

(b) dealing with authority;

(c) learning to deal with uncertainty and ambiguity;

(d) developing personal standards, values, and a sense of purpose;

(e) developing a mature sexuality;

(f) developing feelings of security and competence;

(g) establishing personal identity and attaining prestige and esteem; and

(h) managing emotions

(Astin, 1977; Chickering, 1969; Farnsworth, 1969). Further, their roles of students and entertainers frequently make the transition from childhood to adulthood more complicated (Ferrante, Etzel, & Lantz, 2002). Therefore, it is most helpful to cast a broad therapeutic net and to view their experience of athletic injury and disability within the context of their uniquely demanding lifestyles and developmental position.

Clearly, our position underlines the importance of taking a holistic approach, grounded in evidence-based practice, to the treatment, rehabilitation, and aftercare of injured and disabled student-athletes. We believe that the student-athlete is a *person* first, and it is from this "person-ness" that the athletic, academic, developmental, and career needs evolve. Accordingly, athletic injury can be regarded as both an obstacle and a threat to the realization of long- and short-term needs and goals. Injury and disability can leave student-athletes vulnerable to distress that can complicate and inhibit the process of physical and psychological rehabilitation (Petrie & Perna, 2004). These difficult trials can also offer an opportunity for significant personal growth (Perna, Ahlgren, & Zaichkowsky, 1999). We believe that injured or disabled student-athletes can best be served by understanding their unique needs within the context of their individual histories, personalities, current experiences, and aspirations.

The Unique Consequences of Incurring an Injury for College Student-Athletes

The ways that people characteristically respond to sport-related injury and the theoretical concepts that help us understand why they respond in these ways have been discussed in previous chapters of this book and in other resources (Astle, 1986; Brown, 2005; May & Seib, 1987; Rotella & Heyman, 1986; Silva & Hardy, 1991; Taylor & Taylor, 1997; Tunick, Etzel, & Leard, & Lerner, 1996); therefore, we will not review them here. There are, however, several points that we believe can help the reader understand how college student-athletes respond to injury and/or disability and how to better assist them as they struggle to cope with their losses.

The novelty of loss. When student-athletes' physical capacities are suddenly or progressively not what they have been throughout life, it may simply be the first time they have encountered such a situation. They typically have been successful, highly functioning people: the world of injury and loss is foreign territory for many student-athletes. Indeed, many 18–21-year-olds often have a limited, if any, history of significant losses. They may have little appreciation of the finite nature of human capacities. When student-athletes are not capable of doing what they have taken for granted all their lives, it can be a very frustrating, unwanted revelation. For adults in a position to assist injured or disabled young athlete—adults who usually own a more extensive loss history—it may be difficult to appreciate the magnitude and complexity of the problem. Therefore, it is important that coaches, sport medicine, and helping professionals not underestimate or discount the impact of injury on student-athletes. So, when first meeting with these clients during an initial interview or intake, it is important to sensitively inquire about that person's loss history in sport and outside of sport (e.g., moving, death of relatives or pets, relationship breakups, etc.), which may provide insightful links to healing from physical loss of functioning.

The effects of changed status. As is the case with non-athletes, when student-athletes become injured or disabled, their lives may change in various ways psychosocially. While many injured athletes have uncomplicated adjustment, some do not adjust well. Suddenly or over time, these student-athletes often become isolated and alienated from their peers, experience changes in their social status, and may encounter new academic/developmental concerns (Ermler & Thomas, 1990; Pearson & Petitpas, 1990; Tunick et al., 1996). Student-athletes who cannot take part in day-to-day athletic activities (e.g., conditioning, practicing, traveling, and competing) become separated from their teammates, coaches, and others with whom they normally interact. They become regular "customers" of the sports medicine staff. Because they can no longer function in their customary roles, injured people may become gradually or suddenly estranged from their previously predictable and supportive social network. Sadly, they sometimes are intentionally or unintentionally ignored, set aside, or criticized for being injured by insensitive coaches or peers (which somehow implies that one is weak, less valuable, or not committed enough to "tough it out"). Blaming the victim (i.e., injured athlete) is quite common. The time once spent on the field or in the weight room is now spent in the care of athletic trainers in the athletic training room, with some time sitting on the bench watching others do the now impossible and perhaps traveling with their team. One disabled client succinctly described the confusion and frustration of being in this unfortunate situation in the following way: "It's like I'm on the team, but I'm really not. I don't know what else to do."

Other relationships can and do change for injured or disabled student-athletes. Although their visible physical conditions often make them the focus of public attention for a while, as time passes they fade from the spotlight. Their sport "war stories" become old news, as healthy others take their places on the field or the court or in the pool. Other students on campus and media do not pay as much attention to the student-athlete as they did in the past. Social opportunities often become fewer for the formerly popular athlete. There are no fascinating tales to relate about the upcoming game or meet, only recollections of bygone accomplishments and the unglamorous rehabilitation process are left to tell. Special status is lost or at least diminished. Mental health professionals need to inquire about and be sensitive to this unsettling social transition, taking into consideration individual, gender, and cultural differences associated with changing relationships and status.

Confronted with the reality of assuming a sometimes radically different, usually unanticipated, lifestyle change, injured and disabled student-athletes face different academic situations and social changes. More free time is sometimes available to fortunate injured student-athletes whose rehabilitation activities do not consume a large part of the day, although the opposite may be true in cases of injured yet still active players who require many hours of rehabilitation daily to stay in playing condition. In such situations, academic priorities can come more to the forefront and serve as a "blessing in disguise" for those who have neglected their studies by choice or because of the demands of their active lifestyles. Those working with this group of clients may also hear them report that they have not really been invested much in academics and feel overwhelmed at the prospect of doing so. Previously flexible professors who do not appreciate the need for accommodation, however, may become less sympathetic to the impaired student-athlete who may still need occasional special arrangements in view of the demands and inconveniences of the rehabilitation process (Tunick et al., 1996). Such challenges often need to be addressed and appreciated by mental health professionals to best help student-athletes make decisions, establish or alter priorities, and regain or maintain balance both in and out of the classroom.

For student-athletes with disabilities, especially those whose condition is career ending, academic priorities and career paths will probably need to be closely reexamined in a timely fashion. For many of those faced with this fundamental and usually unprecedented life transition, school and other interests gradually assume a higher priority. The opposite may be true, too, as one's identity and life purpose are contested. These rather "disoriented" ex-athletes are often retention risks who can benefit from a reassessment of purpose, interests, skills, and abilities. On-campus helping professionals who are trained in career-vocational testing and counseling can be great assets in such cases. (See Petitpas et al., 1997, and Riffee & Alexander, 1991, for a discussion of career counseling strategies for student-athletes.) In the case of disabled student-athletes, educational-vocational counseling and supportive psychotherapy can be undertaken concurrently and interactively because there is usually considerable overlap in the concerns seen in such cases (Pinkerton, Etzel, Rockwell, Talley, & Moorman, 1990).

Injured and disabled student-athletes may benefit from combined psychological interventions that address questions about changing **personal identity** (i.e., confidence in maintaining a sense of continuity and sameness of the self) (Chickering, 1969) and a shift in "athletic identity" (Brewer, 1993) to one centered outside of sport. (The reader will recall that developing a sense of personal identity is one of the central developmental life tasks of college students.) When impaired student-athletes are forced to examine who they are, and realize that they cannot be who they once were, they are often left with an overwhelming sense of confusion and numbness. These natural feelings of loss regularly trigger questions about one's identity. This is particularly true for college students as Grayson (1989) observed. Kir-Stimon's (1977) discussion of the mindset of severely disabled persons at the onset of emotional rehabilitation is very similar to what we often hear injured and disabled student-athletes say to themselves:

Who am I?
I am different than I was.
I don't like me.
Nobody likes me.
I am not worthwhile.
Perhaps I never was worthwhile.
Who was I?
I have no real identity anymore.
I have changed. Nothing is the same as before.
My friends, my family, the world about me has changed.
I am lost.

(Kir-Stimon, 1977, p. 365)

Addressing the question of "Who am I if I'm not an athlete?" can be very difficult because some student-athletes have "foreclosed" on their identities early in life (Marcia, 1966). That is, many have learned to identify themselves as athletes at a young age and so act in ways that are consistent with their self-perceptions (Brewer, 1993; Brewer et al., 1995; Chartrand & Lent, 1987; Petitpas et al, 1997). Therefore, it can be quite unsettling to student-athletes (especially for the alarming number of male baseball, basketball, and football players who expect to become professionals) when the self view of being an athlete must be involuntarily abandoned. Indeed, some research suggests that student-athletes may be less mature than their non-athlete peers in terms of being able to make educational and career plans and decisions (Blann, 1985; Kornspan & Etzel, 2004; Sowa & Gressard, 1983. (It is one author's observation in reviewing over 20 years of work with this population that a very small number of student-athletes engage in career counseling.) Nevertheless, encouraging an injured and disabled young person to obtain professional assistance for personal-social and/or educational-vocational concerns in post-injury/disability transition is often very timely from developmental and practical standpoints. Furthermore, universities typically have career development and counseling centers that offer such services for free or for very low cost.

Providing Psychological Assistance to Injured or Disabled Student-Athletes

Although there appears to be a slowly growing trend to involve mental health providers in athletics, only a small number of universities today have professionally trained psychologists, counselors, or psychiatrists whose duties specifically involve providing direct psychological service to student-athletes. Most of these institutions appear to utilize professionals who are members of counseling services, allied mental health centers, or in some instances private practitioners. A select few schools have a staff member who serves as a liaison with the athletic department and links to **CHAMPS/Life Skills programs**: these NCAA programs provide models for programming and assistance to student-athletes that have considerable potential for networking with student-athletes. A very small number of schools appear to have a professional who is affiliated with both the athletic department and a mental health service (Ferrante & Etzel, 2002). Whatever the administrative arrangement, on-campus helping professionals who are interested in or who have been hired to provide assistance to student-athletes in general, and in particular those who are injured and disabled, face many professional challenges.

As mentioned above, several barriers serve to separate helping professionals from injured or disabled student-athletes who could benefit from their expertise. To begin to bridge the gaps that exist, the helping professional interested and trained to help this population will greatly benefit from the support of the athletic director, the chief student affairs officer, the team physician, and sports medicine staff. This influential network of people can assist the helping professional in initial efforts to establish credibility within the often closed athletic community. These people have the ability to create an inroad to the coaching staff and student-athletes that the helping professional may otherwise never develop alone. Some of these people are also crucial to making referrals of injured athletes for psychological assistance.

Given a crack in the door, the helping professional must begin the process of educating the athletic community about the potential usefulness of psychological assistance to injured and disabled student-athletes. This is a constant challenge within intercollegiate athletics community. In general, coaches, student-athletes, sports medicine staff, and administrators do not appear to readily understand how such services can be helpful (or they may be resistant for reasons mentioned earlier). Establishing credibility is a long-term process that can be quite frustrating. Indeed, one of the authors of this chapter was reminded by an athletic department administrator: "Remember, 95% of the people here don't care about what you do."

Meeting with coaches, sports medicine staff, and each team on a regular basis, (i.e., at the beginning of the academic year when NCAA compliance and sports medicine introductory sessions are conducted) is an effective way of introducing the professional to potential referral sources and consumers of services. With the permission of coaches and sports medicine staff, regularly attending practices and visiting athletic training rooms are also effective ways of familiarizing people with the helping professional and the services available to injured and disabled student-athletes. These practices may also serve to undo some of the stigma associated with psychologists and psychological consultation (e.g., "Dr. X is an okay person who is interested in helping us and who can be trusted").

Offering workshops as part of CHAMPS/Life Skills outreach programming is a promising practice. Brochures, posters, and flyers about helping services strategically placed in athletics training rooms and athletics facility bulletin boards are sometimes helpful in advertising the helping services available to student-athletes. Marketing that promotes the confidentiality of this help is important. Offering these services for free or at low cost will facilitate client referrals and self-referrals.

Finally, the Internet offers a powerful, broad-based approach to increasing awareness of psychological assistance for student-athletes and staff that has many advantages to traditional call-in information or service requests (Zizzi & Perna, 2003). Web-based information about counseling and related services is often part of the athletic department website. Internet savvy student-athletes can readily access information about psychological services on campus associated with athletics that can be helpful to them. These sites are confidential gateways to receiving assistance when needed. (See http://www.wvu.edu/~sports/services/ as an example). In the end, the best source of referral appears to be past clients of support service providers who have benefited from psychological consultation.

Although there are many "players" in the athletic community, perhaps the single most important relationship to establish and nurture is the one between athletic trainers and the mental health professional. Athletic trainers historically have a very special relationship with coaches and student-athletes (Compton & Ferrante, 1991; Roh & Perna, 1999). They are perhaps the most trusted people within the athletic community. Indeed, their services are clearly understood, needed, and utilized by numerous rehabilitating athletes on a daily basis. In contrast, this is typically not the case with mental health professionals and their services, unless such services have been used for some time. Developing essential, close relationships with the athletic training staff appears critical to accessing of injured and disabled student-athletes. These relationships can enhance the extent to which helping professionals are accepted and trusted by the athletic community. Also, athletic trainers can be good referral sources of student-athletes who have been injured or who have other difficulties of which the athletic trainer becomes aware (e.g., personal-social problems, substance use, performance decrements, learning disabilities). Making presentations to student trainers about mental health issues, psychological aspects of injury and disability, communication skills, and referral methods can help develop good working relationships with helping professionals and the athletic training staff and their trainees. Student athletic trainers can be or become effective and trustworthy points of contact and referral for needy student-athletes.

Finally, another method of facilitating the provision of psychological assistance to injured or disabled student-athletes is to conduct needs assessments and other surveys. For example, collecting data on the psychological responses to loss of functioning can help establish and reinforce the need to provide counseling or therapeutic services. Undertaking research in collaboration with interested sports medicine staff members can provide a wealth of useful information as well as promote the cooperative efforts of athletic trainers and helping professionals.

Assessment and Intervention

Various authors have commented on ways to assess the psychological status and needs of the injured or disabled person (Heil, 1993; Brewer & Petitpas, 2005; Ray & Wiese-Bjornstahl, 1999). At very least, conducting a clinical interview seems essential to the assessment process. Karg and Wiens (2005) provide a list of suggestions about clinically proven and empirically validated interview content and practices for use in an initial interview. The Sport Clinical Intake Protocol (SCIP) also has considerable utility in these instances (Taylor & Schneider, 1992). One student-athlete instrument that practitioners may want to consider using since it casts a broad net of inquiry is the Life Events Survey for College Athletes (LESCA) (Petrie, 1992).

A general approach to counseling that has proven effective with this group of clients, especially those who may be in an early stages of change (i.e., "resistant"), new to counseling, or somewhat uncomfortable with the notion of referral to a mental health professional post injury, is motivational interviewing (Miller & Rollnick, 2002). These approaches often guide the client in less direct ways by helping them explore their own personal reasons for engaging in particular behaviors prior to "prescribing" interventions such as goal setting, rehabilitation exercises, or other techniques. Ultimately, activity associated with this early phase of treatment should enable a good understanding of the biopsychosocial impact of injury on clients, as well as a sense of their ability to cope with the condition and their motivation for rehabilitation. Accomplishment of all of these should ultimately generate clear and meaningful treatment goals and productive counseling over the course of adjustment and recovery.

The Impact of Injury and Disability on College Student-Athletes: Two Case Examples

The following two case examples are offered to provide further insight into the psychological impact of sport injuries and the role of psychological services in the treatment and follow-up of injured and disabled student-athletes. Each case describes the general course of counseling with an NCAA Division I-A student-athlete. Because of ethical considerations, these cases are presented in composite form to protect the confidentiality of clients.

Case 1

Ann was a highly motivated, 20-year-old diver who was in her sophomore year at the university. She had been moderately successful in her relatively new sport, which she had turned to in high school after participating in gymnastics since age 5. Despite her relative inexperience, under the tutelage of a competent and encouraging young coach, Ann had become quite skilled. While preparing for an upcoming meet one early morning, perhaps not fully awake, she attempted a rather routine back dive and struck the back of her head on the board and crashed into the diving well dazed. Her athletic trainers pulled her, still conscious, from the water, and called 911. Ann was quickly transported to the university emergency department. She was evaluated by the ED staff, who administered a CT scan and subsequently released her later that day, although she felt slightly disoriented. She was diagnosed with a grade 2 mild traumatic brain injury (MTBI) (i.e., "concussion").

The team physician met with Ann in the late afternoon. She determined that Ann was not capable of training and barred her from such activity, to include the upcoming weekend meet. Her parents were immediately contacted; her mother traveled from the family home about 3 hours away by car to care for her. The team physician set a follow-up appointment with Ann for the next afternoon.

Unfortunately, that night Ann had considerable difficulty sleeping, she complained of a persistent headache, felt "cranky," and found herself crying on and off "for no reason at all" during the night. When she met with the team physician the next afternoon with her mother in tow, Ann's affect seemed rather flat and she was intermittently tearful again when with the team physician. Her physician directed Ann to check in with the head athletic trainer each afternoon for a week until she had no symptoms. She would then meet with her again to determine if she could return to participation.

After a week away from training, Ann was functioning better for the most part. She passed an exertion test. With the consent of the head athletic trainer and team physician Ann was cleared to return to train. However, she reported to her athletic trainer that she felt "kinda unhappy," had experienced some difficulty concentrating in class, and could not remember as much as she normally would from lectures and reading. The decision to participate in the weekend conference meet was left up to her and her coach. They both decided to go ahead and let her compete, even though she had not trained much. Unfortunately, she did not perform well at all and returned home on the Monday following the meet discouraged.

Over the course of the next two weeks, Ann continued to train in preparation for the upcoming conference championships. While her diving improved a bit, she was not the same athlete she had been. Ann privately felt uncomfortable on the board and continued to experience mood and academic difficulties. She did not really want to let on that this was happening given her commitment to competing for her team. Ann eventually confided in her athletic trainer, who decided to refer her to a counseling center psychologist associated with athletics. Her initial evaluation revealed that Ann was struggling with moderate depression and mild generalized anxiety, as well as lingering cognitive problems (e.g., attention and memory) that continued to affect her academic performance. It was also learned that Ann had acquired some anxiety associated with the act of diving. Ann met with her new psychologist twice more. They decided that it would be helpful for her to be referred for a psychiatric evaluation to inquire about the usefulness of psychotropic medication and an evaluation at the counseling center for learning difficulties.

A university health service psychiatrist prescribed a small amount of an SSRI that in the short run improved her mood. The learning disability evaluation did not reveal the existence of a diagnosable disorder. Ann continued to see her psychologist through the end of the spring semester (eight more sessions). They worked together on her performance anxiety with learning challenges. During the summer she stopped taking her SSRI after having consulted with her family physician. Ann returned to the university and the diving team in the fall. She followed up with her psychologist and the sports medicine team at the beginning of the academic year and was cleared to participate in her sport.

Case 2

A student-athlete was referred for consultation and recommendations by the director of sports medicine following extensive neurological and other medical examinations. Several months prior to the referral, the student-athlete had experienced a number of symptoms including paresthesias (i.e., numbing and tingling sensations in the hands and feet and part of the face) with accompanying motoric changes, blurred vision, and generally decreased coordination. Results of subsequent examinations revealed that the student-athlete had experienced a demyelinating episode, a phenomenon that is seen in several disorders of unknown etiology. Of these, multiple sclerosis (MS) is the most prominent. The diagnosis of MS becomes quite difficult in that it requires the occurrence of a second demyelinating episode; remission can be quite long-term (e.g., up to 25 years). Consequently, a firm diagnosis could not be made. However, the student-athlete was provided with information to help better understand his general medical situation as it existed. Then, he was referred for psychological services to assess his current psychological functioning and to obtain emotional support and decision-making assistance.

In the initial session, the student-athlete complained of feeling frustrated, discouraged, and intermittently angry and sad. He also reported feeling anxious in view of the "incomplete diagnosis," its potential limitations regarding the questions of his continued sport participation, and uncertainties regarding his personal functioning in the future. Further exploration of the situation revealed that his parents appeared to be denying the implications of the medical examinations. Stating that they "didn't raise a quitter," they were pressing him to continue to participate in his sport. He was also afraid of disappointing his teammates and coach and felt threatened by the possibility of not meeting their expectations. Unfortunately, the student-athlete was physically incapable of performing at the high skill level that he had previously achieved and, as a result, was experiencing considerable dissonance.

In consultation with the referring physician, it was agreed that a treatment team would be formed consisting of the physician, an athletic trainer, and a clinical/counseling sport psychologist. The treatment team plan involved the following: (a) monitoring the student-athlete's medical progress and providing information about the condition; (b) developing and implementing a "controlled" workout/training regimen; and (c) providing supportive counseling/psychotherapy to help him cope with various stressors and assist with decision making relative to the situation.

The student-athlete's participation in regular counseling provided a confidential, professional setting in which he was continually encouraged to explore his concerns and feelings. Over the course of several months, he received help dealing with the personal-social stress surrounding the need to make important decisions (e.g., whether he should prematurely end his sports career, how to interact with his coaches and parents) without the aid of a firm diagnosis. With the assistance of the psychologist, he also was able to resolve issues surrounding his parents and their expectations, as well as the pressures of his coach and teammates.

The role of the athletic trainer and the controlled workout/training regimen held special, strategic significance to the process and outcome of the case. More specifically, the student-athlete faced a number of difficult decisions—each without the benefit of a concrete diagnosis, information that would have made decisions more clear-cut. The controlled workout setting allowed for the development of progressive training goals and the monitoring of any physiological distress, if it occurred. In that setting the student-athlete was encouraged to test progressive limits comfortably, away from the coach's watchful eye and any teammate pressures. With the support of the athletic trainer, the student-athlete was able to gain confidence and experience-based insight into his current level of functioning by seeing gradual increases in performance with or without symptoms. Having made significant progress in the controlled training program, he ultimately rejoined his team with the permission of the physician. Although it was gratifying for him to be a part of his team again, he had experienced ongoing discouragement for some time in view of the fact that his athletic abilities were still well below their previous level. As a consequence of this dissatisfaction, following the conclusion of his season, he announced to his psychologist that he had decided to pursue a medical release and resign from the team—something he had considered and processed in counseling. His plan was to focus on academics and to continue with other campus and community involvements. The student-athlete continued his counseling relationship for some time and obtained assistance with concerns surrounding his premature retirement from sport, as well as issues concerning his personal adjustment to a different lifestyle.

Summary

The preceding chapter has been an attempt to share information about the struggles of injured and disabled student-athletes and ways to provide psychological support to a group of young people who experience unique personal challenges during their college years. We believe that to assist more fully their coping with and recovery from injury and disability, it is important to understand

(a) their distinctive lifestyles,

(b) the shared and idiosyncratic "mix" of developmental tasks that they must confront, and

(c) the considerable athletics system barriers that exist that can prevent or discourage them from seeking and/or obtaining helping services.

The authors hope that our experience-based observations and suggestions will prove useful to readers who want to better understand and more effectively lend a hand to the growing number of student-athletes who experience sport-related losses in functioning each year.

References

American Institutes for Research (AIR). (1988). *Summary results from the 1987-88 national study of intercollegiate athletes* (Report No.1). Palo Alto, CA: Center for the Study of Athletics.

Astin, A. (1977). *Four critical years.* San Francisco: Jossey-Bass.

Astle, S. (1986). The experience of loss in athletes. *Journal of Sports Medicine, 26,* 279-284.

Blann, F. (1985). Intercollegiate athletic competition and student's educational and career plans. *Journal of College Student Personnel, 26,* 115-118.

Booth, W. (1987), Arthritis institute tackles sport. *Science, 237,* 846-847.

Brewer, B. (1993). Athletic identity: Hercules muscles or Achilles heel? *International Journal of Sport Psychology, 24,* 237-254.

Brewer, B., Linder, B., & Phelps, C. (1995). Situational correlates of emotional adjustment to athletics injury. *Clinical Journal of Sport Medicine, 5,* 241-245.

Brewer, B., & Petitpas, A. (2005). Returning to self: The anxieties of coming back after injury, (pp. 93-108). In M. Andersen (Ed.), *Sport psychology in practice.* Champaign, IL: Human Kinetics.

Brown, C. (2005). Injuries: The psychology of injury and rehab. In S. Murphy (Ed.), *The sport psych handbook.* (pp. 215-235). Champaign, IL: Human Kinetics.

Chartrand, J., & Lent, R. (1987). Sports counseling: Enhancing the development of the student athlete. *Journal of College Student Personnel, 66,* 164-167.

Chickering, A. (1969). *Education and identity.* Washington, DC: Jossey-Bass.

Compton, R., & Ferrante, A. (1991). The athletic trainer-helping professional relationship: An essential element for the enhanced support programming for student-athletes. In E. Etzel, A. Ferrante, & J. Pinkney, (Eds.), *Counseling college student-athletes: Issues and interventions* (pp.221-230). Morgantown, WV: Fitness Information Technology.

Courtenay, W. (1998). College men's health: An overview and a call to action. *Journal of American College Health, 46,* 6, 279-290.

Eldridge, W. (1983). The importance of psychotherapy for athletic related orthopedic injuries among adults. *Comprehensive Psychiatry, 24,* 271-277.

Ermler, K., & Thomas, C. (1990). Interventions for the alienating effect of injury. *Athletic Training, 25,* 269-271.

Etzel, E. (1989). *Life stress, locus of control, and sport competition anxiety patterns of college student-athletes.* Unpublished doctoral dissertation, West Virginia University, Morgantown.

Farnsworth, D. (1966). *Psychiatry, education, and the young adult.* Springfield, IL: Thomas.

Ferrante, A., Etzel, E., & Lantz, C. (2002). Counseling college student-athletes: The problem, the need 1996. In E. Etzel, A. Ferrante, & J. Pinkney (Eds.), *Counseling college student-athletes: Issues and interventions* (2nd ed., pp.3-26). Morgantown, WV: Fitness Information Technology.

Friedman, S., & Fanger, M. (1993). Expanding therapeutic possibilities: Getting results in brief therapy. Lexington, MA: DC Heath.

Grayson, P. (1989). The college psychotherapy client. An overview. In Grayson, P. & Cauley, K. (Eds.) *College psychotherapy* (pp. 8-28). New York: The Guilford Press.

Hardy, C., Burke, K., & Crace, K. (1999). Social support and injury: A framework for support-based interventions with injured athletes. In D. Pargman (Ed.), *Psychological based of sport injuries* (2nd ed., pp. 175-198). Morgantown, WV: Fitness Information Technology.

Heil, J. (Ed.). (1993). *Psychology of sport injury*. Champaign, IL: Human Kinetics.

Karg, R., & Wiens, A. (2005). Improving diagnostic and clinical interviewing. In G. Koocher, J. Norcross, & S. Hill (Eds.), *Psychologist's desk reference* (2nd ed., pp. 13-16). New York: Oxford University Press.

Kir-Stimon, W. (1977). Counseling with the severely handicapped: Encounter and commitment. In R. Marinelli & A. Del Orto (Eds.), *Psychological and social impact of physical disability* (pp. 363-369). New York: Springer.

Klossner, D. (2005). Mental health in sport. Paper presented at the meeting of the Annual Association for the Advancement of Applied sport Psychology, Vancouver, Canada.

Kolt, G. (2000). Doing sport psychology with injured athletes. In M. Andersen (Ed.), *Doing sport psychology* (pp. 223-236). Champaign, IL: Human Kinetics.

Kornspan, A. & Etzel, E. (2004). What do we know about the career maturity of college student-athletes? A brief review and practical suggestions for career development work with student-athletes. Athletic Academic Journal, 17, 15-33.

Kushner, H. (1981). *When bad things happen to good people*. New York: Avon.

Lanese, R., Strauss, R., Leizman, D., & Rotondi, A. (1990). Injury and disability in matched men's and women's intercollegiate sports. *American Journal of Public Health, 80*, 1459-1462.

Lynch, G. (1988). Athletic injuries and the practicing sport psychologist: Practical guidelines for assisting athletes. *The Sport Psychologist, 2*, 161-167.

Marcia, J. (1966). Development and validation of ego-identity status. *Journal of Personality and Social Psychology, 3*, 551-558.

May, J., & Seib, G. (1987). Athletic injuries: Psychological factors in the onset, sequelae, and prevention. In J. May & M. Asken (Eds.), *Sport psychology: The psychological health of the athlete* (pp.157-185). Great Neck, NY: PMA.

Miller, W., & Rollnick, S. (2002). *Motivational interviewing* (2nd ed.). NewYork: The Guilford Press.

National Collegiate Athletic Association (2006a). Summary of NCAA sports sponsorship and participation rates data related to the decline of sponsorship of Olympic sports. Retrieved February 23, 2006 from http://www.ncaa.org/library/research/participation_rates/1982-2003/olympic_sports_supplement.pdf

National Collegiate Athletics Association (2006b). NCAA injury surveillance system methods. Retrieved February 15, 2006, from http://www1.ncaa.org/ membership/ed_outreach/health-safety/iss/methods

National Collegiate Athletics Association (2006c). Sport specific injury data 2004-2005. Retrieved February 16, 2006 from http://www1.ncaa.org/membership/ed_outreach/healthsafety/iss/Reports 2004-05.

National Collegiate Athletic Association (2006d). Sports medicine handbook. Retrieved February 23, 2006 from http://www.ncaa.org/library/sports_sciences/sports_med_handbook/2005-06/2005-06_sports_medicine_handbook.pdf

Newcomer, R. R., & Perna, F. M. (2003). Features of posttraumatic distress among adolescent athletes. *Journal of Athletic Training, 38*, 163-166.

Pascarella, E., & Terenzini, P. (2005). *How college affects students: A third decade of research*. San Francisco: Jossey-Bass.

Pearson, R., & Petitpas, A. (1990). Transitions of athletes: Developmental and preventive perspectives. *Journal of Counseling and Development, 69*, 7-10.

Perna, F. M., Ahlgren, R. L. & Zaichkowsky, L. (1999). The influence of career planning, race, and athletic injury on life satisfaction among recently retired collegiate male athletes. *The Sport Psychologist, 13(2)*, 144-157.

Perna, F. M., Antoni, M. H., Baum, A., Gordon, P. & Schneiderman, N. (2004) Cognitive behavioral stress management effects on injury and illness among competitive athletes: A randomized clinical trial. *Annals of Behavioral Medicine, 25*, 66-73.

Petitpas, A., Champagne, D., Chartrand, J., Danish, S., & Murphy, S. (1997). High school. *Athlete's guide for career planning: Keys to success from the playing field to professional life* (pp. 23-42). Champaign, IL: Human Kinetics.

Petrie, T. (1992). Life events survey for college athletes (LESCA). *Behavioral Medicine, 18(3)*, 127-138.

Petrie, T. A., & Perna, F. M. (2004). Psychology of Injury: Theory, Research and Practice. In T. Morris and J. Summers (Eds.), *Sport Psychology: Theories, Applications and Issues 2nd Edition* (pp. 547- 571). Milton, Queensland, Australia: John Wiley & Sons.

Pinkerton, R., Etzel, E., Talley, J., & Moorman, J. (1990). Psychotherapy and career counseling: Toward an integration for use with college students. *Journal of American College Health, 39,* 129-136.

Pinkerton, R., Hinz, L., & Barrow, J. (1987). The college student-athlete: Psychological considerations and interventions. *Journal of American College Health,37,* 218-226.

Ray, R., Terrell, T., & Hough, D. (1999). The role of the sports medicine professional in counseling athletes. In R. Ray & D. Wiese-Bjornstahl (Eds.) *Counseling in sports medicine.* (pp. 3-20). Champaign, IL: Human Kinetics.

Ray, R., & Wiese-Bjornstahl, D. (Eds.). (1999). *Counseling in sports medicine.* Champaign, IL: Human Kinetics.

Remer, R., Tongate, R., & Watson, J. (1978). Counseling the underprivileged minority. *The Personnel and Guidance Journal, 56,* 626-619.

Riffee, K., & Alexander, D. (1991). Career strategies for student-athletes: A developmental model. In E. Etzel, A. Ferrante, & J. Pinkney (Eds.), *Counseling college student-athletes: Issues and interventions* (pp. 101-120). Morgantown, WV: Fitness Information Technology.

Roh, J. & Perna, F. M. (2000). Psychology/counseling: A universal competency in athletic training. *Journal of Athletic Training, 35(4),* 458-465.

Ross M. J, Berger R. S. (1996). Effects of stress inoculation training on athletes' postsurgical pain and rehabilitation after orthopedic injury. *Journal of Consulting and Clinical Psychology, 64,* 406-410

Rotella, R., & Heyman, S. (1986). Stress, injury, and the psychological rehabilitation of athletes. In J. Williams (Ed.), *Applied sport psychology: Personal growth to peak performance* (pp.343-364). Palo Alto, CA: Mayfield.

Silva, J., & Hardy, C. (1991). The sport psychologist: Psychological aspects of injury in sport. In F. Meuller & A. Ryan (Eds.), *The sports medicine team and athlete injury prevention* (pp.114-132). Philadelphia: F. A. Davis.

Sowa, C., & Gressard, C. (1983). Athletic participation: Its relationship to student development. *Journal of College Student Personnel, 26,* 236-239.

Sperber, M. (1990). *College sports inc.: The athletic department vs the university.* New York: Henry Holt.

Taylor, J., & Schneider, B. A. (1992). The Sport-Clinical Intake Protocol: A comprehensive interviewing instrument for sport. *Professional Psychology: Research and Practice, 23,* 318-325.

Taylor, J., & Taylor, S. (Eds.). (1997). Psychology of the rehabilitation process. In *Psychological approaches to sports injury rehabilitation* (pp. 35-55). Gaithersburg, MD: Aspen Publishers.

Tunick, R., Etzel, E., & Leard, J., & Lerner, B. (1996). Counseling injured and disabled student-athletes: A guide for understanding and intervention. In E. Etzel, A. Ferrante, & J. Pinkney (Eds.), *Counseling college student-athletes: Issues and interventions* (2nd ed., pp. 157-184). Morgantown, WV: Fitness Information Technology.

Wiese-Bjornstal, D., Smith, A., Shaffer, S., & Morrey, M. (1998). An integrated model of response to sport injury: Psychological and sociological dynamics. *Journal of Applied Sport Psychology, 10(1),* 46-69.

Zemper, E. (1989). Injury rates in a national sample of college football teams: A 2-year prospective study. *The Physician and Sportsmedicine, 17,* 100-102,105-108,113.

Zimbalist, A. (1999). *Unpaid professionals: Commercialism and conflict in big-time college sports.* Princeton, NJ: Princeton University Press.

Zizzi, S. J., & Perna, F. M. (2003). Impact of a brief workshop on stages of change profiles in athletes. *Athletic Insight: Online Journal of Sport Psychology, 5(4),* online at: http://www.athleticinsight.com/vol5iss4/impactofbriefworkshop.htm

Assessing and Monitoring Injuries and Psychological Characteristics in Intercollegiate Athletes: A Counseling/ Prediction Model

Michael L. Sachs, Michael R. Sitler, and Gerry Schwille
Temple University

One of the consequences of participation in intercollegiate athletics for almost all athletes at some point during their careers is injuries. Although not all athletes are injured severely enough to miss practices and/or games, virtually all intercollegiate athletes sustain injuries at least one or more times during their careers to the extent that medical treatment is required. These injuries may be due to any number of factors, which include, but are not limited to,

- contact with another player or equipment,
- overuse,
- equipment failure,
- previous injury,
- exposure to injury, and
- conditioning.

Introduction

One area that has been examined more extensively is the effect of psychological factors on injuries. In particular, the area of life stress is one that applied sport psychologists find especially important. Although life stress may not lead directly to injuries in intercollegiate athletes, dealing with stress (or, more precisely, not dealing effectively with stress) may indirectly affect the athlete. Life stress resulting from factors both within the athletic context (e.g., concern about upcoming games, conflicts with teammates or coaches, and pressure to perform) and, particularly, outside the athletic domain (e.g., family problems, difficulties with significant others, and academic problems) may negatively affect the person physically (immune system responses, excessive fatigue) and psychologically (distraction).

A proactive approach to dealing with life stress would encompass periodic monitoring, through established psychological inventories, interviews, and other approaches, of the athlete's psychological well-being. Those athletes who appear to demonstrate some degree of psychological distress could be offered counseling to help them deal with the stress. Reducing/eliminating the stress would then facilitate restoration of psychological well-being and concomitant physical well-being, thereby reducing one key factor that may result in injuries. While injuries will occur during participation in the sporting environment, an important underlying factor may be the stress experienced by the individual.

Athletic trainers are key individuals in the athletic environment, given their regular interaction with many athletes and their frontline contact with and responsibilities for the care and well-being of the athletes. Although other medical professionals, such as physicians and nurses (Gregory & Van Valkenburgh, 1991), have roles to play with injured athletes, athletic trainers are, in many ways, potentially the staff most likely to hear about concerns of the athletes and/or spot physical and related mood changes in athletes. As part of a proactive model in dealing with stress, athletic trainers must be involved in a significant way. Research (Wiese, Weiss, & Yukelson, 1990) indicates that athletic trainers are aware of, and supportive of, the key role of sport psychology in athletics, particularly in the injury rehabilitation process.

Background

On first examination it appears reasonably clear from the literature that life stress has a significant impact on injuries in athletes. Kerr and Minden (1988) examined elite female gymnasts and found that stressful life events were significantly related to both frequency and severity of injuries. Hardy and Riehl (1988) found that total life change and negative life change significantly predicted frequency of athletic injury (although not severity) among non-contact sport participants. Similar results with football players were found by Blackwell and McCullagh (1990). Injured players had higher scores on life stress factors and competitive anxiety, and lower scores on coping resources, than did uninjured players.

Other research, however, suggests that the relationship of life stress to injuries may be more complicated than first thought. Smith, Smoll, and Ptacek (1990) found that, in considering the variables of life stress, social support, and coping skills, these factors must be considered together rather than separately. They describe this as conjunctive moderation, "in which multiple moderators must co-occur in a specific combination or pattern to maximize a relation between a predictor and an outcome variable," (p. 360) as opposed to disjunctive moderation, "in which any one of a number of moderators maximizes the predictor-criterion relation" (p. 360). The authors found that, for adolescent sport injuries, social support and psychological coping skills acted in a conjunctive manner—a significant relationship between stress and injury was found only for athletes low in both coping skills and social support.

Work in this area may also be found with children (for those who work with athletes younger than collegiate or even high school levels). A number of studies have found connections between temperament and personality and the risk of unintentional injury in children (Schwebel, 2004; Schwebel & Barton, in press; Schwebel & Plumert, 1999).

In attempting to clarify the life stress, coping skills, and social support interaction, a model of stress and athletic injury may be helpful. Andersen and Williams (1988) developed a theoretical model of stress and athletic injury that includes

- cognitive,
- attentional,
- behavioral,
- physiological,
- intrapersonal,
- social, and
- stress history variables.

A comprehensive view of the stress-injury relationship requires this type of multivariate approach. Previous studies (with the exception of Smith, Smoll, and Ptacek, 1990) have tended to examine only components of this model with comparatively small groups of athletes. Advancement in theory, research, and practice (i.e., potential application) in this area would be aided by examining an array of factors within the model with a much larger group of athletes, across a variety of sports, for an extended period of time.

Monitoring

A basic component of a counseling/prediction model would be the development of a data base of key physical and psychological characteristics of the athlete, to track changes in the athlete that might alert the sport psychologist to potential stress. The physical (including demographic) components would include a number of factors:

- age
- gender
- height
- weight
- percent body fat
- years and level of participation in sport
- previous history of injuries

A battery of psychological inventories (see Table A and discussion in the section on psychological tests) dealing with a number of different psychological states and traits suggested in the model—life stress, mood, anxiety, coping skills, etc.—would, in this model, be administered to all intercollegiate athletes at a given university during the period set aside for physical examinations at the start of the school year. This could also be done, of course, with interscholastic athletes at a high school, members of a club

Table A.

List of Psychological Inventories

Profile of Mood States (POMS) (McNair, Lorr, & Droppleman, 1971)
Incredibly Short POMS (Dean, Whelan, & Meyers, 1990)
Sport Anxiety Scale (SAS) (Smith, Smoll, & Schutz, 1990)
Eating Disorders Inventory-2 (EDI-2) (Garner, 1991)
Health Attribution Test (HAT) (Lawlis & Lawlis, 1990)
Coping Resources Inventory (CRI) (Hammer & Marting, 1988)
Life Experiences Survey - Athletes (LES-A) (Hardy, 1989)
The Exercise Salience Scale (TESS) (Morrow & Harvey, 1990)

team, etc. These results would provide baseline data from which to work with athletes during the school year. Some of the tests could be scheduled for administration several times during the semester. The complete battery could also be administered again prior to the start of the spring semester, to increase the likelihood that psychological problems that might have arisen since the earlier testing points would be detected.

The information obtained would be used in three ways:

- First, if the results indicated a clinically significant level of psychological distress on one of the inventories, the athlete would be counseled to seek assistance, either at the university counseling center or with one of the sport psychologists (preferably a clinical sport psychologist, rather than an educational sport psychologist) working with athletes at the university. In some cases the model will be used within the context of a research study examining psychological factors and injuries. Although advising athletes to seek assistance would potentially confound the research component of such a study, it represents a proactive approach based on the desire to ensure maximum psychological mental health and well-being of the athlete and, concomitantly, readiness to practice and compete in intercollegiate athletics. In this case, ethical principles would suggest that applied concerns outweigh research considerations. Follow-up information would be obtained on each athlete to ascertain adherence to recommendations to seek counseling and readministration of appropriate psychological inventories to measure potential changes on the psychological measure of concern.

- Second, the results could be used in a model to attempt to predict occurrence of athletic injuries during the course of the year. These injuries might be suffered as a result of practices or games, or in other settings (e.g., basketball players playing on their own before practice for the season can officially begin). This model might be useful at other universities as well or may be found to be specific to the university where testing takes place (e.g., perhaps due to peculiarities in environmental conditions).

- Third, it is possible that some of the psychological factors measured may allow prediction of which athletes will return to practice and competition most quickly. Delineation of factors related to adherence to a rehabilitation regimen and a return to participation may be an added outcome of this model, although not a primary focus.

It is important to emphasize that all information obtained through the testing procedures would be kept confidential. The information is designed to be used in an individual, counseling/prediction approach by sport psychologists. Coaches and athletic administration personnel would not have access to the information unless written permission was obtained from the athlete. Indeed, one problem encountered is reluctance on the part of some athletes (and teams in general) to complete a battery of standardized inventories. One will most likely find that participation in the program will be less than 100%. However, those motivated to participate will probably find the process useful, and this may "sell" the program to others who initially are hesitant to participate.

Injury Definition and Documentation/Guidelines

Important to psychological intervention studies in athletic settings is defining the term "injury." It is from this most fundamental level that the incidence of injury can be determined and interpretation of findings and comparison of results between studies can be made more reliably.

The most basic elements in the establishment of an injury definition encompass the need for detail, explicitness, and ease of interpretation (Wallace & Clark, 1988). A set of inclusive and exclusive criteria are needed that allow for differentiation between those who have been injured and those who have not been injured. To date, however, no universally agreed upon definition of what constitutes an injury has been established, although three generally accepted classification criteria include

(a) time loss from participation,

(b) anatomical tissue diagnosis, and

(c) medical consultation.

Each of the definitions available has its own strengths and weaknesses and, as such, varies in its ability to meet research objectives.

One way we have found most helpful is to define an injury as

(a) being sports related,

(b) resulting in a player's inability to participate one day after injury, and

(c) requiring medical attention (university athletic training staff, physician, emergency room), including concussions, nerve injuries (regardless of their time loss), eye injuries, and dental care

(Noyes, Lindefeld, & Marshall, 1988). This definition has the advantage of comprising a multidimensional approach and is relatively sensitive to the broad spectrum of injuries encountered in the athletic setting. This does not include, however, occurrences of the flu, colds, and other related illnesses that would not be seen as sports related per se but could still be due, in part, to psychologically induced stress/depression resulting in a weakened and potentially more susceptible bodily state. Research on psychoneuroimmunology (Carlson & Seifert, 1991; Friedman, Specter, & Klein, 1991; Husband, 1992) supports this point of view and may lead to a change in how we define injury in the future.

Injury frequency is determined by the total number of occurrences encountered during the course of testing (e.g., a season, a year). Injury frequency can then be expressed as a function of the exposure to injury, resulting in determination of an injury rate. The injury rate (see Figure 1) comprises a numerator, the number of events (i.e., injuries) under study, and a denominator, the number of persons at risk of a specific occurrence or event, providing for a determination of risk. A useful way of expressing the denominator is to base it upon every 1,000 athlete-exposures. Athlete-exposures are defined as the frequency with which an athlete is exposed to the potential of injury, and every player at a practice or game is counted as one athlete-exposure. While this determination involves a fair amount of record keeping, much of this information is already being kept by athletic training staff and may only require a systematic organization of the record-keeping process.

Figure 1.
Injury Rate and Determination of Risk

$$\text{Injury Rate} = \frac{\text{Definition of Injury}}{\text{Population-at-risk}}$$

Injury severity is defined by the significance of the injury sustained. Here again, no universal definition exists, although time-loss from activity has been used in several nationally based sports injury epidemiology studies (Alles, Powell, Buckley, & Hunt, 1979; Powell, 1988). The utility of a time-loss definition is that it is relatively easy to measure and is based on the functional consequences of participation (or not participating!) following the injury. When more objective criteria are needed, as is frequently necessary with ligamentous and muscle-related injuries, categorization in accordance with the injury severity index established by the American Medical Association's *Standard Nomenclature of Injuries* (1968) can be used.

Injury data can be prospectively collected by the medical staff assigned to the study. This includes the university's intercollegiate athletic training staff and student athletic trainers who are enrolled in the National Athletic Trainers' Association Approved Undergraduate Athletic Training Program.

Psychological Tests

There are numerous psychological inventories that can be administered to athletes. Ostrow (1996), for example, edited a *Directory of Psychological Tests in the Sport and Exercise Sciences* with information on 314 psychological tests specifically related to sport and exercise. There are many inventories that could be used in a battery of tests, including ones on injury as well as self-efficacy, athletic identity, commitment to exercise, hardiness, and so on. Duda (1998) is also a good source for information on measurement in this area. There are a number of inventories (see Table A) that may be of particular interest in applying the counseling/prediction model:

Profile of Mood States (POMS). The POMS (McNair, Lorr, & Droppleman, 1971) is a 65-adjective rating scale, derived through factor analysis, that measures six dimensions of mood states:

- Tension—Anxiety
- Depression—Dejection
- Anger—Hostility
- Vigor—Activity
- Fatigue—Inertia
- Confusion—Bewilderment

The POMS has excellent psychometric properties (established validity and reliability). Instructions request respondents to indicate how they have been feeling during the past week, but it can be used to ask how respondents have been feeling for longer (e.g., past month) or shorter (e.g., daily) periods of time. Ideally, athletes would have comparatively high scores on Vigor-Activity and comparatively low scores on the other five factors, providing what has been termed an iceberg profile (Morgan & Pollock, 1977), with a peak of vigor and "submerged" levels on the other factors.

The POMS is an excellent means of regularly measuring mood, and is used frequently in applied and research contexts, but can become burdensome if administered too frequently; although 65 items is not a great number, too frequent administration may be undesirable. One way around this problem may be an instrument termed the Brief Assessment of Mood (BAM) (Dean, Whelan, & Meyers, 1990), which has reduced the 65-item POMS to six items. Concurrent validity appears acceptable and this instrument has been used effectively in athletic contexts (Fritts, 1992). One advantage found with administration of the BAM on a regular basis is that respondents develop the habit of completing the form at a regular time in their schedule in a matter of only 10–15 seconds, placing little burden on their time and energy. However, we have also found that coaches are hesitant to have athletes complete even the BAM on days when competition is scheduled, for fear of having the athletes focus too much on their mood states, particularly, of course, if the mood state is negative.

It should be noted that the POMS is currently (spring 2006) being revised and the POMS-R may be available in late 2006/early 2007. Check with the publisher (Multi-Health Systems at www.mhs.com) for more information.

Sport Anxiety Scale (SAS). The SAS (Smith, Smoll, & Schutz, 1990) is a sport-specific measure of cognitive and somatic trait anxiety. Current thinking in sport psychology suggests the advisability of using sport-specific measures as well as instruments that address both cognitive and somatic components of anxiety, such as the SAS. Individual differences in somatic anxiety and two classes of cognitive anxiety—Worry and Concentration Disruption—are measured. The SAS has excellent psychometric properties.

Eating Disorders Inventory-2 (EDI-2). The EDI-2 (Garner, 1991) is a 91-item self-report inventory that assesses an array of factors related to anorexia nervosa and bulimia nervosa. Eleven subscales make up the EDI:

- Drive for Thinness
- Bulimia

- Body Dissatisfaction
- Ineffectiveness
- Perfectionism
- Interpersonal Distrust
- Interoceptive Awareness
- Maturity Fears
- Impulse Regulation
- Social Insecurity
- Asceticism

The EDI-2 has excellent psychometric properties. A new symptom checklist provides additional information about the frequency and severity of symptoms important in considering a diagnosis of an eating disorder, a problem area particularly prevalent in some athletic populations (e.g., gymnasts, runners, divers, and wrestlers). Those interested in this area may also wish to review the EDI-3 (revised version of the EDI-2). See www.parinc.com for more information.

Health Attribution Test (HAT). The HAT (Lawlis & Lawlis, 1990) is a 22-item test that evaluates an individual's health locus of control. Attributions for control of one's health may be made to internal factors, powerful others, and chance. The HAT has excellent psychometric properties. This scale provides an excellent measure for attempting to develop a predictive profile for recovery time for individuals who are injured.

Coping Resources Inventory (CRI). The CRI (Hammer & Marting, 1988) is a 60-item inventory that assesses one's resources for coping with situations. Coping resources can be defined as "those resources inherent in individuals that enable them to handle stressors more effectively, to experience fewer or less intense symptoms upon exposure to a stressor, or to recover faster from exposure" (Hammer & Marting, 1988, p. 2). The CRI measures resources in five domains:

- cognitive
- social
- emotional
- spiritual/philosophical
- physical

Hammer and Marting identify seven uses for the CRI, two of which are particularly relevant to the application of the model: "as a research instrument to investigate coping resources in various populations" and "as a tool for identifying individuals who might be at-risk, in need of counseling, or in need of medical intervention" (p. 2). The CRI has excellent psychometric properties.

Life Experiences Survey - Athletes (LES-A). The LES-A (Hardy, 1989) is an 80-item survey that attempts to determine if any of a variety of life experiences have occurred to the athlete within the past 12 months *and* the perceived impact of the event on the person at the time the event occurred. The survey provides a framework within which to potentially understand moderate to high levels of stress that athletes might be experiencing.

The Exercise Salience Scale (TESS). The TESS (Morrow & Harvey, 1990) measures a number of factors that determine dependence upon exercise. Athletes who are more dependent upon exercise may be more likely to persist in participating in athletics in spite of negative life stress. The TESS has strong psychometric properties.

It is important to emphasize that these are not the only psychological inventories, nor the only psychological constructs, that can be used. Different researchers/practitioners have other areas and other tests they have found meet their needs more effectively. For example, Bergandi and Wittig (1991) found that attentional style was related to frequency of athletic injury with some athletes (in one sport, women's softball), but not others. The Test of Attentional and Interpersonal Style (TAIS) (Nideffer, 1976) could, therefore, be used to measure this construct, particularly if one considers sport-specific versions of the TAIS. Other approaches, looking at other variables (Nideffer, 1989), may prove attractive for different needs in different athletic settings.

Assessment may also call for a broader approach, incorporating tests/measures as well as interviews and other approaches. Gardner and Moore (2006) provide some helpful thoughts on assessment in sport psychology that may be worth considering. Additional helpful information may be found in Leffingwell, Durand-Bush, Wurzberger, and Cada (2005).

Model Application

As noted earlier, the battery of inventories would be administered before the fall semester begins or before the first practice in the case of sports (i.e., football) that begin their season before school is in session. This initial baseline also provides an indication of psychological problems that may have arisen during the summer, when contact with athletes may have been minimal. Intervention can then occur if the sport psychologist feels that the test scores indicate this course of action.

This type of model already exists in many schools with respect to concussions. Covassin (2003), for example, examined gender differences and neuropsychological impairments of concussions among intercollegiate athletes. All athletes took the ImPACT test battery, which provides neuropsychological information, prior to the start of their athletic season. If a concussion occurred, the initial ImPACT information was available to aid in assessing the effect of the concussion on the athlete and providing important information on recovery and potential return to play.

Injury data are then collected throughout the course of the year, through the competitive season and practices, as well as recreational periods (i.e., basketball before the "official" practice date). Some inventories may be readministered on a regular basis to monitor potential changes. This is particularly important for those measures addressing issues that are state, rather than trait in nature. Trait measures will tend to remain stable over time, and administering such measures twice a year may be sufficient. State measures, however, by definition, will change, even on a daily basis. Administering these measures, such as the BAM, on a more frequent basis is therefore desirable. Of course, scoring of these inventories must be done quickly to ensure opportunities for intervention if this is so desired.

At the end of the year, data from the psychological inventories and the injury data can be analyzed to assess potential relationships of theoretical and applied importance, as well as detect changes over time if this is an ongoing process. It is important to note that the process of administering the psychological inventories would ideally have the cooperation of the coach and the athletes. There will be coaches and athletes who would choose not to participate (and human subjects guidelines at universities may require that this non-participation option be present), and some schools may decide that this must be respected. Other schools might decide that, because this process is designed to enhance the well being of the student athletes, all student athletes would be required to participate. Each school must decide how it wishes to proceed.

In applying the model, there are a number of potential uses, as noted earlier. Perhaps the most important, from a clinical/proactive perspective, is the case wherein the results indicate a clinically significant level of psychological distress on one of the inventories. For example, Jane Doe, athlete on team sport x, provides a POMS with a "negative" or inverted iceberg profile, with high scores on tension, depression, anger, fatigue, and confusion, and a low score on vigor. This suggests that something may be going on in Jane's life; this something could "simply" be overtraining (Morgan, Costill, Flynn, Raglin, & O'Connor, 1988) or could reflect other problems, such as interpersonal relationships, academic difficulties, or family matters. The athlete would be counseled to seek assistance, either at the university counseling center or with one of the sport psychologists working with athletes at the university. Providing the athlete with a choice and maintaining confidentiality are important elements in this process. Ingram (2006) addresses some of these issues with respect to eating disorders, an area that is ideal for proactive intervention on the part of athletic departments.

In Jane's case, the POMS, as well as the BAM, could be used to follow up progress in the weeks following the beginning of counseling. Some of the inventories, such as the POMS, may prove quite useful as well in working with athletes who are recovering from an injury (Smith, Scott, O'Fallon, & Young, 1990), and "facilitate the athlete's optimal rehabilitation and a safe return to participation in sports" (p. 38).

This approach provides for a unique partnership of the sport psychologist and athletic trainer. Both groups of individuals have the physical and psychological well-being of the athlete as their greatest concern. Interventions as described in the above model provide a means for facilitating the help we give our athletes in achieving their goals as individuals, students, and athletes.

Summary

Although injuries are a fact of life in intercollegiate athletics, it is extremely desirable to minimize injury frequency and severity. The impact of physical and psychological factors on the frequency and severity of injuries is critical, and is worthy of in-depth investigation. A counseling/prediction model is proposed as an effective means of working with athletes and providing important information for theory and research in this critical area of study.

References

Alles, W., Powell, J., Buckley, H., & Hunt, E. (1979). The national athletic injury/illness reporting system: 3-year findings of high school and college football injuries. *Journal of Orthopedic and Sports Physical Therapy, 11*, 103-108.

American Medical Association. (1968). *Standard nomenclatureof injuries.* Chicago, IL: American Medical Association.

Andersen, M. B., & Williams, J. M. (1988). A model of stress and athletic injury: Prediction and prevention. *Journal of Sport & Exercise Psychology, 10*, 294-306.

Bergandi, T. A., & Wittig, A. F. (1991). *Attentional style as a predictor of athletic injury.* Unpublished manuscript, Spalding University, Louisville, KY.

Blackwell, B., & McCullagh, P. (1990, Spring). The relationship of athletic injury to life stress, competitive anxiety and coping resources. *Athletic Training, 25*, 23-27.

Carlson, J. G., & Seifert, A. R. (Eds.) (1991). *International perspectives on self-regulation and health.* New York: Plenum Press.

Covassin, T. (2003). *Gender differences and neuropsychological impairments of concussions among collegiate athletes.* Unpublished doctoral dissertation, Temple University, Philadelphia, PA.

Dean, J. E., Whelan, J. P., & Meyers, A. W. (1990). *An incredibly quick way to assess mood states: The Incredibly Short POMS.* Paper presented at the annual meeting of the Association for the Advancement of Applied Sport Psychology, San Antonio, TX.

Duda, J. L. (1998). (Ed.). *Advances in sport and exercise psychology measurement.* Morgantown, WV: Fitness Information Technology.

Friedman, H., Specter, S., & Klein, T. W. (Eds.) (1991). *Drugs of abuse, immunity, and immunodeficiency.* New York: Plenum Press.

Fritts, S. (1992). *Psychological factors that predispose athletes to injury.* Unpublished master's thesis, Temple University, Philadelphia, PA.

Gardner, F., & Moore, Z. (2006). *Clinical sport psychology.* Champaign, IL: Human Kinetics.

Garner, D. M. (1991). Eating Disorder Inventory-2 manual. Odessa, FL: Psychological Assessment Resources, Inc.

Gregory, B., & Van Valkenburgh, J. (1991). Psychology of the injured athlete. *Journal of Post Anesthesia Nursing, 6*(2), 108-110.

Hammer, A. L., & Marting, M. S. (1988). *Manual for the Coping Resources Inventory (research edition).* Palo Alto, CA: Consulting Psychologists Press.

Hardy, C. J. (1989). *Life Experience Survey - Athletes.* Chapel Hill, NC: Department of Physical Education, University of North Carolina.

Hardy, C. J., & Riehl, R. E. (1988). An examination of the life stress-injury relationship among noncontact sport participants. *Behavioral Medicine, 14*, 113-118.

Husband, A. J. (Ed.) (1992). *Behavior and immunity.* Boca Raton, FL: CRC Press.

Ingram, Y. M. (2006). *Prevalence rate of eating disorder behaviors in NCAA female athletes and the use of a body image awareness program to affect this prevalence rate.* Unpublished doctoral dissertation, Temple University, Philadelphia, PA.

Kerr, G., & Minden, H. (1988). Psychological factors related to the occurrence of athletic injuries. *Journal of Sport & Exercise Psychology, 10*, 167-173.

Lawlis, J., & Lawlis, G. F. (1990). *Health Attribution Test manual.* Champaign, IL: Institute for Personality and Ability Testing.

Leffingwell, T. R., Durand-Bush, N., Wurzberger, D., & Cada, P. (2005). Psychological assessment. In J. Taylor & G. Wilson (Eds.), *Applying sport psychology* (pp. 85-100). Champaign, IL: Human Kinetics.

McNair, D. M., Lorr, M., & Droppleman, L. F. (1971). *Manual: Profile of mood states.* San Diego, CA: Educational and Industrial Testing Service.

Morgan, W. P., Costill, D. L., Flynn, M. G., Raglin, J. S., & O'Connor, P. H. (1988). Psychological monitoring of overtraining and performance. *British Journal of Sports Medicine, 21*, 107-114.

Morgan, W. P., & Pollock, M. L. (1977). Psychologic characterization of the elite distance runner. *Annals of the New York Academy of Sciences, 301*, 382-402.

Morrow, J., & Harvey, P. (1990). *The exercise salience scale.* Unpublished manuscript, New York, NY.

Nideffer, R. M. (1976). Test of Attentional and Interpersonal Style (TAIS). *Journal of Personality and Social Psychology, 34*, 397-404.

Nideffer, R. M. (1989). Psychological aspects of sports injuries: Issues in prevention and treatment. *International Journal of Sport Psychology, 20*, 241-255.

Noyes, R., Lindefeld, T., & Marshall, M. (1988). What determines an athletic injury (definition): Who determines an injury (occurrence)? *American Journal of Sports Medicine, 16* (Suppl.), 134-135.

Ostrow, A. C. (1990). *Directory of psychological tests in the sport and exercise sciences.* Morgantown, WV: Fitness Information Technology, Inc.

Powell, J. (1988). National high school athletic injury registry. *American Journal of Sports Medicine, 16*(Suppl. 1), 55-56.

Schwebel, D. C. (2004). Temperamental risk factors for children's unintentional injury: The role of impulsivity and inhibitory control. *Personality and Individual Differences, 37,* 567-578.

Schwebel, D. C., & Barton, B. K. (in press). Temperament and children's unintentional injuries. To appear in M. Vollrath (Ed.), *Handbook of personality and health.* New York: Wiley.

Schwebel, D. C., & Plumert, J. M. (1999). Longitudinal and concurrent relations among temperament, ability estimation, and injury proneness. *Child Development, 70,* 700-712.

Smith, A. M., Scott, S. G., O'Fallon, W. M., & Young, M. L. (1990). Emotional responses of athletes to injury. *Mayo Clinic Proceedings, 65,* 38-50.

Smith, R. E., Smoll, F. L., & Ptacek, J. T. (1990). Conjunctive moderator variables in vulnerability and resiliency research: Life stress, social support, and coping skills, and adolescent sport injuries. *Journal of Personality and Social Psychology, 58,* 360-370.

Smith, R. E., Smoll, F. L., & Schutz, R. W. (In press). Measurement and correlates of sport-specific cognitive and somatic trait anxiety: The sport anxiety scale. *Anxiety Research.*

Wallace, R., & Clark, W. (1988). The numerator, denominator, and the population-at-risk. *American Journal of Sports Medicine, 16* (Suppl. 1), 55-56.

Wiese, D. M., Weiss, M. R., & Yukelson, D. P. (1990). *Sport psychology in the training room: A survey of athletic trainers.* Paper presented at the annual meeting of the American Alliance for Health, Physical Education, Recreation, and Dance, New Orleans, LA.

Chapter Eleven

Counseling Athletes with Permanent Disabilities

Keith P. Henschen
University of Utah

Gregory A. Shelley
Ithaca College

In this chapter, two actual vignettes of athletes experiencing permanent disabilities are presented, and information concerning the transitional period as well as the general reaction pattern to injuries is discussed. Next, a number of general guidelines to which the sport psychologist should adhere during the various stages of the psychological rehabilitation are presented. Finally, psychological interventions that would be beneficial in each scenario are discussed. A team approach to handling athletes with permanent disabilities is advocated.

Vignette 1

On a snow covered football field in mid-December an all-pro wide receiver streaks down the sideline, concentrating intently on the long, arching pass headed in his direction. As the ball gently nestles into the receiver's soft hands, a defensive player's helmet is planted in the middle of the receiver's back with unbelievable force. The force of the two players colliding is analogous to that of two cars crashing head-on at about 30 miles per hour with neither applying the breaks. At the instant of impact, the receiver suffers a severing of the spinal cord and is immediately transformed into a paraplegic.

Vignette 2

On a stormy summer night an Olympic, world-class pistol shooter is involved in a tragic automobile accident. She is severely injured, with numerous broken bones and a deep concussion that leaves her in a coma for about two weeks. After awakening from the coma, she continues to experience migraine headaches and blurred vision. It is determined that the neurological damage is permanent and that her vision impairment is uncorrectable. She will remain, throughout her lifetime, legally blind in one eye.

These vignettes describe true-life experiences that create a variety of special circumstances that must be handled by the medical science specialist. Of particular interest are the problems or challenges that these situations create for the sport psychologist. What are the similarities the sport psychology consultant must be cognizant of in both scenarios? What are the obvious and subtle differences? How, when, and where should counseling and intervention techniques be applied in each situation? Also, what are the major concerns that need to be addressed before total reintegration into society can be achieved? In the remainder of this chapter an attempt will be made to provide salient information about how to proceed in each of these cases, as well as discuss the challenges and problems that might confront the sport psychologist.

To begin our discussion, it should be understood that a trauma resulting in permanent termination from sport participation often initiates a life crisis for which very few athletes are prepared. When injury occurs to elite athletes in particular, typically a great deal of publicity and support are generated; however, the injury soon becomes "yesterday's news." The athlete is eventually left to deal with the trauma with only the help of his or her family or intimate support group.

Since high-level athletic participation is no longer probable, the athlete's entire quality of life is in jeopardy. Permanent physical damage may significantly impede the athlete's pursuit of a productive, fulfilling life and may severely limit possible career options (Oglivie & Howe, 1986). Counseling interventions are often indicated at this point to assure functional transitions and achievement of "a new normalcy in life."

The Transition Period

Irrespective of the specific cause of injury-related athletic termination, as illustrated by the presented vignettes, each trauma victim must address a crucial period of adjustment. The demands of this transition are specific to the individual and handled differently by all of those forced to experience it. Any injury is mentally, emotionally, and behaviorally challenging, and the athlete's state of mental health prior to the injury will influence how the athlete reacts to it (Evans & Hardy, 1999). At this time vital issues, such as permanent retirement, identity crises, and the transition from athlete to ex-athlete status emerge. In general, how athletes handle these difficult adjustments is dependent upon the strength of their identification with sport, their perceptions about self-worth, and the importance they place on the expectations held for them by others. For many, the identity of being an athlete is an important part of their feelings of self-worth and interpersonal needs.

A heavy investment in the "sport identity" may be troublesome for those transitioning from athlete to non-athlete; since such individuals have undoubtedly thrived on the recognition and accolades derived from competition-related achievements. When deprived of such reinforcements, injured athletes suffer serious loss because their opportunity for skill development in other areas may be limited (Brewer, 2001). A single-minded commitment to the athletic life has been cultivated within them, and elite athletes are typically encouraged to invest heavily in training and maintain an almost exclusive focus on sports.

In making a smooth and healthy transition from athlete to nonathlete status, the injured athlete's perceptions of self are crucial. Many athletes, even world-class competitors, do not have high levels of self-worth and therefore require much positive reinforcement from significant others (Brewer, 1993; Henschen, 1992). Cessation of such reinforcement, heretofore provided by successful competitive experiences, may result in further decreases in self-worth and difficulty in coping with the demands of transition. Injured athletes who believe they are worthwhile and important persons exclusive of their involvement in sport are likely to adjust more easily to their status change than are those with low self-worth. It should be noted that perceptions of help-lessness regarding the physical self may undermine the entire concept of self.

Loss of recognition and status, as well as the unavailability of what was an exciting lifestyle, may complicate the injured athlete's transition to non-athlete status. Injured athletes are no longer acknowledged in the same manner by other athletes, peers, significant others, and the media. Often, so-called "close friendships" fade, and the injured athlete must rely on primary bases of support—namely, family members. Unfortunately, members of the immediate family are also obliged to confront serious interpersonal, financial, and time-management challenges related to injury of one of its members. Consequently, the adjustment to the injury (the transitional period) may be difficult for athletes due to the need to relinquish center stage, the "roar of the crowd and the smell of the greasepaint," and the loss of opportunity to showcase their talent. They still must deal with unfair expectations that they have been exposed to for years: the expectation that they must "be tough," "play with pain," "never quit," etc. In addition, debilitating injury to a professional athlete may result in serious loss of family income in the face of increased medical expenses.

Emotional Response Factors Affecting Sport Injury

In response to a lack of empirical support for the stage models of adjustment to athletic injury (i.e., athletes proceeding through a sequential series of recovery stages), Heil (1993) argued in favor of cognitive appraisal models in providing a foundation for conceptualizing the process of coping with sport injury. Rather than a predictable set of discrete emotional responses, affective responses to sport injury appear to be more varied across athletes (Heil, 1993). At the core of these models is the athlete's cognitive appraisal (interpretation) of the injury. How athletes interpret the injury then determines their emotional response (e.g., frustration, anger, sadness, relief), and ultimately their behavioral response (e.g., isolation, tardiness, adherence). In short, appraisal (perception) influences emotions, which then influence behaviors. Although the injury is considered the primary stressor, the way in which the injury is perceived is most important. The fact that the injury has occurred is less important than its meaningfulness. Accordingly, one's cognitive appraisal is influenced by the interaction of both personal and situational factors. Several examples of each follow.

Personal Factors

Cognitive appraisal can be affected by any number of personal factors. For example, the athlete's age, injury history, self-esteem, and self-motivation can have an impact upon appraisal. In addition, the degree to which athletes are psychologically invested in their sport, their level of introversion/extroversion, and their tendencies toward neuroticism can influence injury appraisal. Finally, the athlete's overall coping skills influence the degree to which they manage their injury, deal with its long-term effects, and adhere to the rehabilitation regimen.

Situational Factors

There are also a number of situational factors that bear upon the athlete's cognitive appraisal and adjustment to injury, such as the time of season (or point in career), playing status, social pressures to perform, and general life stresses. Obviously, the diagnosis, prognosis, injury severity and duration, and degree to which daily activities and sport performances are impaired also affect appraisal interpretations. And finally, it is important to assess the amount of social support available to the athlete from the coaches and sports medicine team members, because it determines how well recovery is progressing to a meaningful extent. Critical to the cognitive appraisal models is the focus on individual differences in coping with sport injury. Just as each athlete is unique, so is his or her response to sport injury. Suffice it to say that an athlete's cognitive appraisal of sport injury will depend upon

(a) his or her prior psychological level of functioning;

(b) the meaning of the disability;

(c) the nature, location, severity, and duration of the injury; and

(d) the resulting changes in the individual's lifestyle

(Ford & Gordon, 1999). Whenever possible, sports medicine team members should provide hope to the athlete throughout the duration of the rehabilitative process.

Vignette 1: Spinal Cord Injury to a Professional Football Player

Putting aside the questionable sociable acceptability of such sport violence, the issue becomes how to work most effectively with the injured athlete in order to facilitate his transitional period. This football player must overcome two major issues:

(a) retirement from athletics

(b) adjustment to permanent disability

The first issue is relatively meaningless in this scenario since retirement is inevitable, and the athlete will come to this realization almost immediately upon awakening from surgery. The crucial issue is not becoming a productive ex-athlete, but rather dealing with a permanent disability. It is not even an issue of the injury's severity, because it is so severe that it threatens any semblance of a normal future life.

In this case, rehabilitation should involve a medical team approach with special emphasis placed on three stages:

- preoperative
- postoperative
- long-term recovery

Prior to discussing the three stages of rehabilitation for this scenario, it should be made abundantly clear that the most effective procedures will indeed be accomplished by a team approach. No individual can provide all of the services necessary for this athlete as he struggles with rehabilitation. The team should consist of family, friends, teammates, athletic trainers, medical personnel, and the sport psychologist. Each of these individuals has significant contributions to make to the injured athlete and his reintegration into society. Let us examine these contributions in reverse order from the way in which they were presented previously.

In reality, the most crucial portion of the medical rehabilitation team is the sport psychologist. This person will be the only individual remaining in close, personal contact throughout all the stages of rehabilitation. The sport psychologist, because of the professional relationship he or she establishes with the athlete, will also be the sole member of the sports medicine team who can provide compassionate but objective evaluations and reinforcement to the injured athlete in an unbiased fashion. Specific procedures and techniques used by the sport psychologist will be presented as the stages of rehabilitation are discussed.

The second part of the team includes all the medical personnel: the operating surgeons, the attending physician, and the physical therapist. These professionals are experts at what they do; however, they typically are not trained in counseling techniques, essential in this scenario. That is why the sport psychologist must have the confidence and cooperation of the medical staff in order to be effective.

The athletic training staff is normally a crucial element in most injury rehabilitation situations, but this vignette is slightly different. After the initial on-the-field treatment for the injury, the athletic trainers will really have little contact with the athlete; but they can be invaluable to the sport psychologist. They can be a source of much-needed information concerning the personal aspects of the athlete that will be needed in counseling. Nideffer (1983) identified several personality characteristics in athletes that interact with the personalities of the sports medicine team:

- information-seeking
- self-confidence
- self-esteem
- extroversion or introversion tendencies

Athletic trainers can provide the sport psychologist with this personal information about the athlete, thus saving him or her time and energy.

Friends and teammates can also provide the injured athlete with an enormous amount of social support and should strive to be a source of help for an extended time frame. As the severity of the disability becomes apparent, though, these same individuals may become conspicuously absent. Their visits will be frequent in the beginning, but diminish and ultimately become nonexistent over time. Many persons feel uncomfortable in the presence of disabled individuals, and the easiest solution is "out of sight, out of mind." Although sometimes difficult for the injured athlete to accept, friends and teammates have full agendas and committed lives of their own. It is often difficult for active people to spend time with inactive individuals, especially disabled ones. In addition, friends, relatives, and former teammates may be burdened with psychological fears and limitations that inhibit their interaction with permanently disabled persons. The sport psychologist should therefore prepare the injured athlete for this "abandonment" as the rehabilitation process proceeds.

Perhaps the most important members of the team approach are family members who may be as directly affected by the disability as the injured person. The family goes through the initial trauma of the accident, the slow transition period, and the long-term rehabilitation. Family members' lives may be influenced by the disabling injury. The sport psychologist must be prepared to counsel family members through their transitional periods. This may prove to be very difficult. Emotions such as anger, depression, and resentment will be prevalent. In fact, the sport psychologist should recommend general family counseling in all cases involving permanent disability. A number of guidelines should be adhered to during psychological rehabilitation:

1. The athlete should enter counseling as soon as possible.
2. The counselor should establish a positive relationship with all family members.
3. The athlete should receive as much positive support as possible.
4. The same counselors should provide continuity of care.

Constantly changing counselors, for whatever reasons, often sends an inappropriate message, and should be avoided.

Preoperative Stage

It is very important that counseling begin immediately after the injury and prior to surgery. A great deal of psychological preparation for surgery and other invasive procedures is almost always necessary. Fear of surgery is very common, and dealing with pain is difficult. The sport psychologist can prepare an injured athlete for surgery by providing accurate information about what is to happen and what to expect. Fear is often associated with the unknown, and by virtue of providing explanations of the forthcoming surgical experience, the counselor may alleviate this emotion. Training in anxiety reduction and relaxation skills is also frequently appropriate at this time. It would seem appropriate for medical personnel to provide such services to patients, but for various reasons this normally fails to occur. It is wise for the sport psychologist to anticipate providing counseling services that the medical staff is not providing to athletes with disabilities.

Postoperative Stage

In this vignette, surgery resulted in return of all bodily functions with the exception of motor activity. In other words, the football player was ultimately able to do almost everything except walk. The mandate facing the sport psychologist is to deal with the general reaction of this athlete to his tragic locomotive inability and to guide him through the period in which he accepts his serious liability. This is a difficult and time-consuming challenge. One positive psychological aspect is that in the postoperative context, problems are more accessible, closer to the surface, and more likely to be revealed. Again, postoperatively, the sport psychologist needs first to handle the transition of the athlete and then to lay the foundation for reintegration into society.

Long-Term Stage

The long-term stage of counseling has two purposes:
- helping the athlete deal with disability, and
- reintegrating him or her into society.

Although these two are interrelated, learning to deal with the disability is the most crucial. If coping with the disability is accomplished, then reintegration is likely. The sport psychologist must assist in the cognitive restructuring of many aspects of the injured athletes' perceptions. The athlete must be convinced that he or she is still a viable, productive, and important individual, even though no longer a sports hero. Ogilvie & Howe (1986) stated that once athletes are resigned to the facts of retirement, they will experience an interesting shift in values. Instead of valuing such things as being first, traveling, having money, and being popular, they will redirect their emphases to reflect higher value being placed on family and friends. The counseling should focus on what the reality of the disability actually is and what the athlete will be able to do. The counselor should always present this information in a positive fashion.

It is our contention that the athlete described in Vignette 1 will respond positively to the challenge of rehabilitation. He has, since childhood, flourished in competition and has been exposed to conflict and conflict resolution challenges in the sports arena. Challenges and competition are integral parts of his life and can be used in his rehabilitation. This athlete must be convinced that even though physical participation in sport as once experienced is no longer possible, there is still the challenge to channel many of his abilities and skills towards successful rehabilitation. The object of competition now becomes himself, his own muscles and nervous system, instead of other football players.

Counseling this individual should include some, if not all, of the following interventions:
- cognitive restructuring
- visual imagery
- thought stopping
- panic mitigation
- relaxation
- goal setting
- positive self-talk

Exactly how to employ these with this particular disabled athlete is dependent upon a variety of factors, such as personality, previous psychological training, and progress through the transition phases. Rather than describe these skills here, we refer to other authors who have advocated and offered detailed descriptions of programs using these techniques (Henschen & Shelley, 1999; Pearson & Pepitpas, 1990). The counseling in this scenario may continue for years.

Vignette 2: Neurological Damage to an Olympic Pistol Shooter

This case is totally different from the last one. Here the high-level competitor is not faced with an obvious lifetime disability and in fact can function very effectively in society with her impairment. Counseling in this case must focus primarily on retirement from competition rather than on dealing with a restrictive permanent disability. Again, two stages of counseling are recommended: (a) the postoperative stage; and (b) the long-term stage.

Postoperative Stage

The athlete in Vignette 2, as is the case with almost all injured individuals, will experience the same general reaction pattern during the transition. The emphasis during the postoperative stage will be to regain a normal level of health and to involve her husband, family, and friends in the transition period. Due to the visual demands of pistol shooting, this athlete will need to accept the termination of her competitive shooting career. She will be able to continue as a recreational shooter, but intense high-level competition is improbable. The athlete's motivation and readiness for rehabilitation and counseling in this stage will be determined by what she thinks happened, how she feels about what happened, and what she plans to do about the accident (Taylor & Ogilvie, 2001). Once she is physically healthy, it is quite likely she will attempt to shoot again, but understandably with poor results. The counselor must be ready for the anger and frustration that will follow. After she has proven to herself that she is no longer physically capable of competitive pistol shooting, the long-term stage of counseling will commence.

Long-Term Stage

Counseling in this scenario should focus on retirement from competitive athletics. In this case the key people in the athlete's total reintegration efforts will be the counselor and the athlete's spouse. If there are "significant others" in this athlete's life, they will also be important factors. Through interaction with the athlete, the counselor must locate the influential variables that are causing her to experience frustration in the retirement process.

Previous research has identified the following factors that frequently influence the "stress" of retirement from the active life:

- degree of marital satisfaction,
- the personality of the athlete,
- level of self-esteem and self-concept,
- self-motivation and self-direction,
- social and emotional support,
- value orientation,
- life satisfaction,
- education level,
- present and future financial situations, and
- perceived career opportunities.

This list is not exhaustive but provides many of the most common factors necessary to consider when dealing with forced athletic retirement. Again, the counselor must address some of the aforementioned variables but also can aid the athlete's readjustment by teaching her a number of psychological skills. These skills are taught with the intent of providing a greater quality of life. The following psychological skills could be beneficial to this athlete:

- relaxation
- imagery
- cognitive restructuring
- hypnosis
- positive self-talk
- concentration training

The long-term objectives for counseling this athlete involve having her accept the termination of her competitive athletic career and helping her to proceed with her life in a positive manner. This injured athlete should be encouraged to remain socially integrated with her former teammates in terms of personal needs. Also, her coach should maintain a relationship with the athlete even though she may never compete again. The athlete should be allowed to move away from her sport (pistol shooting) at a pace commensurate with her emotional reintegration.

Common Fears

All injured athletes experience various fears in the different stages of rehabilitation that must be addressed and worked through prior to full reintegration into the sporting world and/or society in general. Counseling to address the following common fears of injured athletes is imperative, especially in the long-term stage:

(a) losing their position on the team;

(b) being treated differently by coaches, teammates, or peers;

(c) losing attention/recognition from others;

(d) being isolated from the team;

(e) re-injuring themselves after returning to competition;

(f) not recovering fully; and

(g) not knowing whether they will ever play again.

These fears are real to the person experiencing them, although they can be either rational or irrational. A competent counselor can use a variety of techniques to help athletes confront their fears:

1. Facing the fear. The fearful athlete gradually approaches the fear-evoking situation (initially in a safe and reassuring atmosphere), and then in more direct and demanding conditions.

2. Accepting. The athlete is helped to feel more comfortable in allowing the fear to occur without strongly reacting to it.

3. Flooding. The fearful athlete is exposed to the fearful situation for a protracted period of time to provoke intense fearful feelings.

4. Systematic desensitizing.

5. Modeling.

How athletes react to and overcome their fears depends upon their personalities. A generalization may be permissible at this point, however, that may be helpful to both counselors and injured athletes: self-confidence can counteract fear.

Summary

Counseling athletes with permanent disabilities is indeed a formidable challenge because each athlete's response to injury is unique. Sport trauma is real, and often initiates a life crisis for which very few athletes are prepared. Counselors should recognize the importance of the transitional period and the many psychological factors that affect readjustment. Also, the general reaction pattern phases (denial, anger, depression, grief, and reintegration) must be worked through appropriately prior to successful readjustment. Counselors also need to recognize that the way in which athletes respond to permanent disability is dependent upon their physical, emotional, and psychological foundation. An athlete's adjustment to injury is dependent upon

(a) prior psychological functioning;

(b) the meaning of the disability to the athlete;

(c) the nature, location, severity, and duration of the injury;

(d) the resulting changes in the individual's lifestyle; and

(e) how fears are addressed and mitigated.

We advocate a team approach to handling athletes with permanent disabilities. Sport psychologists, medical personnel, athletic trainers, family, friends, and teammates are all important contributors to the team approach. Each of these groups has significant influences during the preoperative, postoperative, and long-term stages of rehabilitation.

References

Brewer, B. W. (1993). Self-identity and specific vulnerability to depressed mood. *Journal of Personality,* *61*(3), 343-364.

Brewer, B. W. (2001). Psychology of sport injury rehabilitation. In R. N. Singer, H. A.Hausenblas & C. M. Janelle (Eds.), *Handbook of sport psychology* (2nd ed., pp. 787-809). New York: John Wiley & Sons, Inc.

Evans, L. & Hardy, L. (1999). Psychological and emotional response to athletic injury:Measurment issues. In D. Pargman (Ed.), *Psychological bases of sport injuries*(pp. 49-64). Morgantown, WV: Fitness Information Technology, Inc.

Ford, I. W., Gordon, S. (1999). Coping with sport injury: Resources loss and the role of social support. *Journal of Personal and Interpersonal Loss, 4,* 243-256.

Heil, J. (1993). *Psychology of sport injury.* Champaign, IL: Human Kinetics.

Henschen, K. (1992). Developing the self-concept in track and field athletes. *Track and Field Quarterly,* *92*(1), 35-37

Henschen, K. P., & Shelley, G. A. (1999). Counseling athletes with permanent Disabilities. In D. Pargman (Ed.), *Psychological bases of sport injuries* (2nd ed., pp. 255-27). Morgantown, WV: Fitness Information Technology, Inc.

Nideffer, R. M. (1983). The injured athlete: Psychological factors in treatment.*Orthopedic Clinics of North American, 14,* 373-385.

Ogilvie, B., & Howe, M. (1986). The trauma of termination from athletics. In J. M. Williams (Ed.), *Applied sport psychology* (pp 365-382). Palo Alto, CA: Mayfield.

Pearson, R. E., & Petipas, A. J. (1990). Transitions of athletes: Development and Preventive perspectives. *Journal of Counseling and Development. 69,* 7-10.

Chapter Twelve

Using Counseling Groups in the Rehabilitation of Athletic Injury

Trent A. Petrie
University of North Texas

Millions of athletes, from recreational to competitive levels, become injured every year (e.g., Kraus & Conroy, 1984). In areas where sport participation is high, such as high schools and colleges, over 30% of student-athletes will be injured in any given year and hundreds of millions of dollars will be spent on treatment (Meeuwisse & Fowler, 1988; NCAA, 1992; Requa, 1991). Further, injury rates have been found to be almost five times higher during competitions than during training or practices or during play of unorganized sports (Van Mechelen, Twisk, Molendijk, Blom, Snel, & Kemper, 1996). Contact and high-risk sports, such as football, gymnastics, wrestling, and soccer, can have injury rates two to five times higher than those found in noncontact sports, such as baseball and softball (NCAA, 1992). Although early research showed that boys had a greater incidence of injury than girls (Kraus & Conroy, 1984), women's increasing participation in sports has led to higher rates of injury, equaling or exceeding men's in many instances (Elias, 2001; Menckel & Laflamme, 2000).

Injuries are serious health problems that affect a large number of athletes each year. Although the physical, medical, and financial concerns associated with injury have long been evident, sports medicine professionals (in which I include sport psychologists, athletic trainers, and physiotherapists) now are acknowledging the psychological costs that injured athletes bear and recognizing that these responses can impede rehabilitation and recovery and delay return to competition even for athletes who are physically healed (Gould, Udry, Bridges, & Beck, 1997b; Kolt, 2000; Larson, Starkey, & Zaichkowsky, 1996; Podlog & Eklund, 2006; Wiese-Bjornstal, Smith, Shaffer, & Morrey, 1998). Based on this recognition, sports medicine professionals are integrating psychosocially based interventions, such as goal setting, positive thinking and confidence, social support, and counseling, into rehabilitation protocols in hopes of improving attitudes toward rehabilitation, increasing adherence, and facilitating recovery (Brewer, Jeffers, Petitpas, & Van Raalte, 1994; Larson et al., 1996).

This chapter examines the use of groups (a psychosocially based modality for intervening) for addressing the psychological responses of injured athletes and improving rehabilitation and recovery.

- First, the chapter provides a brief overview of a model that describes athletes' responses to injury and then reviews the psychological reactions that athletes typically have when injured.

- Second, the chapter addresses the ways in which athletes typically cope when injured and overviews the commonly endorsed psychological skills and strategies used when assisting in injury recovery. This section introduces social support as a key construct in injury recovery and reviews the types of support typically needed by injured athletes.

- Third, the chapter introduces the idea of groups as an effective and efficient modality for addressing the psychosocial needs of injured athletes, and it presents two specific types of groups that can be used to facilitate injury rehabilitation—psychoeducational and counseling.

Psychological Responses to Injury

According to Wiese-Bjornstal et al.'s (1998) integrated model of response to sport injury, athletes' emotional and behavioral reactions result from their primary ("How stressful is being injured to me?") and secondary ("How well can I cope with being injured?") cognitive appraisals of the injury. This appraisal process does not occur in isolation; rather, it is influenced by personal factors, such as

- athletic identity,
- age, and
- injury severity,

and situational factors, such as

- time in season,
- social support, and
- playing status.

For example, a college gymnast who views gymnastics as the most important part of her life, who wants to qualify for the NCAA championships and who is living far from home and thus has limited family support, suffers an anterior cruciate ligament (ACL) tear during the middle of her junior year season. As a result of these personal and situational factors, she may view the injury as incredibly stressful and herself as not having the resources to cope effectively. These appraisals, in turn, influence how she responds emotionally (e.g., feels depressed, anxious) and behaviorally (e.g., does not adhere to rehabilitation schedule, puts forth minimal effort during rehabilitation). Her appraisal process will not be static, but rather is a dynamic interplay between her cognitions, emotions, and behaviors. So, as time passes, she will make new appraisals of her situation (e.g., injury status, rehabilitation progress, surgery), which in turn will lead to new emotional and behavioral responses, which in turn will influence future appraisals.

Although cognitive appraisals are central in understanding athletes' responses to injury and thus determine the specific psychological reactions individuals have, athletes commonly experience a range of emotional responses when injured. Researchers, in both quantitative and qualitative studies, have found that athletes can feel depressed/sad, anxious/worried, frustrated, confused, angry, afraid, self-pitying, denying, guilty, doubtful, and isolated/alienated (e.g., Leddy, Lambart, & Ogles, 1994; Podlog & Eklund, 2006; Tracey, 2003; Udry, Gould, Bridges, & Beck, 1997). In addition, some athletes will experience what are labeled "positive" emotions, such as relief, optimism, and acceptance, or may view a season-ending injury as a benefit, something that allows them to grow personally (e.g., learn to manage time better, develop outside interests, clarify priorities) and/or become psychologically tougher (e.g., increase motivation, improve confidence) (Udry et al.).

It is not enough, however, to simply acknowledge these common emotions or label them as "positive" or "negative." Four other factors must be considered to understand fully athletes' psychological reactions to injury:

1. As discussed previously, athletes' emotional reactions result from cognitive appraisals that are influenced by their specific situations and personalities, and thus reactions will vary from person to person and from situation to situation. For example, an elite runner who highly identifies with that role may have a more extreme emotional reaction than a recreational jogger who is not so singularly defined. Or, a basketball player might experience more distress if a serious injury happens in the middle of the competitive season than if it occurs during the off-season when there is time for rehabilitation and recovery.

2. Emotional reactions can vary over time; some research indicates that negative mood is highest immediately following the injury and surgery and then dissipates as recovery unfolds (e.g., Rock & Jones, 2002) and other studies suggest that emotions may vary over the course of rehabilitation (e.g., Wiese-Bjornstal, 1998). For example, a swimmer who has undergone surgery may experience an increase in frustration and depression throughout the course of rehabilitation every time he does not meet a physical therapy goal.

3. "Negative" emotions, such as anger or frustration, actually may be facilitative in the recovery process and should not be viewed as something that must be alleviated (Wiese-Bjornstal, 1998). For example, a skier might use her feelings of anger and frustration as a source of motivation during the long and difficult rehabilitation of a torn ACL.

4. Athletes' levels of psychological distress can negatively influence their rehabilitation, in particular their attendance at sessions (Daly, Brewer, Van Raalte, Petitpas, Sklar, 1995). For example, a diver who is feeling highly frustrated, tense, and anxious about his back injury may avoid his rehabilitation sessions and thus limit the important physical conditioning he needs to do to fully recover.

Specific cognitions and sources of stress in relation to injury also have been identified and fall under the category of psychological responses (Gould et al., 1997b; Podlog & Eklund, 2006; Tracy, 2003). For example, in a study of elite skiers, Gould et al. (1997b) identified seven areas of stress/concern in relation to the season-ending injuries they had experienced. The athletes' primary stressors were psychological and social in nature, including

- fear of re-injury,
- social isolation,
- losing a spot on the team, and
- watching teammates compete.

Although less frequent, the skiers reported

- physical concerns (e.g., pain, inactivity),
- medical concerns (e.g., seriousness of injury, dealing with slow progress in rehab), and
- career and financial concerns (e.g., lost sponsorships).

Following injury and during the return to competition, Podlog and Eklund (2006) found that athletes experience stressors including

(a) dealing with fears about returning to competition, such as

- variability in pain,
- fear of re-injury,
- fear of not reaching pre-injury performance levels, and
- self-presentational concerns about performing poorly in front of others,

(b) handling adversity, such as

- adapting to increased levels of training and competition,
- lower levels of confidence,
- not making the team, and
- injuries in other parts of the body.

Such stressors can influence how athletes think about their situations, affect their emotions, and have an impact on how they respond behaviorally.

An athlete's reaction to injury is a complex, dynamic process that is influenced by situational and personal factors and stressors in the environment. At its core are the athlete's cognitive appraisals of the injury and of his or her ability to cope successfully. Resulting from these appraisals are emotional and behavioral responses that can either facilitate recovery or interfere with an athlete's rehabilitation process. When responses are debilitating, the coping strategies used by an athlete or the psychosocial interventions introduced by sports medicine professionals become the key factor in determining how successfully an injured athlete recovers.

Psychosocial Interventions and Coping with Injury

Researchers have identified a range of coping resources, behaviors and personal characteristics, and psychosocial interventions that assist athletes in their rehabilitation and recovery from injury (Brewer et al., 1994; Cupal, 1998; Gould, Udry, Bridges, & Beck, 1997a; Larson et al., 1996; Meyers, Peyton, & Jensen, 2004; Podlog & Eklund, 2006; Rock & Jones, 2002; Udry, Gould, Bridges, & Tuffey, 1997). For example, Gould et al. (1997a) identified four key categories of coping strategies that skiers reported using to handle their season-ending injuries:

1. Driving through was characterized by striving for high levels of personal motivation, setting goals, and focusing on rehabilitation. These coping strategies emphasized taking control of the situation and stressed an intrinsic orientation.

2. Self-distraction, such as keeping busy and participating in a variety of activities, was important because all of the athletes' time was not taken up by rehabilitation or training.

3. Managing emotions and thoughts was accomplished by using mental imagery, keeping a positive focus (e.g., using positive self-talk), sharing emotions, and taking it slow in rehabilitation (i.e., not giving in to internal or external pressure to return to competition prematurely). These strategies underscore the importance of actively addressing the emotions associated with injury and of cognitively reframing a negative into a positive.

4. Using social resources, such as seeking support from friends and teammates and using other injured athletes as role models and sources of motivation, was also employed. These strategies underscore the importance of support in rehabilitation.

In comparing those skiers who successfully came back from their injury with those who did not, Gould et al. (1997a) found that successfully managing emotions and thoughts, in particular using mental imagery and taking it slow, differentiated the two groups.

Although not labeled as coping strategies, Larson et al. (1996) surveyed athletic trainers to determine the behaviors and characteristics of athletes who do and do not successfully handle their injuries. Athletes who cope successfully comply with their rehabilitation program, maintain a positive attitude about their injury and life, are motivated to work hard during rehabilitation, are determined to return to competition, set goals for themselves, are self-confident, and remain involved with their teams. Less successful athletes do not comply with treatment protocols, experience a wide range of negative emotions, are unmotivated, externalize, withdraw from team and others, lack self-confidence, and communicate poorly with coach and others. Overall, athletes seem to cope most effectively when they

- manage their emotions,
- keep a positive attitude,
- use goals and other psychological strategies to remain motivated,
- are instrumental in their approach to rehabilitation,
- are self-confident, and
- seek out and communicate with supportive others.

Paralleling the coping strategies reportedly used by athletes, sports medicine professionals have recommended several different psychosocial interventions to facilitate injury rehabilitation and recovery. For example, Larson et al. (1996) found that athletic trainers, in helping athletes cope, kept them involved with the team and helped them improve their social support, used goal setting, focused on positive thinking and self-confidence, and communicated effectively with them. Others (e.g., Shaffer & Wiese-Bjornstal, 1999) have advocated using positive thinking (cognitive restructuring), mental imagery (in particular that focused on healing the injured body part, maintaining sport skills, and achieving rehabilitation tasks), relaxation, goal setting, and improving social support in the treatment of injury, viewing these as key skills that sports medicine professionals should possess and be able to implement with injured athletes.

Researchers also have examined the credibility and effectiveness of these psychosocial interventions and coping strategies. For example, physical therapy patients viewed goal setting, imagery, and general counseling (facilitating discussion of thoughts and feelings) as credible means for assisting in injury rehabilitation (Brewer et al., 1994), whereas college football players perceived behaviorally based approaches (positive self-talk, relaxation, goal setting) and counseling (empathy, support, catharsis) as acceptable interventions for dealing with concomitant psychological reactions to injury (Meyers et al., 2004). Concerning effectiveness, in-depth longitudinal examinations of injured athletes have suggested that counseling (listening, emotional support), cognitive-behavioral strategies (imagery, goals), and improving social support can assist athletes in

- managing their negative emotions,
- handling setbacks in rehabilitation,
- maintaining and enhancing motivation, and
- adhering to rehabilitation programs

(Evans et al., 2000; Rock & Jones, 2002). Cupal (1998), in her review of psychological interventions in sport injury rehabilitation, concluded that counseling and psychosocial interventions are effective, particularly in terms of increasing physical functioning, reducing pain and anxiety, and facilitating earlier strength gains. Although there are a variety of credible psychosocial interventions, a key to their effectiveness is matching the strategy to the individual athlete's specific concerns, reactions, or issues. For example, an injured soccer player who is surrounded by family and friends and believes he is receiving a sufficient level of emotional support may not benefit from an intervention aimed at increasing either his support network or his perception of support received. He might, though, benefit from setting goals with his physiotherapist so as to increase his motivation and focus during rehabilitation.

Podlog and Eklund (2006) suggested that self-determination theory was a useful model for understanding athletes' experiences, from the time they are injured through their recovery and return to play. In the same vein, this model can explain how these psychosocial interventions and coping strategies assist injured athletes in handling their psychological reactions. Self-determination theory posits that when individuals feel

- competent (instrumental, effective),
- autonomous (owning one's behaviors, internal locus of control), and
- related (connected to others),

their functioning is optimal as defined by enhanced well-being, intrinsic motivation, and better relationships with others (Podlog & Eklund, 2006; Ryan & Deci, 2000). Unfortunately, as a result of being injured, many athletes have diminished feelings of competence, autonomy, and/or connectedness, and thus may not adequately invest in rehabilitation or feel sufficiently confident to return to high-level competition when they are physically healed. As Podlog and Eklund (2006) noted, athletes' return to competition may be facilitated by environments, including those created by the sports medicine professionals, that assist them in regaining an internal locus of control, a feeling of connection to and support from others, and a sense of overall effectiveness in their lives.

The general focus of the psychosocial interventions discussed in this section are (a) instrumental (developing new skills and strategies that can enhance coping), and (b) relational (receiving emotional support and care from supportive others).

In terms of self-determination theory, instrumental approaches (cognitive behavioral interventions such as positive thinking, imagery, setting goals, or relaxation) may assist injured athletes by giving them strategies to retake responsibility for their rehabilitation, motivating themselves from within, and increasing their belief that they can recover and return to play. Relational approaches (counseling, such as listening empathically), on the other hand, can give injured athletes a forum for expressing their emotions, connecting with other people, and reframing their experience as positive and one from which they can learn. These interventions, if targeted appropriately, can help injured athletes redevelop their lost sense of competence, autonomy, and relatedness and optimize their emotions and behaviors with respect to returning successfully to competition.

Group as a Modality for Intervention with Injured Athletes

Although it is no longer a question of whether psychosocial interventions should be a part of injury rehabilitation programs (Cupal, 1998), the issue remaining concerns the mode of delivery. There are two primary modalities for delivering the psychosocial interventions discussed in this chapter: individual and group. In an individual format, the injured athlete meets alone with the sports medicine professional for a certain period of time (e.g., 45 minutes) at a specific level of frequency (e.g., once per week). During meetings, the sports medicine professional, depending on the focus of the intervention (i.e., relational and/or instrumental), educates the athlete on psychosocial skills and strategies that are essential to rehabilitation, and/or provides support, active listening, and empathy, encouraging the athlete to discuss his or her thoughts and emotional reactions to the injury and recovery process. In the group modality, the athlete meets concurrently with the sports medicine professional and other injured athletes. During these meetings, which have a specific duration and frequency of occurrence as individual meetings do, athletes benefit not only from the knowledge, experience, and skills of the group leader but also from one another.

Although researchers and sports medicine professionals have reported on the effectiveness of individual counseling in their work with injured athletes (e.g., Evans et al., 2000; Kolt, 2000; Rock & Jones, 2002), group is an effective and efficient modality that may offer some benefits over the individual format. Across a wide range of client, counselor, and treatment variables, groups consistently have been shown to be as effective as individual in treating many types of psychopathology (e.g., Bovasso, Eatin, & Armenian, 1999; McRoberts, Burlingame & Hoag, 1998). Given that the general effectiveness of this modality is not in question, what are the unique aspects of group that make it superior in some instances in the delivery of psychosocial interventions with injured athletes? There are three characteristics to highlight:

1. Group is an efficient means for delivering services to athletes. In an individual format, intervening with eight injured athletes could require up to eight hours of a sports medicine professionals' time each week, depending on duration of contact.

Compared to 60–90 minutes per week if that professional worked with the eight athletes in a group format, the time savings are substantial.

2. Because of the unique therapeutic factors that exist, issues such as increasing support and reducing alienation, learning how other injured athletes have coped, accepting the injury and reframing challenges in recovery, and improving communication with others may be better suited to a group format. For example, the group format provides the mechanism for learning that

   (a) others often experience many similar emotions and fears (universality),

   (b) how we behave influences how others perceive and respond to us (interpersonal learning), and

   (c) we can improve ourselves by simply observing how others with similar concerns/issues handles their situation (vicarious learning).

3. Athletes have a strong sense of independence, such that asking for help is often uncomfortable (Tracey, 2003), and they may hold a negative bias toward those who seek individual assistance from a psychologist (Ferrante, Etzel, & Lantz, 1996). Participating in a group of one's peers, however, particularly when it has been sanctioned by coaches, athletic directors, sports medicine personnel, or sport organizations, may lessen the bias and increase the willingness to seek assistance.

There are many group formats, ranging from self-help to therapy, yet there are two in particular that are well-suited for delivering psychosocial interventions and assisting injured athletes: psychoeducational and counseling.

1. Psychoeducational groups focus on developing members' affective, cognitive, and behavioral skills and strategies through a series of structured presentations that revolve around a specific theme (e.g., recovery from injury) (Corey & Corey, 2006). Through these presentations, members can increase awareness about their current life situations and learn new skills and strategies to cope more effectively. These groups make use of didactic learning, structured activities (e.g., role-playing), in-session practice of skills, homework assignments, and discussion. They may be particularly effective with adolescents and young adults because of their similarity to the classroom learning environment (Corey & Corey). Although psychoeducational groups may serve a relational purpose, their primary focus is instrumental.

   Psychoeducational groups have been used with athletes with some success. For example, freshmen student athletes, through eight different sessions, were introduced to issues such as stress management, study skills, careers, life as a student athlete, and sexual responsibility to help them make a successful transition during their first semester in college (Harris, Altekruse, & Engels, 2003). Based on feedback provided, the researchers concluded that the group experience helped the student athletes adjust to college and reduce their stress. Although generally not referred to as a psychoeducational group, this format is the foundation through which performance enhancement skills are taught to teams and groups of athletes, and thus represents an approach with which most sport psychologists are familiar and skilled.

2. Counseling groups, which are less structured and more relational in their focus, are ideal for treating injured athletes (Corey & Corey, 2006).

   - First, they are focused on helping individuals deal with current, conscious issues that are interfering with daily living. As such, they emphasize becoming more aware of how current emotions and ways of thinking and behaving are blocking goal attainment and problem resolution, such as how athletes' emotional reactions to injury may be influencing their behaviors in rehabilitation.

   - Second, problems are viewed in a developmental context with an emphasis on growth and capitalizing on strengths. Not all problems or concerns are indications of pathology nor do they require deep intrapsychic change. Many problems are normative and can be solved by reconnecting with the strengths and resources within the athletes themselves and their environment, such as when athletes come to understand that they have cognitive control over their reactions to their injuries and that they can motivate themselves from within to accomplish their rehabilitation goals.

   - Third, they emphasize skill acquisition, behavioral change, and transfer of learning to other life areas. For example, athletes may be asked to set goals, learn new skills (e.g., how to effectively talk with their coach), or try a behavior in a new environment (e.g., share emotions with friends/family as opposed to just in group), all of which are familiar processes.

   Overall, counseling groups provide the opportunity

   - to express emotions,
   - receive support,
   - receive feedback on current thoughts and behaviors,
   - practice new skills,
   - clarify communication patterns,
   - increase self-awareness and understanding,
   - solve problems, and
   - behave, think, and feel more positively and effectively outside the group session.

   The subsequent two sections outline how the psychoeducational and counseling group formats may be applied in the treatment of injured athletes. Under the psychoeducational approach, a six-session group is presented that includes the psychosocial skills/strategies shown to be effective in assisting athletes post-injury. Because it is not within the purview of this chapter to provide an indepth presentation of each one, readers are referred to other sources (e.g., Andersen, 2000, 2005; Van Raalte & Brewer, 2002; Williams, 2006) to learn more about these skills, including their underlying theory, empirical basis, and application. Because the counseling group is a more open, less structured format, this text takes a less prescriptive approach, introducing instead key therapeutic factors that exist within the group context and examining how these factors can contribute to the treatment of and recovery from injury.

A Psychoeducational Group Approach

In a psychoeducational group with injured athletes, it is important to keep in mind the major issues, reactions, stressors that they experience post-injury/surgery, such as a range of deleterious emotions, social isolation/alienation, the perception of being unable to effectively change situations or actively engage in the rehabilitation process, lack of motivation, diminished self-confidence, and negative appraisals of situations/experiences. They may feel lost, unsure, disconnected, and lack efficacy regarding rehabilitation, training, and return to competition. Thus, psychoeducational sessions need to present information on and give opportunities to practice the skills and strategies that will allow athletes to effectively cope with their reactions and develop greater feelings of self-efficacy about and ownership of their rehabilitation, as well as greater feelings of connection with important people in their lives.

The six-session format outlined in this section includes presentations on

(a) introduction to injury,

(b) setting goals and improving motivation,

(c) imagery,

(d) confidence and positive thinking,

(e) relaxation, and

(f) enhancing support and improving communication.

Although these are important skills and strategies for assisting with injury rehabilitation, they are not the only ones a sports medicine professional may want to consider. Depending on the rehabilitation context, the professional, and/or the injured athletes themselves, a different set of topics might be selected or a longer or shorter framework chosen. For example, it might be that the major issue for a set of injured athletes is motivation and staying on track with rehabilitation goals. In such a case, the set of presentations might focus primarily on those topics by going into more depth on each one, as opposed to presenting information on five or six other important but not as relevant issues.

Session One. The main purpose of the first session is to provide a normative context in which the athletes can understand their psychological reactions to injury. Following injury, many athletes experience intense (which generally are labeled as negative) emotional reactions that are confusing and distressing in their own right. These athletes often lack information about what is normal, whether in regards to their emotional and other reactions or to the process of recovery. Thus, sports medicine professionals might discuss common emotional, physical, cognitive, and behavioral responses to injury, and in doing so present information in lay terms on current models of injury response (e.g., Wiese-Bjornstal et al., 1998). In addition, they might address the stressors and challenges athletes face during the course of recovery. Covering these topics can help athletes understand the dynamic nature of injury recovery and how their thoughts play a central role in determining their reactions.

Session Two. In the context of understanding what normally occurs following injury and during rehabilitation, the primary purpose of this session is to refocus athletes on what they want to achieve in rehabilitation and give them the practical strategies for doing so. Most athletes are used to setting and working toward goals in their sports, but they may not have thought to apply this approach in relation to their recovery from injury or they may not feel able to do so because of their current emotional and cognitive state. Providing injured athletes with a system for effectively setting goals (e.g., Gould, 2006; Marchant, 2000) and then helping them set goals for their current situation gives them something concrete they can focus on and do, and it sets the stage for increasing efficacy and motivation. In presenting this topic, sports medicine professionals also might address the issue of motivation more directly, covering attribution theory (in particular the locus of causality) in the discussion. When injured and emotionally down, athletes may externalize their successes and lose the opportunity to build efficacy and motivation. Through a discussion of the attribution process, athletes can learn how their interpretations of success strongly influence their motivation and future behaviors. In other words, they can reclaim their successes as their own and begin the process of redeveloping an internal locus of control.

Session Three. Tension, pain, inability to sleep, and worry all can interfere with rehabilitation, yet athletes may not know how to effectively minimize the negative effects of these responses. Thus, the primary purpose of this session is to introduce athletes to relaxation and provide them with techniques for relaxation outside of session. In covering this topic, sports medicine professionals might provide a brief background on how individuals' bodies respond physically to stress and how relaxation provides a means for effectively handling those responses. In particular, athletes should be given the opportunity to practice in session the relaxation approaches introduced to them. Such practice provides the leader with the opportunity to make corrective feedback in the athletes' techniques and helps the athletes feel more confident in their ability to use the skill outside of session. Because imagery can be enhanced when in a relaxed state, this session serves as an important prelude to session four.

Session Four. Because most athletes are familiar with imagery as it relates to sport performances, they may respond positively to the introduction of this strategy. Taking into account the injured athletes' existing imagery knowledge-base, sports medicine professionals might teach them about how imagery works and the benefits that can accrue through its use. The main purpose of this session, though, is to help athletes generalize their imagery knowledge to the rehabilitation process. In particular, sports medicine professionals might focus on how imagery can help injured athletes

- regain (or maintain) confidence,
- promote healing in the injured area,
- improve effectiveness of rehabilitation,
- enhance relaxation,
- increase motivation for rehabilitation and recovery,
- learn new athletic skills or stay sharp with those already developed, and
- practice tactical aspects of their sport (e.g., a skier imaging specific runs on a mountain, or a basketball player imaging running the team's offense against different opponents).

Although sport-skill practice may be familiar to injured athletes, including it in this session reminds them that, even though their current physical training may be limited, there still are things they can do to stay mentally and physically sharp. In addition, helping athletes develop their own individualized imagery program and learn how (and when) to apply it during rehabilitation and recovery will be a key part of this session.

Session Five. The primary purpose of this session is to address the negative thinking that often exists following injury and that can undermine motivation, confidence, and recovery. Depending on the severity of the injury, rehabilitation may be a long, painful, difficult process that is marked by obstacles that must be overcome if the athlete wants to fully recover and return to competition. Over such a long journey, it can be a challenge to remain positive and motivated toward rehabilitation, yet having such an attitude is important for coping successfully. Thus, sports medicine professionals might present information on how thoughts influence emotions and subsequent behaviors (which is an extension of the appraisal information presented in session one), and thus help athletes understand that their reactions generally are under their control (or result from how they talk to themselves). They might help athletes identify the situations in which negative thinking tends to occur, become aware of the negative thoughts that arise in those situations, and develop more positive, rational ways of thinking about and talking to themselves. A key element in this session is having athletes, out of session, self-monitor their thinking and actively practice substituting positive statements to enhance their emotional and behavioral functioning.

Session Six. Because injured athletes can feel alienated and isolated from primary supports (e.g., teammates) due to geography, personality, and/or emotional state, the primary purpose of this session is to help athletes identify sources of support and then establish connections so they may receive what they need. In covering this topic, sports medicine professionals might introduce the concept of support, delineate the types of support that may be available to individuals, and help athletes determine what support they want and from whom they want to receive it. Not all athletes want the same type of support (e.g., emotional comfort vs. task challenge), nor do they want it in the same amount or from the same people. In fact, some athletes view too much support as a source of stress (Gould et al., 1997b). Thus, decisions about support need to be made individually, and this session can help athletes begin to identify their best sources of support. For many athletes, friends and family may represent good sources of emotional support, whereas sports medicine professionals and coaches may be best for obtaining information about their injury, their rehabilitation, or other technical aspects of their training and return to competition. In this session, sports medicine professionals also might teach injured athletes about communication and give them opportunities to practice asking for support and dealing with the responses they may receive.

Summary. A psychoeducational approach offers sports medicine professionals an effective and efficient way to present important information and teach necessary skills and strategies to injured athletes. Whether the sessions include the topics outlined in this section or the professional addresses other issues that are more relevant to their situations, what is more important is that the presentations provide the athletes with

(a) concrete practical information on the topic,

(b) opportunities to practice the skill or strategy in session and to develop plans for how it generalize to their daily lives,

(c) chances to ask questions and seek feedback, and

(d) assignments to complete during the subsequent week of rehabilitation and training.

If the presentations do so, then the athletes will be more likely to develop their competence and autonomy and feel more connected to others, whether in the group or in their outside environment.

A Counseling Group Approach

Counseling groups are less structured and less formulaic than their psychoeducational counterparts. Whereas in the psychoeducational format injured athletes learn and change by obtaining information through didactic presentations, practicing new skills and strategies during structured in-session opportunities, and completing homework assignments designed to generalize learning, theoretically, change occurs in the counseling format through the presence and interplay of key therapeutic factors (Yalom, 1995). According to Fuhriman and Burlingame (1990), clinician interventions, such as

- reflection,
- experiential activities,
- confrontation,
- interpretation,
- self-disclosure,
- exploration,
- guidance,
- focus on affect and cognition, and
- encouragement

are effective if they act as a catalyst for the development of therapeutic factors, such as universality, altruism, and interpersonal learning. If they do, then these interventions are likely to produce desired psychosocial outcomes, such as improvements in emotional, cognitive, and behavioral functioning.

The therapeutic factors represent, in many ways, the objectives of talking therapies (Fuhriman & Burlingame, 1990). They are what ultimately brings about change and improvement in the client. Yalom (1995) identified 11 primary therapeutic factors that he viewed as essential aspects of the change process, including

- instillation of hope,
- universality,
- imparting information,
- altruism,
- corrective recapitulation of the primary family group,
- development of socializing techniques,
- imitative behavior,
- interpersonal learning,
- group cohesiveness,
- catharsis, and
- existential factors.

Although other constructs have been labeled as therapeutic factors, this discussion will focus on the factors identified by Yalom.

Although discussed as independent constructs, therapeutic factors are interdependent, existing and working together to facilitate change. According to Yalom (1995), although these therapeutic factors exist in every group,

(a) their importance and interrelatedness may vary considerably from group to group,

(b) their relative importance may differ from member to member, and

(c) they represent different parts of the change process, from something members learn to something members do to how much members express their emotions.

For example, in an injury group, one member may benefit most from knowing that other athletes are having similar emotions in relation to the injury experience whereas another may find that learning to talk more effectively with her coaches is most helpful. In another injury group, members might benefit most from having the opportunity to talk through and understand what their injuries mean to them in the context of their lives and to develop a close set of relationships with one another.

Although Yalom (1995) has identified 11 therapeutic factors, there are nine that are particularly relevant in a counseling group with injured athletes, for three primary reasons:

- First, philosophically, these nine are consistent with and likely to exist in a counseling group whose focus is on developing strengths, solving problems, establishing support, expressing emotions, and learning new skills and strategies. This type of present-oriented, solution-focused approach will resonate with athletes and increase the likelihood of their remaining in group counseling and benefiting from the therapeutic factors.

- Second, interventions and coping that have been suggested as helpful in the psychological treatment of injured athletes, such as expressing emotions, accepting the injury, and using other injured athletes as role models, are consistent with these factors.

- Third, psychological reactions to injury that have been documented among injured athletes (e.g., Gould et al., 1997b) would likely dissipate or be improved from the presence and interplay of these factors within a counseling group.

The remainder of this section is an overview of each therapeutic factor and an examination of its importance in relation to an injury group. Each factor is presented independently, but as Yalom (1995) expresses, the factors are interrelated and often exist simultaneously in group counseling.

1. *Instillation of hope.* The hope or expectation that things will get better, communicated by group leaders or members, defines this construct. Having hope is essential early in treatment because it keeps injured athletes connected to and involved in the group long enough for other therapeutic factors to come into play (Yalom, 1995). Some of this hope will come from the sports medicine professionals' statements about the efficacy of treatment and about their experiences in assisting athletes in recovering from injury and returning to competition, and initially should be communicated to potential members during pre-group screening meetings. These meetings serve the purposes of answering athletes' questions about the group, reducing their anxiety about being a member of a group, setting expectations for

their involvement in the group, and instilling the hope that they will improve as a result of their involvement in the counseling group. The meetings are an essential part of the group counseling approach, particularly if the group will be "closed." (See next section for more information on group status). But hope also is communicated, both directly and indirectly, by the members themselves. Invariably, some of the athletes in the group already will have been through injury rehabilitation and know the landscape, will be further along in their current physical rehabilitation, or just will be thinking and feeling more positively about their return to sport than other group members. Through discussions facilitated by the leaders, comments made by the members, and even just observations of the other members, the athlete learns that recovery does occur and things do improve. Leaders can facilitate the development of this factor by encouraging discussion about injury status and rehabilitation, directly pointing out similarities among group members in terms of injury, rehabilitation, and recovery, and by sharing their own optimism about treatment and the work the members are doing in group.

2. *Universality.* Injured athletes often report feeling isolated and alienated from important supports, which can only exacerbate a general belief that they are unique in their situation, alone in their suffering, and unable to connect with others (Yalom, 1995). By talking with other injured athletes in the group, they have the opportunity to learn that others experience many of the same problems, not to mention the exact same thoughts and feelings, as they do. This knowledge that there is a commonality to their problems, thoughts, and feelings and that they are not uniquely alone, wretched, or unlovable (Yalom, 1995), provides a tremendous sense of relief. For example, a basketball player, who has just had surgery on a season-ending injury, enters an injury counseling group believing that no one else has gone through the physical pain and emotional distress he is experiencing. As he listens to the other athletes in the group, however, he comes to understand that they too have felt the anger, loneliness, fear, and uncertainty that he has, often using the same words he does to describe the experiences. This understanding lessens his psychological distress and allows him to open up and share more in the group. By encouraging member self-disclosure about their injuries and the emotions and thoughts connected to them, leaders can help to bring about this therapeutic factor, which has been shown to be particularly important early in the group experience because of its influence on the development of member connection, trust, and cohesion (Kivlighan & Goldfine, 1991).

3. *Imparting information.* According to Yalom (1995), this therapeutic factor occurs through didactic instruction by the leaders or direct advice offered by the members. Although instruction or advice is not the main purpose in a counseling group, there will be times when injured athletes can benefit from information provided directly by the leaders. In such instances, the injured athletes may simply have inaccurate information (e.g., about their physical injury) or insufficient knowledge about an important topic (e.g., how to set goals effectively). In either situation, the leader can provide accurate information for the benefit of the members. For example, during a group counseling meeting, the athletes are discussing

their lack of motivation toward rehabilitation and the fact that they are frustrated in their attempts to set goals concerning their recovery. Upon inquiry, the leader discerns that the athletes are missing key steps in setting their goals and offers concrete instruction on how they might improve their goal setting, including homework assignments to help them apply this strategy in their daily rehabilitation.

Information also is shared when members give each other advice or guidance on how to handle whatever situation or emotion is being discussed. Advice giving often occurs early in a group's development and, although the "what" that is offered (the content) is usually not that useful to the recipient (e.g., it is not uncommon for group members say "Yes, but…" to such offerings of advice), the process of offering the advice is important, conveying connection, concern, and care (Yalom, 1995). Leaders may want to watch for this phenomenon early in the group's development and encourage the injured athletes to give voice to the message that underlies the advice, communicating directly the care and concern they feel toward the other group member. Interestingly, Kivlighan and Goldfine (1991) found that, although the amount of advice given across a short-term group likely remains unchanged, members view it as more important in the latter phases of the group's development. They suggested that, as the members become more familiar with and connected to one another, the quality of the advice changes, becoming more personal and thus meaningful to the recipient.

4. *Altruism.* Injured athletes may feel demoralized, unimportant, and lacking in the belief that they can effect change in their lives. Through their participation in group counseling, however, they have the chance to offer support, encouragement, guidance, and understanding, to engage in the intrinsic act of giving, and to provide relief and healing to another (Yalom, 1995). Although powerful in its effects, altruism is not something that most group members initially appreciate. As Yalom noted, group members wonder how they can help one another: How can one emotionally distressed injured athlete assist another? Yet, they do and the results of their giving are felt not just by the other group members. Injured athletes whose support, caring, advice, or understanding makes a difference in another member's life often feel empowered, connected, and efficacious. Through their giving, they have made a difference; they have effected change and made a personal connection with another person. Thus, leaders may want to encourage member interaction and giving in hopes of facilitating such interchanges.

5. *Modeling (Vicarious learning).* The observation and modeling of others is a powerful mechanism for change, yet one that is often overlooked in counseling (Yalom, 1995). Through observation, injured athletes have the opportunity to learn new and more effective ways of thinking about themselves and their situations, solving problems in their lives, handling the daily stressors and obstacles associated with a long recovery, and behaving more positively in rehabilitation and with important others. Early in a group's development, injured athletes may look to identify with more "senior" members and subsequently be open to these members' perspectives and ways of handling their injury. Even if the imitation of others is short-lived, Yalom suggested that it has the potential to establish an adaptive spi-

ral in which injured athletes become increasingly open to trying new ways of thinking and behaving based on what they see others do in session and hear about what occurs outside of group. For example, an injured lacrosse player identifies with another group member (soccer player) and begins to "try on" that athlete's behaviors in group, such as being personally disclosing about his fears of re-injury and asking questions of other group members. In time, the lacrosse player's behaviors become less a direct imitation of his peers, and now the player is more open to other experiences that he sees occurring among the other members, such as seeking support from family and investing more energy in physical therapy. The reality is that injured athletes may be more open to their peers' ideas and experiences than to what the leaders have to say. Thus, leaders may want to encourage self-disclosure early in group and to purposefully label the behaviors and thoughts shared by members that are adaptive and positive. Doing so helps athletes know what is positive and thus what they may want to emulate.

6. *Development of social skills.* In all groups, opportunities exist for members to learn basic and more advanced social skills, though how direct this learning is depends on the group's purpose and the leader's style (Yalom, 1995). In injury groups, social learning can take many forms, from direct instruction by the leaders on how to listen, ask for feedback, or talk with a coach, to more indirect ways, such as labeling and reinforcing positive communication that occurs during group sessions. For example, an injured football player may be given the opportunity to role play talking with his coach about his status on the team, whereas another may be told by the leader that she really liked the way the athlete was supportive when another member shared her emotional distress. Although many athletes possess basic social skills, their injuries and their psychological reactions to them may have disrupted the implementation of those skills and contributed to the social isolation they are experiencing. By reconnecting with what they already know and by learning new ways of communicating with and behaving toward others, injured athletes can improve their relationships with important people in their lives, feel more efficacious, and take more responsibility for their rehabilitation and recovery. Thus, in group, leaders can assess informally the injured athletes' level of social skills and then give them opportunities, either in group or through out-of-session homework, to make improvements.

7. *Catharsis.* Simply put, catharsis is the release of unexpressed emotions in relation to unwanted thoughts, unexpressed pain, or unconscious fears and anxieties that have become known (Corey & Corey, 2006; Yalom, 1995). For many injured athletes, particularly those who are experiencing considerable psychological distress and do not have sufficient or acceptable supports with whom they can talk and share, the expression of emotion in and of itself may bring considerable relief. For example, a baseball player, whose severely torn rotator cuff will require surgery and keep him out for the entire season, has kept his emotions in check at all times, not allowing himself to express his sadness and anger about his injury. Although he has presented himself to others as "fine," he has not been sleeping well, has been experiencing headaches, and has lost his appetite. In group counseling, though, his pain

overwhelms him one day and he expresses all the feelings that he has been holding inside. Although embarrassed at first by his emotional "outburst," as he receives support and understanding from the other group members he begins to feel like a huge weight has been lifted off of his shoulders. In the days that follow, many of his physical symptoms dissipate. Disclosures such as this can facilitate trust and cohesion among group members and establish the norm of reciprocal emotional sharing (Corey & Corey, 2006). Although some athletes may disclose during initial group sessions, it is likely that catharsis will occur more frequently and in more meaningful ways as the group develops (Kivlighan & Goldfine, 1991).

Although important, particularly for those who may be socially isolated and experiencing intense negative emotions, direct expression alone is insufficient to promote lasting change. Injured athletes also need to reflect on their emotional expression so that they can gain insight into their experience and ultimately make positive changes in how they are thinking and behaving. Thus, leaders of injury counseling groups can encourage emotional expression among their members but should make sure that the injured athletes also are provided with opportunities to gain a cognitive understanding of their expression (e.g., "Why am I feeling so sad, scared, angry, etc.?"). Without movement to the cognitive and behavioral, little of substance will change in their lives and the injured athletes may end up experiencing the group simply as "venting" time. If injured athletes do make the connections between their thoughts and feelings, though, they will come to understand that they have control over their experiences and can take responsibility for behaviors that may have seemed initially to be outside of their control.

8. *Existential factor.* Although the label "existential" may suggest that this factor is incompatible with a present-oriented, growth-focused counseling group, the reality is that the ideas underlying it (Yalom, 1995) parallel the issues and stressors that many injured athletes report experiencing, including that

   (a) being injured may seem unfair and unjust ("Why did I get injured?"),

   (b) athletes must take responsibility for their behaviors and choices, such as how they are going to approach their rehabilitation,

   (c) being injured can be physically and emotionally painful and this pain must be faced, and

   (d) no matter how much assistance and support is available, each athlete must face and overcome the injury by himself or herself.

   For example, an injured field hockey player's lack of motivation for rehabilitation may be directly related to her questioning the fairness of her situation and the arbitrariness of her suffering, and to her being mired in self-doubt and despair as she compares herself to teammates who are not injured. Although there is no timeframe in which such issues may be raised during group or specific interventions that will lead directly to their emergence, leaders need to be aware that these factors are likely present, to some degree, in all injured athletes and to look for opportunities to facilitate discussion about them. Through their resolution, that is a cognitive understanding and acceptance of their situation, injured athletes can increase their commitment, internal motivation, and connection to others.

9. *Interpersonal learning.* According to Yalom (1995), psychological distress and symptoms occur as a result of problematic interpersonal relationships. Thus, the purpose of group counseling is to provide individuals with the opportunity to
   (a) receive feedback on their way of relating to others,
   (b) develop new insights into and awareness of their emotional, cognitive, and behavioral patterns, as well as interpersonal strengths and weaknesses,
   (c) understand the impact they have on other people,
   (d) understand that individuals are responsible for the interpersonal worlds they create,
   (e) accept personal responsibility for changing their interpersonal behaviors, and
   (f) begin the process of behaving differently in group and generalizing those behaviors to relationships in the outside world. Although this factor is complex and unfolds over the course of group counseling, in any given session, injured athletes may engage in any of these aspects of interpersonal learning. For example, the injured athlete who receives feedback from other group members that his negative attitude and complaining are annoying and result in members feeling emotionally distant from him may realize that this is the reason none of his teammates are hanging out with him any more. Through that feedback, he has learned that he has created his current social isolation through his behaviors and that he has the opportunity to alter that by changing how he expresses himself when around his teammates.

By actively encouraging
(a) self-disclosure,
(b) dynamic and spontaneous interchanges among members,
(c) the expression of and openness to direct and honest feedback,
(d) a cognitive understanding of how others perceive us and experience our behaviors, and
(e) the identification and application of new ways of behaving, leaders can facilitate all aspects of interpersonal learning and bring about profound changes within injured athletes and their existing relationships.

Summary. A counseling group for injured athletes is a less structured, more dynamic approach than that found in a psychoeducational group. As such, there is no one prescribed way to lead this type of group, with many different theoretical orientations and counseling styles being acceptable. Yalom (1995) and other group theorists (e.g., Corey & Corey, 2006), though, have suggested that emotional, cognitive, behavioral, and (ultimately) interpersonal change occurs within individuals as the result of the presence and interplay of specific therapeutic factors. Thus, sports medicine professionals who lead counseling groups for injured athletes may want to think in terms of how their interventions influence the development and maintenance of these therapeutic factors. For when present, these factors can bring about important changes in the athlete, including
   • increased self-awareness,
   • emotional expression,
   • development of new interpersonal connections,

- more effective ways of communicating,
- increased self-responsibility in life, and
- increased motivation.

Other Issues to Consider When Running Injury Groups

The previous two sections outlined two types of groups that can be integrated into rehabilitation programs for injured athletes, examined the topics that might be covered, and (in the case of counseling groups) reviewed the therapeutic factors that would be associated with change. Sports medicine professionals need to consider, in the context of implementing injury groups, five other important issues that apply to both group formats:

(a) confidentiality

(b) informed consent

(c) group status,

(d) group timing

(e) leader training

This section provides an overview of each issue.

1. *Confidentiality.* In general terms, confidentiality concerns the imperative that what is shared in the context of a professional relationship will be kept secret and not disclosed to others. Depending on the education, training, and affiliation of sports medicine professionals, confidentiality is likely to be codified in professional ethics and/or sanctioned by legal statute, providing direct guidance concerning the limits of and protections to the conversations held with clients. In most cases, sports medicine professionals are not allowed to disclose what is shared in the context of working with injured athletes, except under specific circumstances, such as a court order, threat of harm to self or others, abuse of child or older adult, or release from the patient allowing such disclosures. The presence of confidentiality facilitates the development of trust in the patient-professional relationship, which is the foundation for effective treatment.

    Although sports medicine professionals may have to follow legal and ethical guidelines concerning confidentiality when leading psychoeducational and counseling groups, the injured athletes themselves are under no such mandates. Thus, it is imperative that the group leaders discuss the issue of member confidentiality at the beginning of the group. Doing so provides injured athletes with the opportunity to express their ideas about how information shared in the group should be treated (e.g., members will not disclose names or other identifying information about one another) and to learn that they have some control over their treatment. Confidentiality is essential in counseling groups where emotional expression and personal disclosure are encouraged because, without it, athletes are not likely to develop the necessary level of trust to engage in open and honest discussions about themselves, their injuries, their fears, and their goals.

2. *Informed consent.* Another important ethical issue is informed consent, which refers to patients/clients being provided with sufficient information so they can understand the parameters of treatment and then voluntarily agree to participate

in it. According to Corey and Corey (2006), such consent should include information on confidentiality and its limits; the leader's background, training, and qualifications; the purpose and goals of the group; the roles and responsibilities of the leaders and members; and if applicable, the leaders theoretical orientation. If relevant, consent forms also should include information on whether or not participation is voluntary (e.g., whether athletic department is mandating participation in the group), whether there are any fees associated with participation, whether the group is open (i.e., new members may join any time) or closed (i.e., once the group begins, no new members may join), and whether the group will be recorded (e.g., videotaped), and whether the leaders can be contacted in between sessions and, if so, how. It is important that such information be provided in writing and that members sign the forms at the beginning of treatment. This discussion of informed consent assumes that the members are adults. If the injured athletes are minors, then other issues, such as communicating with parents, must be addressed. (See Corey & Corey, 2006, for more information).

3. *Group status.* Group status refers to whether the group will be open or closed to new members once it begins. Each approach has its benefits and limitations, and sports medicine professionals must determine the best approach, taking into account their own training and personalities, the rehabilitation environment in which treatment will be delivered, and the athlete clientele themselves. For example, open groups allow newly injured athletes to enter at any time, recognize the reality of a dynamic rehabilitation process in which athletes do not recover on schedule, and increase the likelihood of having sufficient numbers of members each week. On the other hand, open groups, by virtue of their shifting membership, make it harder to develop trust and may discourage commitment and adherence. Closed groups are beneficial in that membership is set from the start, which helps trust and commitment, and members have the opportunity to develop relationships and new support systems. Because of their set nature, though, closed groups may not meet the needs of newly injured athletes, unnecessarily delaying their access to treatment.

4. *Group timing.* Group timing comprises three different issues:
   (a) What will be the length of each group session? Although counseling (and many psychoeducational) groups generally last 75–90 minutes, this time frame might be too long in some settings or for some athletes and thus can be changed to fit the needs of the situation.
   (b) What will be the duration of the group? In many cases, counseling groups are offered within a short-term model (e.g., Burlingame & Fuhriman, 1990; Piper & Joyce, 1996), with closed groups generally lasting 8–12 sessions. Psychoeducational groups, like the one described in this chapter, may be shorter in duration. Again, decisions about duration need to be made in the context of the treatment venue and clientele. For example, at a university, a 12-week injury counseling group might make sense given that most academic terms are 15 weeks in length. However, at a sports medicine clinic, a more

realistic time frame might be 6–8 weeks, which coincides with the average time patients are seen in physical therapy.

(c) When will the group start? Should the groups start after injury but before surgery? Should the groups be tailored to begin or to allow injured athletes to enter only following surgery? For example, in a treatment setting where the average time between injury and surgery is four weeks, it might be beneficial to have groups open to athletes pre-surgery. In settings where surgery closely follows injury, groups might be timed such that injured athletes enter in the days immediately after. The key is to make the groups available to the athletes during the times when they are in need.

5. *Leader training.* If they have taught college courses, given professional presentations, or worked with sport teams doing psychological skill training, sports medicine professionals will have most of the skills and experiences to successfully develop and lead a psychoeducational group. The same, however, cannot be said for counseling groups. As Corey and Corey (2006) noted, leading a counseling group requires specialized training, including coursework and supervised practica in group counseling/psychotherapy, which many sports medicine professionals do not have. Even those who are licensed psychologists may not be ready to lead an injury group if they do not have knowledge and training in the psychosocial processes associated with injury.

Given the complexities associated with running an injury group and the need for training and knowledge not only in group processes but also in the psychology of injury, sports medicine professionals might consider co-leading such groups. In the ideal situation, professionals from psychology (e.g., counseling psychologist) and sports medicine (e.g., athletic trainer or physiotherapist) would join together to develop and implement a group. Such a pairing would be an exciting opportunity for each professional, bringing together the knowledge and skills from each domain to the benefit of both the injured athletes and the leaders themselves. If such a pairing is not possible and the sole group leader is not sufficiently experienced in a particular area (e.g., psychology of injury), it is essential that he or she seek supervision from a qualified professional while leading the group.

Summary

Athletic injury is a complex process that involves physical, emotional, cognitive, and behavioral components. Although athletes generally are well-cared-for physically and medically, research has suggested that their psychological reactions, if unaddressed, can interfere with rehabilitation, delay recovery, and undermine return to competitive play. This chapter presented information on two different group approaches for working with injured athletes:

1. Psychoeducational groups, which generally are didactic and prescriptive, are effective in teaching injured athletes needed psychosocial skills and strategies, as well as giving the athletes opportunities to directly practice the skills and strategies in a structured environment. This type of group represents a particularly effective and

efficient way to deliver information to injured athletes and generally can be led by most sports medicine professionals.

2. Counseling groups, on the other hand, are less structured and emphasize learning through the relationships and interactions among the members. Through the presence of specific therapeutic factors that result from the leader's interventions, injured athletes address and learn to cope successfully with many of the issues and stressors that they face post injury. Counseling groups generally require specialized training, so sports medicine professionals who do not have the necessary background and experience may want to co-lead such groups.

Because both types of groups are effective approaches for bringing about positive change, sports medicine professionals need to determine which group will be most appropriate within their specific environments and with their clienteles of injured athletes.

References

Andersen, M. (Ed.). (2000). *Doing sport psychology*. Champaign, IL: Human Kinetics.

Andersen, M. (Ed.). (2005). *Sport psychology in practice*. Champaign, IL: Human Kinetics.

Bianco, T., & Eklund, R. (2001). Conceptual considerations for social support research in sport and exercise settings: The case of sport injury. *Journal of Sport & Exercise Psychology, 23*, 85-107.

Bovasso, G., Eaton, W., & Armenian, H. (1999). The long-term outcomes of mental health treatment in a population-based study. *Journal of Consulting and Clinical Psychology, 67*, 529-538.

Brewer, B., Jeffers, K., Petitpas, A., & Van Raalte, J. (1994). Perceptions of psychological interventions in the context of sport injury rehabilitation. *The Sport Psychologist, 8*, 176-188.

Burlingame, G., & Fuhriman, A. (1990). Time-limited group therapy. *The Counseling Psychologist, 18*, 93-118.

Corey, M., & Corey, G. (2006). *Process and practice groups* (7th ed.). Belmont, CA: Thomson.

Cupal, D. (1998). Psychological interventions in sport injury prevention and rehabilitation. *Journal of Applied Sport Psychology, 10*, 103-123.

Daly, J., Brewer, B., Van Raalte, J., Petitpas, A., & Sklar, J. (1995). Cognitive appraisal, emotional adjustment and adherence to rehabilitation following knee surgery. *Journal of Sport Rehabilitation, 4*, 23-30.

Elias, S. (2001). 10-year trend in USA Cup soccer injuries: 1988-1997. *Medicine and Science in Sports and Exercise, 33*, 359-367.

Evans, L., Hardy, L., & Fleming, S. (2000). Intervention strategies with injured athletes: An action research study. *The Sport Psychologist, 14*, 188-206.

Ferrante, A., Etzel, E., & Lantz, C. (1996). Counseling college student-athletes: The problem, the need 1996. In E. Etzel, A. Ferrante, & J. Pinkney (Eds.), *Counseling college student-athletes: Issues and interventions* (pp. 3-26). Morgantown, WV: FIT, Inc.

Fuhriman, A., & Burlingame, G. (1990). Consistency of matter: A comparative analysis of individual and group process variables. *The Counseling Psychologist, 18*, 6-63.

Gould, D. (2006). Goal setting for peak performance. In J. Williams (Ed.), *Applied sport psychology: Personal growth to peak performance* (pp. 240-259) New York: McGraw Hill.

Gould, D., Udry, E., Bridges, D., & Beck, L. (1997a). Coping with season ending injuries. *The Sport Psychologist, 11*, 379-399.

Gould, D., Udry, E., Bridges, D., & Beck, L. (1997b). Stress sources encountered when rehabilitating from season-ending ski injuries. *The Sport Psychologist, 11*, 361-378.

Harris, H., Altekruse, M., & Engels, D. (2003). Helping freshman student athletes adjust to college life using psychoeducational groups. *Journal for Specialists in Group Work, 28*, 64-81.

Kivlighan, D., & Goldfine, D. (1991). Endorsement of therapeutic factors as a function of stage of group development and participant interpersonal attitudes. *Journal of Counseling Psychology, 38*, 150-158.

Kolt, G. (2000). Doing sport psychology with injured athletes. In M. Andersen (Ed.), *Doing sport psychology* (pp. 223-236) Champaign, IL: Human Kinetics.

Kraus, J., & Conroy, C. (1984). Mortality and morbidity from injuries in sports and recreation. *Annual Review of Public Health, 5*, 163-192.

Larson, G., Starkey, C., & Zaichkowsky, L. (1996). Psychological aspects of athletic injuries perceived by athletic trainers. *The Sport Psychologist, 10,* 37-47.

Leddy, M., Lambert, M., & Ogles, B. (1994). Psychological consequences of athletic injury among high-level competitors. *Research Quarterly for Exercise and Sport, 65,* 347-354.

Marchant, D. (2000). Targeting futures: Goal setting for professional sports. In M. Andersen (Ed.), *Doing sport psychology* (pp. 93-104). Champaign, IL: Human Kinetics

McRoberts, C., Burlingame, G., & Hoag, M. (1998). Comparative efficacy of individual and group psychotherapy: A meta-analytic perspective. *Group Dynamics: Theory, Research, and Practice, 2,* 101-117.

Meeuwisse, W. H., & Fowler, P. J. (1988). Frequency and predictability of sports injuries in intercollegiate athletes. *Canadian Journal of Sport Sciences, 13,* 35-42.

Menckel, E. & Laflamme, L. (2000). Injuries to boys and girls in Swedish schools: different activities, different results? *Scandinavian Journal of Public Health, 28,* 132-136.

Meyers, C., Peyton, D., & Jensen, B. (2004). Treatment acceptability in NCAA division I football athletes: Rehabilitation intervention strategies. *Journal of Sport Behavior, 27,* 165-169.

National Collegiate Athletic Association (1992). *1991-1992 Women's volleyball injury surveillance system.* Overland Park, KS: Author.

Piper, W., & Joyce, A. (1996). A consideration of factors influencing the utilization of time-limited, short-term group therapy. *International Journal of Group Psychotherapy, 46,* 311-328.

Podlog, L., & Eklund, R. (2006). A longitudinal investigation of competitive athletes' return to sport following serious injury. *Journal of Applied Sport Psychology, 18,* 44-68.

Requa, R. (1991, April). The scope of the problem: The impact of sports-related injuries. *Proceedings from the Conference on Sport Injuries in Youth: Surveillance Strategies.* Bethesda, MD: National Advisory Board for Arthritis and Musculoskeletal and Skin Diseases, National Institute of Arthritis and Musculoskeletal and Skin Diseases, and Centers for Disease Control.

Rock, J., & Jones, M. (2002). A preliminary investigation into the use of counseling skills in support of rehabilitation from sport injury. *Journal of Sport Rehabilitation, 11,* 284-304.

Shaffer, S., & Wiese-Bjornstal, D. (1999). Psychosocial intervention strategies in sports medicine. In R. Ray & D. Wiese-Bjornstal (Eds.), *Counseling in sports medicine* (pp. 41-54). Champaign, IL: Human Kinetics.

Tracy, J. (2003). The emotional response to the injury and rehabilitation process. *Journal of Applied Sport Psychology, 15,* 279-293.

Udry, E., Gould, D., Bridges, D., & Beck, L. (1997). Down but not out: Athlete responses to season-ending injuries. *Journal of Sport & Exercise Psychology, 19,* 229-248.

Udry, E., Gould, D., Bridges, D., & Tuffey, S. (1997). People helping people? Examining the social ties of athletes coping with burnout and injury stress. *Journal of Sport & Exercise Psychology, 19,* 368-395.

Van Mechelen, W., Twisk, J., Molendijk, A., Blom, B., Snel, J., & Kemper, H. (1996). Subject-related risk factors for sports injuries: A 1-yr prospective study in young adults. *Medicine and Science in Sport and Exercise, 28,* 1171-1179.

Van Raalte, J., & Brewer, B. (Eds.). (2002). *Exploring sport and exercise psychology* (2nd ed.). Washington, DC: American Psychological Association.

Wiese-Bjornstal, D., Smith, A., Shaffer, S., & Morrey, M. (1998). An integrated model of response to sport injury: Psychological and sociological dynamics. *Journal of Applied Sport Psychology, 10,* 46-69.

William, J. (Ed.). (2006). *Applied sport psychology: Personal growth to peak performance.* New York: McGraw Hill.

Yalom, I. (1995). *The theory and practice of group psychotherapy* (4th ed.). New York: Basic Books.

Section Four | Issues for Coaches

Section 4 begins with an unusual chapter (13) written by Mark Andersen, who describes lessons learned from his attempts at assisting an injured athlete rehabilitate, only to have his efforts backfire. In chapter 14 Theresa Bianco argues that coaches have critical roles to play in the rehabilitative process and offers suggestions as to how such support may be forthcoming.

In the final chapter of this section (15) Jane Henderson writes about suicide among athletes of various skill levels. She discusses causally related as well as preventive issues, and maintains that the incidence of such self-inflicted injury continues to increase.

Chapter Thirteen | Collaborative Relationships in Injury Rehabilitation: Two Case Examples

Mark B. Andersen
Victoria University, Melbourne, Australia

How do athletes get through rehabilitation after a serious sport injury? What are some of the factors that lead to positive outcomes, and what aspects of the biopsychosocial process of recovery might interfere with timely return to participation? Other chapters in this text address many of these issues including social support, mental toughness, past experience with injury, and coping resources among others. This chapter focuses on one of the central issues in rehabilitation: the collaborative relationships between injured athletes in rehabilitation and the service providers who care for them. Those two key words, "collaborative" and "relationships" form the core of the message in this chapter. Collaboration in a relationship implies a measure of mutual agreement and investment. This stance is in contrast to medical doctor-patient models of care where the unidirectional flow of treatment is from expert practitioner to relatively passive recipient.

Why Study Relationships?

Brewer, Andersen, and Van Raalte (2002) have presented a biopsychosocial model of injury recovery (see Figure 1). Their model includes numerous variables associated with the rehabilitation process grouped into factors such as characteristics of the injury; sociodemographics; biological, psychological, and social/contextual factors; intermediate biopsychological outcomes; and rehabilitation outcomes. This chapter focuses on one small part of the model, the social/contextual factors, and more specifically, rehabilitation relationships.

Recovery from injury, or from illness and training for that matter, does not occur in a vacuum. Recovery occurs within a complex biological, psychological, and social matrix. The interplay of these complex factors is also dynamic in that at any given time certain psychological, social, or biological variables may

Figure 1.

A biopsychosocial model of sport injury rehabilitation.

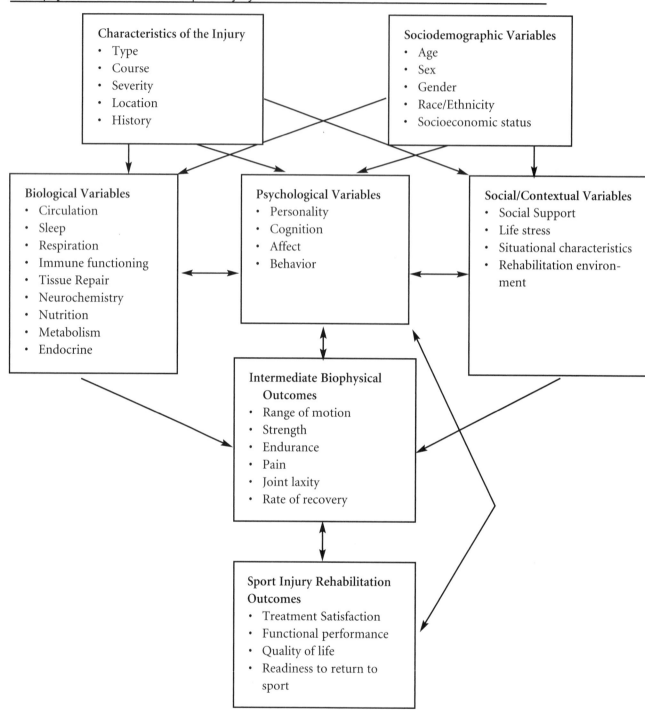

Note:
Brewer, B. W., Andersen, M. B., & Van Raalte, J. L. (2002). Psychological aspects of injury rehabilitation: Toward a biopsychosocial approach. In D. I. Mostofsky & L. Zaichkowsky (Eds.), *Medical and psychological aspects of sport and exercise* (pp. 41-54). Morgantown, WV: Fitness Information Technology.

become more salient than at other times. But the core of effectiveness in recovery is the relationships athletes have in their lives (see Kolt & Andersen, 2004a, 2004b).

In terms of relationships in rehabilitation, we know from psychotherapy research (Sexton & Whiston, 1994) that the type of psychotherapy applied is almost irrelevant in regard to outcomes (outcomes being happiness, or better functioning, or improved quality of life). People tend to get better in psychotherapy. Research has shown repeatedly that it is the quality of the relationship between the caregiver and the client that explains the most variance in psychotherapy outcomes. I think the same can be said for most of the helping professions both in and out of sport. For example, if an athlete and a nutritionist really like each other, enjoy their interactions, and have mutual respect, and the athlete feels cared for, then the athlete is more likely to adhere to the advice of the nutritionist, make healthy changes in diet, reap the benefits, and possibly become happier. And maybe even improve athletic performance.

Human relationships are powerful phenomena, and our collaborative working alliances with athletes can, unfortunately, become misalliances when they steer athletes down roads where recovery and rehabilitation become a problem. For example, an athlete may have a wonderful relationship with his coach whom he views as a father figure. His biological father, an abusive alcoholic, is the "bad father," and the coach represents the "good father" he always desired. Love is in the air, and the athlete wants to please his coach and make him proud. The coach values hard work; most coaches do. So what happens? The athlete works extra hard, is substantially reinforced with attention and praise from the coach, and just keeps on going. The coach is a good coach and checks in with the athlete about his training. The athlete, not wanting to disappoint the coach about all his small pains and soreness and sleeping 11 hours a day, does not report any of these problems, and in the end incurs a serious overuse injury that needs surgery and eventually ends his sporting career. In this hypothetical example, the human relationship had disastrous results in terms of the athlete's career, but we see this scenario played out over and over again. Relationships fuel change, for better and for worse.

In sports medicine and sport psychology many of us are convinced that sport is necessarily a good thing. It may not be, and such prejudicial thinking may influence our work with athlete clients. Moreover, there is an assumption that the return of a rehabilitated athlete to the playing field as quickly as possible is the best conceivable outcome. Perhaps this is not so. When our exclusive focus is upon ankles and limbs, a quintessential perspective may be lost: namely that the injury has more meaning than a brief hiatus from sport. Even the assumption that the athlete also wants to get better fast and return to practice and competition may be incorrect. In some cases an injury is a way out of sport. I have had an athlete say to me, "What I need now is a career-ending injury." Damaging himself was the only way he could see of "legitimately" getting out of a sport that caused him great psychological pain. When we don't explore the meaning of injury, we may end up going down treatment paths that are not fruitful and may actually be counter-therapeutic.

We should also try and determine exactly who the real client is when we render service to an injured athlete. Is it the athlete? Is it the team and its hope for success that is intimately connected to the health of the injured athlete? Is it the coach and his or her aspirations? Is it the administration and the people who pay for our services? The client, oddly enough, may also be us, and in getting the athlete back into play we enhance our status, insure further income, receive kudos, and fulfill our narcissistic needs. Those providing service to athletes need constantly to ask the question "Who is being served by my actions?" If the answer is "Not the athlete," then the answer is wrong. Sometimes we are in blind collusion with exploitative systems. Sport environments are often deeply pathogenic places where people learn really horrible lessons that twist their views of the world and of themselves (e.g., the equation *good performance = good person*). More on psychologist weaknesses will be found in the case example of Emma, later in the chapter.

Relationships in Injury Rehabilitation

When an athlete becomes seriously injured on the playing field, many of his or her current relationships may change dramatically. The athletic trainer, who is usually on the sidelines of the playing fields and has typically prepared the athlete for competition and practice by taping his or her ankles, is usually the first to reach the injured player. The athlete is in pain, in shock, or even in denial that there is anything wrong. The coach may be anxious, angry, confused, or all three. The teammates may be in shock. The athletic trainer, however, is the one "doing" things, talking with the athlete, touching the athlete, and letting the athlete know he or she is in good hands.

With other sports medicine personnel. After the injury has been handled by the trainer, other relationships with sports medicine personnel will start to emerge. In the case of a needed knee reconstruction, the orthopedic surgeon will enter the athlete's world in a significant way. Orthopedic surgeons personae can range from "cold fish," where they are impressed with their own skills and interested only in knees (not people), to caring and loving practitioners of medicine whose focus is much more on the whole athlete than on the body part in question. The former can engender a sense of helplessness and lack of control in the athlete. The latter will most likely be a powerful force in the athlete's recovery. After surgery, a relationship usually starts with a physical therapist. An examination of an athlete-physical therapist relationship, later in the chapter, is presented in the case example of the swimmer, Guillaume.

With coaches and teammates. The range of coach and teammate relationships with injured athletes may extend from behaving in a physically and emotionally embracing, warm manner to shunning the athlete as if a shattered knee cap were contagious. There is no "one-size-fits-all" for how best to deal with injured athletes and their teammates and coaches. From the athlete's point of view, it may be that hanging around with the team, going to practice, and attending team meetings are stressful and remind the athlete that he or she is not participating and contributing. When injured and out of commission, some athletes cannot face being back with the team and sitting on the sidelines. Other athletes actually need to be around the team at practices and competitions to feel like they are still involved. Finding out what athletes need and desire should take precedence over the viewpoints of the coach and teammates. The best solution for the rehabilitating athlete is often idiosyncratic and should reflect analysis and discussion on behalf of all parties.

With significant others (parents, friends, partners, siblings). The literature on the role of social support in rehabilitation is vast (see Udry & Andersen, in press, for a review). Again, supportive relationships seem to have salubrious effects on injury recovery. Social support, however, may have a dark side. Well-meaning others, in their efforts to help, may inadvertently foster dependency and reinforce sick-role behavior in the athlete. For example, parents may be motivated to help their affected child to the extent that they begin to do things for the athlete that the athlete could do for himself or herself. Social support during rehabilitation probably needs to be negotiated so that the support is actually helpful and not a factor that may delay recovery.

Collaborative Relationships

The Physical Therapist, Maps, and the Injured Athlete

In physical therapy treatment, professionals use protocols, or maps. Table 1 is a verbal representation of treatment for a ruptured Achilles tendon rehabilitation, but it is a map nonetheless. It has signposts and directions. It starts from A and goes to B and ends up at C and contains different phases, the exercises that go with those phases, as well as the achievements needed to progress to the next phase. This map is extremely useful, but what is important to bear in mind is that it is still a map (rehabilitation of an Achilles tendon) and not a full representation of the territory itself. The statement "The map is not the territory" bears constant repeating. A big part of professional education is about learning maps. In psychology, and sport psychology in particular, we learn about theories and models of human behavior, in other words, maps. We learn the cognitive-behavioral therapy canon of relaxation, positive self-talk, goal setting,

Table 1.
Achilles Tendon Rehabilitation Protocol

Patient usually NWB (non-weight bearing) for 3-4 weeks unless otherwise indicated. Use heel lift for 2 weeks once bearing weight. PT usually begins at 3-4 weeks post-op unless otherwise indicated. Physician should indicate when to progress phases.

Phase I (at least PWB [partial weight bearing] beginning at 4 weeks post-op)
Gait training (wean from heel lift after 2 weeks if applicable). Soft tissue massage and/or modalities as needed

Exercises:
Towel calf stretch (without pain), Theraband exercises (dorsi and plantarflexion, inversion, eversion). Sitting calf raises, straight leg raises, BAPS in sitting. Bike light if ROM (range of motion) allows. May perform pool exercises also.

Progress to Phase II when:
Tolerates all Phase I without pain or significant increase in swelling, ambulates FWB (full weight bearing). ROM for plantarflexion, inversion and eversion are normal; dorsiflexion is at approximately neutral.

Phase II (Generally 6-8 weeks post-op)
Gait training. Soft tissue work and/or modalities as needed.

Exercises:
Standing gastroc and soleus stretches. Bike—light to moderate resistance as tolerated.
Leg press: quads bilateral to unilateral, calf raises (sub-maximal bilateral to unilateral) Sitting calf raises to standing at 8-10 weeks. BAPS board standing (with support as needed), step ups, step downs. Unilateral stance; balance activities with challenges if appropriate (such as ground clock). Mini-squats – bilateral to unilateral. Stairmaster – short steps 4", no greater than level 4 if no pain or inflammation. May continue pool if appropriate.

Progress to Phase III when:
Cleared by physician, can do each of Phase II activities without pain or swelling, ROM equal bilaterally. Able to do bilateral calf raise without difficulty and weight equal bilaterally, unilateral stance balance equal.

cognitive restructuring, visualization, and so forth that helps us work with athletes on performance enhancement, their personal lives, and the process of their injury rehabilitation. Less commonly in sport psychology circles, psychodynamic psychotherapy is done with athletes, and psychodynamic supervision with sport psychology trainees. Freud's maps of id, ego, and superego, psychosexual development, ego defense mechanisms, and childhood experiences can be used to understand clients' and students' worlds and struggles. But Freud's psychosexual maps, just like cognitive-behavioral theories and the biomedical models of injury treatment used by many physical therapists, are not the territories. In short, they are all incomplete—useful, but incomplete.

This Achilles tendon rehabilitation map represented in Table 1 is helpful but flawed, or at least, incomplete. It is a map of a body part's response to treatment. The territory of that map is actually the owner of the Achilles tendon, his or her experiences, social life, ontogenetic histories, hopes, dreams, and fears. The implication here is not that maps have no value. (See work on psychosocial antecedents of athletic injury in Andersen & Williams, 1988, and Williams & Andersen, 1998, and on biopsychosocial maps of injury rehabilitation in Brewer et al., 2002). Maps, however, have their limitations.

Back in the 14th century, some European maps of the world showed the end of knowledge, often with an edge to fall off of, with the warning inscribed, "Here there be monsters." In the *terra incognita* of injury rehabilitation there may indeed be monsters in the form of debilitating anxiety, depression, histories of sexual abuse by relatives and coaches, and eating disorders. We need better maps and better descriptions of where there may be monsters. Some monsters may just be small gremlins that physical therapists with good helping skills can handle. Other monsters may require vanquishing knights from other professions.

Touch, vulnerability, and trust. Physical therapists, like many sport psychologists, may have relatively long-term intimate relationships with their clients. Psychologists are intimate with clients on the level of their experiences, hopes, fears, dreams, past traumas, and relationships with others. Athletes in physical therapy may also share many of their experiences with their physical therapists in conversations during treatment. The best physical therapists I know are also wonderful lay psychologists. Physical therapists, however, interact with clients in ways psychologists must never interact. They touch their clients, often in ways that place the client in vulnerable positions (e.g., therapy on a groin injury). Touch is powerful, and the laying on of hands has been used in medicine from long before the time of Hippocrates.

Allowing touch and willingly letting another into one's own personal space involves a measure of trust. The more the other enters one's personal space as rehabilitation treatment progresses, the more trust in the other (usually) develops. As trust and comfort increase, some clients become less guarded (the treatment room is safe, as is the therapist) and begin to open up and tell stories about their frustrations, anxieties, hopes, and dreams. This process also happens with hairdressers and bartenders. In the case of the latter, the opening up is not so much because of touch but rather due to lubrication by ethanol, but the process is similar.

If the physical therapist is a naturally skilled helper (see Egan, 2001), then the telling of intimate stories will grow, as in the case of Margaret and Guillaume. There is, however, another feature of touch that helps accelerate this opening-up process. Massage and manipulation of body parts have the potential to evoke strong emotions or memories of past experiences, both good and bad. On the treatment table during massage, a client may suddenly have a strong unexplainable emotional reaction, or a memory of a past trauma, or an image of an event at a birthday party when the client was 8 years old. Almost all physical therapists and massage practitioners have experienced these phenomena with clients (see Nathan, 1999).

The question is: How does the physical therapist respond to the personal stories being told during therapy and the memories and emotions that the therapy itself evokes? The problem is that the question cannot be answered. We don't know. The best physical therapists respond with empathy, concern, care, and unconditional positive regard. Those sorts of responses sound exactly like what a good psychologist does. The best physical therapists also know how to make referrals sensitively when material comes up that appears to need another professional's expertise.

In the rehabilitation of injured athletes, one of the best collaborative (and often one of the most rewarding) relationships is between sport psychologists and physical therapists. In many cases, the physical therapist is on the frontline and is the first person to notice that the psychological aspects of the injury and rehabilitation need attention. In injury rehabilitation, many interested parties (e.g., coaches, orthopedic surgeons) often drop out of the picture, but the physical therapist's presence is usually sustained over an extended period. Moreover, some athletes who are experiencing psychological problems associated with injury and rehabilitation may not need (or desire) the ministrations of a sport psychologist. If they are being treated by a fine physical therapist, then their psychological care will also be handled well by the person who is touching them, massaging them, and listening to their stories.

The Sport Psychologist and the Injured Athlete

During their rehabilitation, athletes may develop relationships with sport psychologists that focus on mental skills such as relaxation or healing imagery (see Graham, 2004). The collaboration between the sport psychologist and the athlete may be directed toward using the down time to work on the mental aspects of the game. In some rare (one hopes) cases, an athlete may enter into relationships with sport psychologists in order to enlist an ally in his or her struggles and frustrations with other sports medicine personnel and the rehabilitation process. In such a case, the working alliance may become a misalliance that increases the risk of athlete unhappiness and collegial rifts among helping professionals.

Interested Parties and Agendas

For many coaches, exercise physiologists, sport physiotherapists, biomechanists, and sport psychologists, the collaborative relationships with athletes are based on agendas that are focused on behaviors. We want to help them get better at their performances. We want them to rehabilitate fully from injury and get back to the playing fields in top form. In some training centers and sports institutes around the world, the sport psychology unit is called Performance Psychology. That name says a lot, but it is problematic in that it implies an emphasis on behavior and not on the person. And unfortunately, it is this behavior that becomes a means to an end; that is, the quest for more medals and goals glorified by the Olympic ideals of *citius, altius,* and *fortius.* Not often enough is the focus on the happiness and personal well-being of the athlete. When collaborating with athletes, sport psychologists often accept their unrealistic needs and thus help them increase their unhappiness.

Some practitioners in the field of sport psychology seem to miss the point being made here. Sport psychologists have been heard to say, "I deal only with performance enhancement (or injury rehabilitation to return to sport), not with personal issues." So the focus is on behavior or recovery and not on the person. The naiveté of saying one works only in performance enhancement or injury rehabilitation and not personal issues is shocking. Performance, especially at the elite level, is a profoundly personal issue for the athlete. Performance is tied to dreams, self-worth, self-esteem, relationships with parents and coaches, and often one's identity. Good performances can lead to elation, joy, and happiness. Poor performance can lead to sadness, despair, and even suicide. So how is performance not a personal issue? When sport psychologists say they deal only in performance enhancement, they are uncoupling the person and the behavior, and that stance is one of the first steps in dehumanization, exploitation, and abuse.

Sport psychology has its historical roots located in coaching, physical education, and skill acquisition models, all of which aim at performance and are legacies from which to *disconnect* in training students to become good psychologists. Agendas in service are broad and have more to do with the happiness and well-being of athletes than with specific sporting behaviors or rehabilitation efforts aimed at getting them to return to competition. Hopefully, in caring, collaborative, and even loving relationships with athletes, students will accept the premise that athlete worthiness is not contingent on performance or even on return to sport after injury. What is vital to understand is that all athletes are worthy. So many of us have been taught, and embrace, the equation mentioned above: *good performance = good person.* That equation is a curious and horrible re-coupling of a person and his or her behavior and teaches the lesson that one's worth is a function of one's performance. There are few more damaging equations in sport and in life.

In an athlete's world, the sport psychologist may be one of a few individuals who do not have a contingent agenda. The sport psychologist may represent the only available haven where weakness, doubt, and fear can be expressed, protected, and cared for. In our collaborative efforts with athletes we should provide a model of what a caring human relationship is and strive to countermand other pathogenic and contingent relationships found in many other areas of sport.

Transference and Countertransference in the Helping Professions

"Transference" and "countertransference" are Freudian terms (Freud, 1912, 1915). Transference is a process that occurs during psychotherapy in which the client begins to respond (on feeling, thinking, and acting levels) to the therapist in ways that reflect patterns of responses to significant others in the client's life. For example, if a young woman had a painful time dealing with a controlling mother, against whom she rebelled, in therapy she may (especially with an older woman) begin to see the therapist as over-controlling and start resisting the therapist's help. The therapist may not be acting objectively in a controlling way, but the pattern for relationships with older females, learned from experiences with her mother, is one of control and resistance. That pattern also gets projected onto the therapist and leads to difficulties and blockages in therapy involving projection of a fantasized love object. As Andersen (2004) has stated:

> For example, children who have been physically or psychologically abused by a parent may begin to build strong fantasies about the good parent they do not have, but fervently wish they did. They may build up this internal picture of the loving, caring, generous, always-there-for-them parent. This fantasized love object may then later get projected onto a parental type figure, such as a therapist, teacher, or coach (see Grant & Crawley, 2002). The fantasized good parent projection is often the source of clients falling in love with their therapists. (p. 74)

Transference processes within clients have a counterpart where the therapist begins to act and respond to clients in similar patterns as he or she has responded to significant others in the past (and present).The term for that process is countertransference (Epstein & Feiner, 1983; Gabbard, 1995; Greenson, 1992; Strean, 1994; Stein, 1986). For example, therapists who are older than many of their clients may get big-sister or big-brother protective feelings about younger clients that come from experiences with their own real or fantasized siblings. As Andersen (2004) stated:

> Transference and countertransference are ubiquitous phenomena and are probably a part of most human relationships. Learning how to use them to positive effect is the role of psychologists, teachers, coaches, supervisors, and physical and manual therapists (see Henschen, 1991; Mann, 1986; Ogilvie, 1993; Petitpas, Giges, & Danish, 1999; Yambor & Connelly, 1991). The world of sport offers many examples of transference and countertransference. It is a common experience for athletes to become deeply attached to coaches. Part of that attachment (or love) may have roots in past parental relationships. If an athlete has had loving, healthy, supportive parents, then the probability of responding well to a caring, sensitive coach, and forming a strong bond that helps the athlete perform better in sport, is quite high. In contrast, if an athlete has been psychologically abused by a parent, then that athlete may gravitate to psychologically abusive coaches because that is the model for relationships with powerful others. Psychologically abusive coaches were probably abused by their coaches. Generally, we coach how we were coached, and we parent as we were parented. A happier connection for an abused athlete is to find a coach who represents the fantasized "good parent" they wished they had. With such a coach, the transference can be quite profound. (p. 74)

The interplay of transference and countertransference will be illustrated in the case examples that follow. "Guillaume" represents a case in which the athlete's relationship with his physical therapist became the foundation of his future professional life. The second example ("The Case of Emma," from this chapter author's own files, illustrates how a well-meaning sport psychologist, oblivious to the athlete's transference issues, can become a damaging influence, despite the best intentions.

Case Examples from Physical Therapy and Sport Psychology

"My PT Is Awesome!" The Case of Guillaume

Guillaume is a 21-year-old French-Canadian swimmer who was coming to the end of his swimming career. He was a good collegiate swimmer, but not quite up to National Team level. He trained most of the time in Western Canada where he was on a university scholarship, and where there were not that many people who spoke French. At the end of what he thought was his next-to-last season, his chronically troublesome shoulder finally gave out, and he needed surgery. He knew that the surgery and the rehabilitation would spell the end of his swimming a year earlier than planned. He had finished his third year of a bachelor's degree in sport sciences and had one year to go. His final year at university would be a year without competitive swimming. The surgical repair to the shoulder went fine, but the rehabilitation would take a long time. Shortly after surgery he started working with a physical therapist (a "physiotherapist" in British Commonwealth countries) named Margaret.

Margaret has been working as a physiotherapist in Western Canada for over 20 years. She is a solid, buxom woman who threw shot-put and discus when she was at university. She has specialized in sport physiotherapy for over a decade. She is a bit of mother to her clients, and she'll occasionally bring in home-baked cookies and give them to the athletes. She is a consummate professional and a warm, caring individual. She has two daughters and is married to a man who coaches track and field. Margaret has what could be called a "therapeutic presence." Despite her somewhat imposing stature, within minutes of meeting her people begin to feel like they do when in the company of a favorite auntie. She sets folks at ease and communicates a sincere interest in others. Her schedule is always full because the athletes know her, and they love her. When Guillaume told one of his friends that he would be starting physiotherapy soon, his friend said, "Ask for Margaret."

Guillaume lost his mother to breast cancer when he was 17. His father is a loving but quiet and busy man. Although not overtly demonstrative, he does show affection and gives encouragement to his son's endeavors. He has not remarried. Guillaume is the oldest of three children and takes after his father. He, like his father, is somewhat laconic, but once he is engaged he can be a personable conversationalist.

When Guillaume met Margaret for his first appointment, her introductory words were "Comment ça va, mon chéri?" (How are you, my dear?) He broke into a smile and responded in French. They carried on a little chit-chat in French, and then Margaret said, "Oh my, I think I have exhausted my high-school French." Guillaume was in an area of the country where he didn't hear a lot of his first language, and his physiotherapist won him over from the start. Margaret had him get up on the treatment table and pulled out an anatomy book from the shelf. Before any physical treatment started, she went over the anatomy of the shoulder and showed him where his damage was and what she would be manipulating. She explained that the treatment was designed to make sure no adhesions got started and that he would regain his strength and full range of motion.

Margaret is a talker, but not a self-centered one. During the treatments (e.g., joint mobilization) she would explain exactly what she was doing, warn him that something rather painful might be coming up, and generally keep him informed during the whole process. As physiotherapy progressed, Margaret and Guillaume told each other stories, and Guillaume began to confide in her about his worries over what he was going to do now that swimming was out of the picture and graduation was less than a year away. He had been thinking of becoming a coach and using his exercise science degree, but lately he had lost interest and had felt both unmotivated and anxious about his future. Margaret, ever the mom, told him, "Oh, chéri, you're just a baby. You have lots of time, and there are loads of interesting things to do with your degree. You'll find something. You're too smart not to." Margaret knew from his stories that he had lost his mother 4 years earlier. She was always motherly to those in her charge, but with Guillaume she fell even more so into the mom role, mostly unconsciously. Her countertransference to Guillaume had roots in not having a son herself and wishing she had a boy to take care of, along with wanting to be a replacement for his lost mother at a time when the boy himself was a bit lost. This loving and caring countertransference met its match in Guillaume's transference needs to have a caring older woman in his life, one he could talk to and who could be a sounding board for his anxieties at a time when he was starting to think about life decisions. He had always talked more with his mom than with his dad and generally felt more comfortable around older women than he did around older men. Guillaume and Margaret are examples of what happens when positive transference and countertransference meet. Even though he was feeling unmotivated and anxious about his future, his transference to Margaret was a major factor in his making every effort to do well in rehabilitating his injured shoulder. He was always proud to show off to Margaret how much strength and range of motion he was getting back. And Margaret, of course, praised him to the hilt (and the cookies would come out).

One day they were talking about Margaret's athletic experiences when she was at university. Guillaume asked what she had majored in at school, and Margaret replied, "Mon chou, I was in jock sciences just like you." They then discussed how sport and exercise science was a great degree for Margaret to use to get into physiotherapy school after her bachelor's. After that conversation, something happened to Guillaume. He became less anxious and started doing some studying on possible professions to pursue after his degree. A few weeks later he asked Margaret about which physiotherapy schools in Canada she thought were good. She mentioned a few in Montreal, Quebec City, and Western Canada.

The complex process Guillaume was starting to go through is called the identification with, and internalization of, the loved object. Margaret was a loving, caring, motherly other who filled a lot of Guillaume's needs way beyond his treatment in physiotherapy. In many ways, he wanted to become like Margaret, one who helps and nurtures others. Many people do internalize and identify with a parent or parental figure. Guillaume began to internalize many of the positive features of Margaret, both interpersonally and professionally. Through his relationship with Margaret, Guillaume began to "find himself," an Eriksonian task of establishing identity (Erikson, 1994).

Physiotherapy with Margaret came to an end part way through Guillaume's senior year, but he still kept in contact with her. When it came time to apply to physiotherapy schools he chose five different programs, one of which was where Margaret had received her training. He asked her to write a letter of recommendation for him for that school. Margaret was flattered and more than happy to write a glowing letter. When Guillaume received his first acceptance letter from a physiotherapy school, Margaret was the first person he told. They went out to dinner to celebrate. Over dinner and a couple glasses of wine, Guillaume said to Margaret, "I can't thank you enough for all you did for me. You are so awesome, and my ideal is to one day become as good a physio as you are." Margaret's eyes began to fill and she leaned over, took his hand, and said, "Oh, mon petit, you're gonna make this old girl cry."

Guillaume was accepted at three of the five schools and chose the one in his home town of Montreal. He is now a physiotherapist in Quebec. He stays in contact with Margaret and even calls her to consult on cases. They see each other at least once a year at physiotherapy or sports medicine conferences. Their tradition now is that he brings her cookies each time they meet.

Reflections

The case of Guillaume and Margaret is a composite example stemming from conversations with a physiotherapist, along with author's own experiences of the power of relationships to influence people lives well beyond the focus of their therapeutic work together.

The issues of transference and countertransference are rarely addressed in formal physiotherapy training, and if they are addressed, it is done so perfunctorily. In sport psychology, not enough attention is paid to relationships and these powerful dynamic processes. This state of affairs exists probably because of the focus on problems and solutions and not on the vehicle for problem solving, the relationship.

One psychologist recalls working, early in his psychodynamic training, with a young man with dysthymia. They had a therapeutic relationship for almost a year. Toward the end of therapy the young man told the counselor that he wanted to become a counselor, too, saying, "I want to be like you." The psychologist knew that the young man had considerable positive transference to him but had not realized the depth of the relationship: "I had before me a young man who had identified with me, internalized me, and wanted to become like me. As much as his identification was flattering and feeding my narcissistic tendencies, his revelation about wanting to become like me brought home, in a frightening and humbling fashion, just how powerful a caring relationship can be."

Transference and identification are not phenomena found only in psychotherapy relationships. One physiotherapist tells stories of clients who, after long-term treatment with her, have decided to become physiotherapists or massage therapists. Identification and internalization of the therapist may occur at more subtle levels than the client choosing to become a therapist. Whether they appreciate it or not, physiotherapists (and psychologists) often become models for clients of how to think, feel, and behave. Physiotherapists model concern, healthy attitudes toward self-care, and positive thinking about recovery (among many other things). These models are communicated and often are taken up by clients, becoming part of the clients' internal landscapes. It is the quality of the relationship that fuels the incorporation of the physiotherapist's values. The process is humbling and daunting, and it speaks to the power of human interaction in the realm of therapy—almost any kind of therapy.

"It's Your Fault" The Case of Emma

My encounter with Emma occurred early in my career (20 years ago) when I was quite naïve. I thoroughly believed in the sport psychology canon of cognitive-behavioral techniques, and I was on a mission to help athletes perform better and recover from their injuries. The goals of the athlete, the sports medicine personnel, and I were to get Emma back out there running as soon as possible.

Emma was an 800-meter runner. She had severe tendonitis in her Achilles tendon. I was working with the athletes at her NCAA Division I university when she first came to my office. She was open and charming, dedicated to her sport. Her Achilles tendon was quite painful and she wanted to work on some pain management strategies. I was convinced that she could benefit from learning some self-hypnosis techniques, so we started her off with some autogenic training. Emma proved to be a wonderful hypnotic subject and learned her autogenics more rapidly than any athlete I could recall. She was amazed at the deep relaxation states she could attain, and we furthered her autogenics into healing imagery to warm up her Achilles and get more blood flow to the area to enhance recovery. We also worked on helping her "send her leg away," a type of dissociative process, which, when added to the autogenics, would anesthetize her lower leg so she could get to sleep without pain and without so many analgesics.

Our relationship grew with each session. She loved doing the mental exercises each week with me in my office and practiced diligently at home. We were both excited about her progress. She fueled my narcissistic needs to be seen as a competent psychologist (so I liked her a lot), and I became, I believe, a substitute for her coach (dangerous interpersonal territory not on many maps of service delivery), in that her coach really did not want to pay much attention to her until she was fit to run again. He was not so much rejecting her as he was handing her over to others. He told her, "You go and get better, then come back and we'll work." He was well meaning, but he probably did not understand her need for counsel, direction, and contact with him. Her physical therapist was a nice guy, but he was also extremely busy and not really the talkative type. Being a psychologist, I am the talkative type, and I think I became the focus of her needs for attention during her recovery.

We would talk about her sport, her worries about her sponsorship from an athletic shoe manufacturer, her boyfriend, her school, her family, and her desires to make it to the NCAA championships. She would tell me things like, "I have learned so much from you. This stuff we're doing is great." Such compliments swelled my already relatively fat head, and I encouraged and massively reinforced her good work. Mutual admiration societies may be fun experiences for those involved, and may help promote change, but they can also blind. My enthusiasm for her progress in self-hypnosis and my basking in her praise blinded me to the true depth of her abilities with autogenics and the dangers it entailed.

She once told me a story of a previous coach she worked with, whom she adored and for whom she would do anything. This coach worked her hard, and she made great gains. He taught her some lessons about "running through the pain." These lessons, at first, seemed to be good ones, but in time she broke down with overuse injuries. She said, "I was so disappointed in myself that I didn't say, 'No, I can't take it,' and I was so disappointed in him that he couldn't see that what he was doing was wrecking me." I did not understand the import of that story until much later, and neither did I realize that it was a disguised warning to me about doing things with her that would lead to damage and disappointment.

I am not sure how many sport psychologists appreciate that autogenics can be learned so well by some athletes that they can induce the effects even in situations not conducive to going into hypnotic or dissociative states. And here is where I made a big mistake. I was so enthralled with Emma's abilities and success that I did not consider the potential negative outcomes of having such skills. I did not give her any warnings about when autogenics should not be used except the usual ones (e.g., not right after a meal, not while driving). Masking pain to get to sleep is one thing. Blocking pain during training is something else altogether. Pain is sending an important message, and blocking that message may have dire consequences. My omission of caveats about blocking pain is partially to blame for what happened to Emma.

Her "coach" (or possibly "big brother" or "father") transference to me seemed to be one of the driving forces behind her mental work, her success with autogenics and healing imagery, and her return to running. She had been at about 90–95% and had run at that level with some pain, but was confident that she could do an all-out run in an upcoming competition. Her coach and her physical therapist seemed to think the same. So did I. Then disaster struck. In the competition where she was going to give 100%, at about the 650-meter mark, her Achilles tendon completely ruptured. I was not at the out-of-town event, but I went to see her a few days after she got home. She was miserable, and we talked about what happened. She seemed distant and aloof. About 10 minutes into our conversation she said, "If *you* hadn't taught me autogenics so well, I wouldn't have blocked the pain. I would have pulled up in the race and not be sitting here with this." I was stunned speechless for a few moments. I was being professionally attacked and blamed for her injury. I felt a defensive wave cross my ego and wanted to say, "I never told you to use autogenics when you were racing," but I stopped myself, because I realized I had never told her not to. And then the story of her coach came back to me. Her work with me was a repetition of her experiences and her relationship with her former coach. She adored me, worked hard for me, and in the end believed she was damaged by me. Her anger at me was a mix of her current situation with roots in past negative experiences with a trusted mentor. I pulled my shattered professional ego back together a little and, in a *mea culpa* sort of way, said, "Emma, I am so sorry. You were doing so well with your mental training and recovery that I just didn't think of warning you not to mask pain when you are running. I should have done that; I can't tell you how sorry I am." Then she said something with so much bitterness and feeling of betrayal that I still can hear it to this day: "Well, it's a little too late for that warning now, don't you think?" I was the trusted mentor who turned into the enemy. I had become the current incarnation of betrayal and abuse.

Reflections

As was the case with both her former coach and her Achilles tendon, my relationship with Emma had ruptured. My enthusiasm, naiveté, and inexperience had led me to deliver incomplete and dangerous, albeit well-meaning, service that contributed to damaging an athlete. I talked with Emma one more time when I saw her on campus a couple of months later. She was polite, formal, and distant. She never called for any more appointments; our professional relationship had died. Emma's story is a tale of how powerful relationships, even with positive transference and countertransference features, can end in pain, disillusionment, and repetition of past trauma.

As she had done with her former coach, I am sure Emma also blamed herself for part of her situation, but her relationship with me and the events surrounding her injury might have been even more confusing. With her coach she knew, quite consciously, that she was training to a point that was not good, but she just couldn't say no. Therefore when injury came, it was not totally unexpected. With me there was no doubt. What we were doing was fantastic (she believed), and she had all the confidence in the world that what she and I were working on was just perfect for her. Her injury, because of my incompetence, may have evoked an even greater sense of betrayal than what she experienced with her former coach. In the end, my involvement with Emma was damaging to her both physically and psychologically. My relationship with Emma happened about 20 years ago, and I still feel guilt, shame, and embarrassment over what happened. One way I have tried to expiate that guilt is to make sure all my students hear the story of Emma and me.

I do not completely hold with the statement by Nietzsche (1889/1998) that "strength increases; vigor grows through a wound" (p. 3). I think that sometimes wounds hurt for a really long time, and, as in the case with Emma, they occasionally get reopened and hurt even more. The best I have done with the wounding of Emma (and myself) is to pass the story on to others and hope that "*knowledge* grows through a wound." And if knowledge is a form of strength and vigor, then maybe Nietzsche was not so far off base.

Final Observations and One More Tale

I have found over the years that what students remember most from classes, readings, and conference presentations are not so much the science, theories, models, and research evidence, but the personal stories that illustrate them. In a true sense, stories are scientific. They reflect, in an empirical real-world, and necessarily messy way, how models can, or should, reflect what we see out in the field when working with real people. Many of my former students have come back to me years later and said, "I was working with an athlete and she reminded me of that story we heard in class." Stories can be powerful, and they may remain with those who hear them for years.

I like models and maps. I hope the biopsychosocial model of injury recovery, as well as the maps of the human experience reflected in the dynamic theories of transference and countertransference, will be examined for their usefulness and applicability to what we do when we work with injured athletes. In closing this chapter, I would like to tell a story about injury, rehabilitation, recovery, training, and overtraining, and how all the good information we have comes up against the real world of sport and gets swept aside when the life of an athlete collides with the pathogenic arena of sport.

Sean is a doctoral student of mine from Canada. I won't disguise him at all, and he has given me permission to tell his story. He has a healthy narcissism and will be chuffed that I am writing about him, his psychopathology, and his experiences of injury, training, and recovery. Sean came from an Olympic family. His father was an Olympic rower who so overtrained for the Mexico City Games in 1968 that he fell seriously ill and almost died. Sean loves his dad, and much of the motivation for Sean wanting to go to the Olympics was fueled by an overwhelming desire to "fix" his dad and make all his dad's disappointment, pain, and regret go away. It doesn't matter that he set himself an impossible task. It is often the lot of children to try to fix their parents.

Sean, a rower like his Dad, trained hard for the Sydney Games in 2000, so hard that he overtrained, did not recover properly, overdid it, injured his wrist, and didn't make it to Sydney. He then entered our doctoral program in sport psychology at Victoria University, and guess what? He wanted to study injury and overtraining. It's funny how many sport psychology students and, I suspect, exercise physiology, biomechanics, and nutrition students, and other students as well, end up studying themselves or some aspect of themselves. Study is often aimed at trying to comprehend one's life and to "fix" oneself.

Sean wanted to understand his experiences in the lead-up to Sydney, and also to understand his dad. Sean had, and still has, a strong streak of perfectionism. He had to be the perfect boy, the perfect son, the perfect rower, and with us at Victoria University, the perfect doctoral student. As is the case with sons (and daughters) who have parents who struggle with various forms of unhappiness, they often try to distract their parents and make them happy through their own accomplishments. Sean's achievements were fueled by a massive motivation to be perfect, to fix his parents, the family unit, and ultimately to fix himself.

After three years of coursework and applied internships working with athletes to become a psychologist (he has turned into a fine one) and after his research aimed at injury, recovery, training, overtraining, self-discovery, and understanding his experiences, he decided that he would go back to Canada and try again for the 2004 Athens Olympic rowing team. This time, however, he was forearmed. He knew bucket loads about injury rehabilitation, overtraining, and recovery. He knew all the signs and symptoms; he knew what balance in training meant. He understood stress, under-recovery, and how to avoid overuse injuries. He knew what proper nutrition for his energy expenditure was. He was bound and determined not to make the same mistakes as he did the last time. Then he came up against the reality of training with the Olympic hopefuls.

When he knew he was reaching his limit and tipping over into dangerous territory and risking injury, he would take time to recover, but this time off was met with odd looks and comments from the other rowers and with subtle and not-so-subtle suggestions from the coach that maybe he didn't have the dedication and drive needed to be an Olympic rower. And his overwhelming desire to "fix" his dad surfaced again. So despite all his knowledge and his intelligence (and he *is* a very smart guy), he succumbed to the "more is better," "train through the pain," and "don't be a sissy" mentality of elite sport. He was conscious the whole time of what he was doing, but the pressures in that environment were overwhelming. He succumbed to the pressures of the training environment, blew up his back this time, and never got to Athens.

Sean's story is a cautionary tale of training, injury, and recovery. If a bright guy, armed with all sorts of knowledge about what is good and not good for him, still succumbs to the Darwinian pressures of elite sport, then what is all our knowledge about injury, rehabilitation, and recovery going to do for us and the athletes in our care, in the face of the pathogenic environment and pressures of elite sport, and the painful and needful ontogenetic dynamic personal histories of our athletes? Our positive collaborative relationships with athletes in rehabilitation may prove to be good experiences, but then they have to go back out there and deal again with many of the problems that may have contributed to their injuries in the first place. Plus ça change, plus c'est la même chose.

There is a footnote to this story: Sean worked hard on his doctoral dissertation, but like most other things in his life, it had to be "perfect." He was often loath to hand in material to me and his other supervisor because it wasn't perfect. With a lot of psychotherapy and some supervisors beating him severely about the head and shoulders, in a caring manner (our collaborative relationship with Sean as a student is a whole other story), trying to pound his self-defeating perfectionism out of his head, Sean had gotten to a place where his dissertation didn't have to be perfect, nor did he have to be the perfect son or the perfect athlete. Now he just has to be "good enough." He will always struggle with perfectionism, but he has acquired the tools to stop and say, "Okay! Just make it good enough." Sean's dissertation is done, examined, and approved. It was good enough. He is now a doctor and a registered psychologist in Australia (equivalent to licensure in the USA).

Sean is my student, but he is also my teacher. I hope the tales told in this chapter, of Guillaume, of Emma, and of Sean have helped illustrate the bewilderingly complex world we encounter when we work with athletes. I learned a great deal from my coursework at university, and I would not want to diminish its impact on my professional development. The most significant learning I have experienced, however, has come from encounters with students and athletes, their stories, their dreams and disappointments, their fantasies, and the collaborative relationships that developed between them and me as we journeyed together across both the familiar and unexplored territories of their lives.

References

Andersen, M. B. (2004). Transference and countertransference. In G. S. Kolt & M. B. Andersen (Eds.), *Psychology in the physical and manual therapies* (pp. 71-80). Edinburgh, Scotland: Churchill Livingstone.

Andersen M. B., & Williams, J. M. (1988). A model of stress and athletic injury: Prediction and prevention. *Journal of Sport & Exercise Psychology 10*, 294-306.

Brewer, B. W., Andersen, M. B., & Van Raalte, J. L. (2002). Psychological aspects of injury rehabilitation: Toward a biopsychosocial approach. In D. I. Mostofsky & L. Zaichkowsky (Eds.), *Medical aspects of sport and exercise* (pp. 41-54). Morgantown, WV: Fitness Information Technology.

Egan, G. (2001). *The skilled helper : A problem-management and opportunity-development approach to helping* (7th ed.). Stamford, CT: Wadsworth

Epstein, L., & Feiner, A. H. (1983). *Countertransference: The therapist's contribution to the therapeutic situation*. Northvale, NJ: Aronson.

Erikson, E. H. (1994). *Identity and the life cycle* (reissue ed.). New York: Norton.

Freud, S. (1912). The dynamics of transference. In J. Strachey (Ed. & Trans.), *The standard edition of the complete psychological works of Sigmund Freud, Vol. 12* (pp. 97-108). London: Hogarth Press.

Freud, S. (1915). Observations on transference-love: Further recommendations on the technique of psycho-analysis III. In J Strachey (Ed. & Trans.), *The standard edition of the complete psychological works of Sigmund Freud, Vol. 12* (pp. 157-173). London: Hogarth Press.

Gabbard, G. O. (1995). Countertransference: The emerging common ground. *International Journal of Psychoanalysis 76*, 475-485.

Graham, H. (2004). Imagery. In G. S. Kolt & M. B. Andersen (Eds.), *Psychology in the physical and manual therapies* (pp. 125-139). Edinburgh, Scotland: Churchill Livingstone.

Grant, J., & Crawley, J. (2002). *Transference and projection: Mirrors to the self*. Philadelphia: Open University Press.

Greenson, R. R. (1992). Countertransference. In A. Sugarman, R. A. Nemiroff, & R. R. Greenson (Eds.) *The technique and practice of psychoanalysis, Volume II: A memorial to Ralph R. Greenson*. Madison, CT: International Universities Press.

Henschen, K. (1991). Critical issues involving male consultants and female athletes. *The Sport Psychologist 5*, 313-321.

Kolt, G. S., & Andersen, M. B. (Eds.). (2004a). *Psychology in the physical and manual therapies*. Edinburgh, Scotland: Churchill Livingstone.

Kolt, G. S., & Andersen, M. B.. (2004b). Using psychology in the physical and manual therapies. In G. S. Kolt & M. B. Andersen (Eds.).*Psychology in the physical and manual therapies* (pp. 3- 8). Edinburgh, Scotland: Churchill Livingstone.

Mann, J. (1986) Transference and countertransference in brief psychotherapy. In H. C. Meyers (Ed.), *Between analyst and patient: New dimensions in countertransference and transference* (pp. 119-129). Hillsdale, NJ: Analytic Press.

Nathan, B. (1999). *Touch and emotion in manual therapy*. Edinburgh, Scotland: Churchill Livingstone.

Nietzsche, F. (1998). *Twilight of the idols: Or how to philosophize with a hammer* (D. Large, Trans.). New York: Oxford University Press. (Original work published in 1889)

Ogilvie B. C. (1993). Transference phenomena in coaching and teaching. In S. Serpa, J. Alves, V. Ferreira, & A. Paulo-Brito (Eds.), *Proceedings of the VIII World Congress of the International Society of Sport Psychology*. Lisbon, Portugal: International Society of Sport Psychology.

Petitpas, A. J., Giges, B., & Danish, S. J. (1999). The sport psychologist-athlete relationship: Implications for training. *The Sport Psychologist 13*, 344-357.

Sexton, T. L., & Whiston, S. C. (1994). The status of the counseling relationship: An empirical review, theoretical implications, and research directions. *The Counseling Psychologist 22*, 6-78.

Stein, M. H. (1986). Acting out – transference and countertransference: Technical considerations. In H. C. Meyers (Ed.), *Between analyst and patient: New dimensions in countertransference and transference* (pp. 63-75). Hillsdale, NJ: Analytic Press.

Strean, H. (1994). *Countertransference*. New York: Hawthorn Press.

Udry, E., & Andersen, M. B. (in press). Psychological aspects of athletic injury and sport behavior. In T. S. Horn (Ed.), *Advances in sport psychology* (3rd ed.). Champaign, IL: Human Kinetics.

Williams, J. M., & Andersen, M. B. (1998). Psychosocial antecedents of sport injury: Review and critique of the stress and injury model. *Journal of Applied Sport Psychology 10*, 5-25.

Yambor, J., & Connelly, D. (1991). Issues confronting female sport psychology consultants working with male student-athletes. *The Sport Psychologist 5*, 304-312.

Chapter Fourteen | Sport Injury and the Need for Coach Support

Theresa M. Bianco
Concordia University

Sustaining and recovering from a sport injury can be an extremely stressful and disruptive event for athletes, particularly when the injury is severe and the athlete is heavily invested in sport (Bianco, Malo, & Orlick, 1999; Heil, 1993; Smith & Milliner, 1994; Sparkes, 1998). In addition to having to cope with the physical stresses of injury, injured athletes must also contend with a host of psychosocial stressors. Chief among these stressors are concerns about the implications of injury on the athlete's sport career. For example, will it be possible to regain pre-injury form and continue to achieve pre-determined athletic goals? The multitude of stressors engendered by injury can place excessive demands on the athlete's coping resources and give rise to a range of adjustment difficulties. One way in which this maladjustment is manifested is through treatment non-adherence. Failure to comply with treatment is problematic because it can impede recovery and increase the risk of additional injury (Brewer, 1998; Doyle, Gleeson, & Rees, 1998; Gould & Udry, 1995). Moreover, outcomes such as these will serve only to exacerbate the athletes' distress and lead to further adjustment problems.

Although the extent of adjustment difficulties experienced by injured athletes will vary, it is clear that most athletes exhibit some form of psychological disruption and thus require assistance (Heil, 1993). One form of assistance that is proving to be particularly useful in helping athletes cope with the stress of injury and recovery is social support—and coach support in particular. Research shows that injured athletes want support from their coaches and that the support provided is instrumental in relieving distress, encouraging adherence, and easing the transition back to full training and competition (Bianco, 2001, 2002; Johnston & Carroll, 1998a; Rees & Hardy, 2002; Shelley, 1999; Udry, Gould, Bridges, & Tuffey, 1997).

Discussion in this chapter, which addresses the role of coach support in recovery from sport injury, is based on published research and studies undertaken in the course of the author's doctoral studies at the University of Western

Australia (Bianco, 2002). The program of research was composed of a series of qualitative and quantitative studies conducted with both elite and professional coaches and athletes regarding coach support in the context of sport injury. The chapter is divided into two major sections:

(a) the stresses of injury and athlete responses to being injured—a logical starting point because the need for coach support is determined in great part by how the stresses of injury affect the athlete; and

(b) coach support and the ways in which it can be of value to the injured athlete.

The coach support process and some of the challenges involved in ensuring that injured athletes get the support they need are then described. The chapter concludes with a list of recommendations for both athletes and coaches.

Part 1: The Injury Experience

The Stresses of Injury

Danish (1986) described sport injury as one of the most stressful events athletes would likely encounter in their careers. A quick scan of Table 1 helps shed light on why this may be so. It is clear from the table that sport injury is an event that has an impact on several aspects of an athlete's life and as a result engenders a wide range of stressors.

Stresses of Rehabilitation

On a physical level, there is likely to be a significant amount of pain and discomfort arising from being injured, both at the time of injury and throughout rehabilitation. These physical symptoms may be transient or persistent, depending on the type and severity of the injury and the treatment protocol. Breaking down post-surgical scar tissue, for example, may require doing exercises that can be very painful (Doyle et al., 1998; Gould & Udry, 1995; Steadman, 1993).

In addition to physical discomfort, the process of rehabilitation presents several motivational challenges. Rehabilitation can be monotonous and under-stimulating, with athletes having to do repetitive exercises at intensities lower than to what they are accustomed. Athletes may also find themselves having to do these exercises on their own. Together, these factors can give rise to boredom, frustration, and de-motivation. John, a professional rugby player, put it this way: "For a person of my calibre, going from doing heavy workloads and working hard to be super fit to doing piddly exercises was just dreadful. The first three months of rehabilitation were the worst time in my life."

Another characteristic of rehabilitation that can be stressful is that the course of recovery is often marked by setbacks and periods of little or no improvement (Rotella & Heyman, 1993; Steadman, 1993; Taylor & Taylor, 1997). Times like these can make it very difficult for injured athletes to remain optimistic. Instead, they can be left feeling rather despondent and anxious about the future. Such feelings are likely to be heightened for those athletes with chronic conditions or complicated recoveries. In such cases, athletes may lose complete faith in the possibility of a full recovery and consider quitting their sport (Smith & Milliner, 1994).

Table 1.

The Stresses of Injury

Stressor Type	Stressor
Stresses of rehabilitation & recovery	Physical aspects - pain - physical rigors of treatment - restricted physical activity Program structure - repetition & monotony of exercise - working at lower intensities - working alone Course of recovery - slow progress in rehabilitation - rehabilitation setbacks - lengthy recovery time
Cognitive Stressors	Consequences of injury on performance - permanent limitations to ability - inability to regain pre-injury form Consequences of absence from sport - losing position on team - being dropped from the team - falling behind others - missing learning opportunities - missing selection opportunities - missing important events - being forgotten by coach Consequences of restricted activity - losing fitness - losing technique/skills
Social Stressors	Isolation - from sport & teammates - from friends Pressure - from coaches - from sport organization - from media
Financial Stressors	Direct costs associated with injury - cost of surgery - cost of rehabilitation - cost of medication + rehab. equipment Indirect costs associated with injury - loss of salary - loss of scholarship - loss of sponsorship contract/opportunity

Note: From Bianco, 2002.

Cognitive Stressors

Being injured is also stressful because it poses a significant threat to the athlete's future. Research shows that injured athletes worry about how the combination of injury, restricted physical activity, and prolonged absence from sport will affect their athletic careers (Bianco et al., 1999; Gould, Udry, Bridges, & Beck, 1997; Johnston & Carroll, 1998b; Rotella & Heyman, 1993). With respect to the injury itself, athletes tend to worry about whether they will recover fully and be able to perform at pre-injury levels. These types of concerns are likely to be most evident among athletes with little or no injury experience or who have chronic injuries. For these athletes, the lack of experience and/or recurrence of symptoms can contribute to great uncertainty about the future (Bianco, 2002).

The forced absence from sport imposed by injury can raise concerns about losing the position on the team or being replaced altogether. Athletes are well aware that competition for spots, particularly at the elite level, is such that there are plenty of talented players available to replace injured ones. They also realize that there is a strong possibility that replacement players will perform well, making it difficult for injured athletes to resume their former positions (Bianco, 2002; Gould et al., 1997).

Being absent from sport also means being out of sight, and injured athletes may worry that their coaches will forget about them or overlook them when opportunities arise. Another implication of being absent is missing out on learning opportunities, such as training and skill development. This can leave athletes feeling that everyone has "leapfrogged" ahead of them and they may fear that, as a result, their coaches will limit their opportunities when they return. Another consequence of being absent is missing out on important events and opportunities. This can be especially difficult if the event is a prestigious one and one that occurs infrequently, such as the Olympic Games (Bianco, 2002; Leddy, Lambert & Ogles, 1994; Taylor & Taylor, 1997).

With regard to restricted physical activity, concerns may arise about losing fitness and skills and not being able to catch up to those who have continued to train and compete. Such concerns tend to be particularly salient among athletes with first-time injuries, whose inexperience often leads them to overestimate the amount of time required to recover lost skills and missed training (Bianco, 2002).

Social Stressors

Other difficulties associated with being injured include isolation from the team and teammates (Bianco et al., 1999; Heil, 1993). As a result, there may be a sense of loneliness and disconnection from the sport. Isolation appears to be more of a strain for those athletes involved in team sports and thus accustomed to being part of a large group. As Chris, a professional football player, put it: "To go from being around 14 guys all the time to being alone was hard to take. I had no one to talk to." Athletes may also find themselves isolated from their friends as their limited mobility may impose restrictions on the types of activities in which they may participate. For example, being on crutches would make it difficult for an athlete to partake in a number of outdoor activities.

Depending on the athlete's status and position, there may be pressure from the coaches or the sport organization to recover quickly (Bianco et al., 1999). One example, reported by several national team skiers, involved an unwritten team policy that any rookie who took more than six months to recover from an injury would be dropped from the team. These athletes felt a tremendous amount of pressure, and many admitted returning to the slopes before being fully recovered for fear of losing their positions. For the individual sport athlete, pressure from the coach can be felt more acutely. John, a national track and field athlete, had this to say about the issue: "As an individual sport athlete, everything is focused on you. You have to try to juggle the coach's expectations and pressures, as well as all your own baggage."

Another source of pressure, particularly for high-profile athletes, is media pressure (Bianco, 2002; Petrie, 1993). Speculations in the media regarding one's recovery status and athletic future can be distressing for an athlete. Chris, a professional soccer player, summed it up this way: "When the media gives you the reputation of being injury-prone, it can be very hard to handle. No one wants to be known as a risk."

Financial Stressors

There may also be financial repercussions to being injured. The costs may be direct and include expenses involved in medical care and rehabilitation. There are also indirect costs associated with injury that may stem from lost wages and revenue from other sources. For example, a football player thought to be "injury-prone" because of a series of injuries is not likely to be sought after for product endorsements. The financial implications of injury are more likely to be of concern in the case of chronic injury, where the costs involved may exceed an athlete's medical coverage and result in significant financial strain (Bianco, 2002).

Clearly, there is a lot to contend with and it is not surprising that some athletes find themselves overwhelmed by the injury experience. Not only are there a lot of related problematic issues, but they are likely to be present over a long period of time. Further complicating the matter is the fact that the challenges associated with injury will vary across time, with some dissipating and some new ones emerging. This ever changing environment requires that the athlete be able to make constant adjustments throughout the injury experience. As Hobfoll (1988) pointed out, the process of coping itself may be stressful, further adding to the person's strain. Thus, for the injured athlete, the impact of injury itself combined with the concomitant demands it engenders can create a significant amount of psychological and emotional strain.

Athlete Responses to Injury

The response to injury can be viewed as occurring at three levels:
- cognitive
- emotional
- behavioral

These clusters of responses are believed to occur in a top-down fashion, with cognition influencing emotions which, in turn, determine behavior. It is important to note, however, that the direction of influence can also be reversed with behavioral outcomes affecting emotions and ensuing cognitions. For example, Lucy, a track and field athlete, sprained her ankle during an Olympic qualifying event. Her immediate thought was that her career was over; she was despondent and neglected to seek medical attention. A few days later, she could barely move her ankle. This made her feel even more despondent and confirmed her belief that indeed her career was over.

Cognitive responses

Cognitive appraisals play a central role in determining the significance of an event and the ensuing emotional and behavioral responses. According to Lazarus & Folkman (1984; 1991), the amount of disruption an individual experiences in response to stress is determined in great part by how the person evaluates the situation. This evaluation occurs at two levels:

- At the primary level, the event is assessed in terms of its significance or meaning and the amount of disruption it is likely to cause.
- This is followed by a secondary appraisal of whether sufficient resources, both personal and social, are available to cope with the demands posed by the event.

Stress results when it is perceived that the demands associated with a particular event exceed available coping resources. The greater the excess of demands, the greater the extent of disruption caused. Thus, an athlete's response to being injured will be determined by the weight given to the event and how the athlete perceives his or her ability to confront the challenges posed by the event.

Cognitive appraisals are not always accurate, however, particularly in times of stress. When stressed, individuals are prone to engaging in cognitive distortions, which are exaggerated or inaccurate views of reality (Beck, Rush, Shaw, & Emery, 1979). These distortions can take on several forms and include: catastrophizing, overgeneralization, personalization, selective abstraction, and dichotomous thinking.

- Catastrophizing involves blowing an event out of proportion. A skier who believes that a torn anterior cruciate ligament automatically means his career is over would be engaging in this form of distortion.
- Overgeneralization involves extending the consequences of the event to other unaffected areas. A football player with an ankle injury who believes he will lose his throwing accuracy as a result of the injury is overgeneralizing.
- Personalization occurs when people see themselves as being victims. A baseball player with a recurrent shoulder injury who asks, "Why me? What did I do to deserve this?" is engaging in personalization.
- Selective abstraction refers to focusing on only those case examples that are consistent with one's negative perspective. A gymnast with a broken wrist who fails to acknowledge examples of gymnasts who have recovered fully but instead fixates on those who never recovered fully is engaging in selective abstraction.
- Lastly, dichotomous thinking is akin to seeing events as being either black or white, with no gray area. A basketball player with an ankle injury who believes he is useless because he can't play is engaging in dichotomous thinking.

Research shows that cognitive appraisals are likely to be influenced by a host of personal and environmental factors.

Personal factors include
- age (Brewer, Linder, & Phelps, 1995),
- injury history (Smith, Scott, O'Fallon, & Young, 1990),
- self-esteem (Leddy et al., 1994),
- optimism (Ford, Eklund, & Gordon, 2000; Grove & Gordon, 1995),
- hardiness (Ford et al., 2000),
- athletic identity (Brewer, 1993; Young & White, 1995), and
- coping skills

(Grove & Gordon, 1995; Rotella & Heyman, 1993).

Environmental factors include
- level of life stress (Brewer, 1993),
- timing of the injury (Bianco et al., 1999; Smith et al, 1990),
- duration of consequences (McDonald & Hardy, 1990; Johnston & Carroll, 2000; Smith et al., 1990),
- impairment of sports performance (Brewer, et al., 1995),
- interactions with treatment team (Pearson & Jones, 1992), and
- availability of social support

(Bianco, 2001, 2002; Gutkind, 2004; Udry et al, 1997; Pearson & Jones, 1992).

Appraisals are important because they drive the choice of coping strategy. As Lazarus and Folkman (1991) pointed out, every situation involves some aspects that are controllable and some that are uncontrollable. Coping effectively involves selecting the strategy that matches the controllability of the situation. Emotion-focused strategies are most appropriate for dealing with uncontrollable aspects of the environment. These strategies are aimed at regulating emotions and include activities such as cognitive restructuring and positive self-talk. When it comes to dealing with the controllable features of a stressor, problem-focused strategies are most appropriate. Problem-focused coping is aimed at managing the problem causing the stress and can include activities such as goal setting, seeking social support, and adhering to rehabilitation. Thus, one avenue to facilitating coping with injury is to ensure that athletes appraise the situation accurately and identify areas in which they can exert some control.

Emotional responses

How individuals appraise an event will have an impact on how they feel about that event. Just as there are individual differences in cognitive appraisals, there will also be variation in emotional responses to being injured. Although emotional responses vary in degree, they tend to follow a typical pattern. Heil (1993) proposed the "Affective Cycle of Injury" model as a means of describing this pattern. As depicted in Figure 1, the model comprises three states that athletes cycle through as they struggle to come to terms with being injured. The distress stage describes the emotional upheaval brought on by injury and includes emotions such as shock, anger, bargaining, anxiety, depression, isolation, guilt, humiliation, preoccupation, and helplessness. Denial refers to the sense of disbelief experienced in response to injury and may occur in varying degrees, including outright failure to accept the severity of the injury. Heil explained that denial could be adaptive in that it allows emotions to be processed slowly and sys-

Figure 1.
The affective cycle of injury model from Heil (1993).

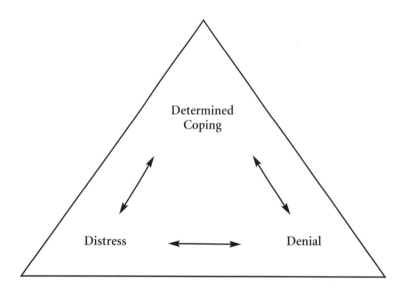

tematically over time, but maladaptive if it interfered with the emotional work of recovery. Finally, determined coping refers to acceptance (to varying degrees) of the severity of the injury and its implications. Determined coping is characterized by proactive efforts aimed at working through the process of recovery.

The research shows that mood disturbances tend to be most prevalent in those who identify strongly with the athlete role and whose injury is severe (Brewer, 1993; Brewer et al., 1995; Smith, et al., 1993; Sparkes, 1998; Young, White, & McTeer, 1994). As Turner and Roszell (1994) explained, the greater the commitment to a particular identity (e.g., athlete identity), the greater the impact on self-image and well-being when that identity is challenged or disconfirmed (e.g., when severely injured). In terms of the pattern of responses, they tend to be transient in nature, generally proceeding from negative to positive affect over time (Johnston & Carroll, 2000; Leddy et al., 1994; Quackenbush & Crossman, 1994; Smith et al., 1990; Smith, et al., 1993). This progression from negative to positive affect tends to be curvilinear, with athletes vacillating between emotional highs and lows, in accordance with perceptions of recovery and progress in rehabilitation (Brewer et al., 1995; McDonald & Hardy, 1990; Smith et al., 1990). A setback in rehabilitation, for example, could cause a shift from feelings of optimism and hopefulness to feelings of frustration and discouragement.

Behavioral responses

The cognitive and emotional adjustment to injury will influence behavior, in that it will affect motivation for rehabilitation (Bianco et al, 1999; Rotella & Heyman, 1993; Taylor & May, 1996). An athlete who can successfully manage the psychological stresses of being injured is likely to be motivated and show good treatment adherence. The athlete who has difficulty adjusting, on the other hand, is likely to experience a motivational deficit and show problems with adherence.

Rehabilitation adherence is the bedrock of an efficacious recovery and includes behaviors such as:

(a) compliance with instructions to engage in appropriate restriction of physical activity (e.g., rest, workout limitations),

(b) completion of home rehabilitation exercises and icing,

(c) compliance with medical prescriptions, and

(d) participation in clinic-based exercises and therapy

(Brewer, 1998; Fisher, 1990). Failure to comply with the treatment protocol can, in the short term, slow recovery and interfere with the healing process. Results such as these will exacerbate the athlete's concerns and give rise to further cognitive distortions. The athlete is likely to then feel frustrated and demoralized and may completely lose motivation for rehabilitation. It is not long before the athlete becomes caught in a downward spiral of non-adherence (as shown in Figure 2). Take Sean, for instance. Sean was a football player who tore his anterior cruciate ligament during a championship game. In the beginning he did all of the exercises the physiotherapist recommended but became frustrated that his knee wasn't healing quickly. He became angry that he was going to miss the rest of the season and started to feel that rehabilitation was a waste of time. He lost interest in going to rehabilitation and instead did exercises at home, but not with the necessary intensity. Recovery reached a plateau and Sean became angry with himself for his lack of discipline, but he could not seem to muster the motivation necessary to carry out the exercises as recommended by his sport therapist.

The long-term consequence of non-adherence that is of great concern is that it can leave the injured area weakened and vulnerable to further injury (Crossman, 1997; Doyle et al., 1998; Gould & Udry, 1995; Steadman, 1993). In their discussion of the rehabilitation of knee injuries, Gould and Udry (1995) explained that the failure to do exercises designed to prevent scar tissue build-up could result in reduced mobility in the knee. This reduced mobility can interfere with the proper execution of sport skills and increase the risk of re-injury.

Figure 2.
Typical pattern of maladjustment in rehabilitation

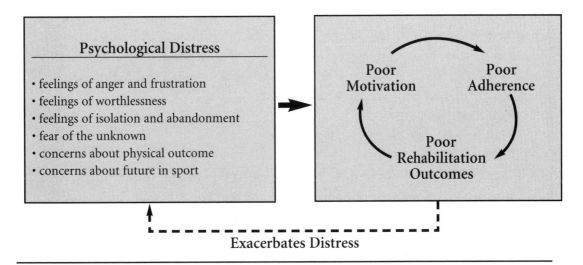

It should be noted that non-adherence refers to both under-adherence and over-adherence. In the latter case, the problem is not one of under-motivation but rather one of being overly motivated. In such cases, athletes may be inclined to try to do too much in an effort to speed up the recovery process. One national team skier, who had had knee replacement surgery, confessed that he was secretly seeing three physiotherapists at the same time in an effort to cut his recovery time! Unfortunately, his plan backfired and he pulled a hamstring, which added an extra 2 months to his recovery time. Clearly, the message here is that more is not always better and athletes sometimes need to be saved from themselves.

Part 2: Coach Support

As demonstrated in the first part of the chapter, sport injury engenders a wide range of stressors. Furthermore, the process of coping with this multitude of stressors can be emotionally draining and give rise to adjustment difficulties that are likely to have an adverse effect on recovery. There is a pressing need to find ways of helping alleviate the athletes' distress and encourage adaptive coping. Coaches are well-positioned to be of assistance in this regard for several reasons. First, coaches are influential in deciding the future of their athletes, and given that injured athletes worry a great deal about their athletic careers, it is reasonable to expect that coach input can play an important role in relieving such concerns. Also, because coaches play the role of motivator in their athletes' sporting life, it is likely that they can also be instrumental in keeping athletes motivated throughout recovery (Heil, 1993). Coaches who know their athletes well, for example, know what to say and do in order to keep them motivated. Applying this knowledge to the rehabilitation setting could reduce motivational deficits and encourage proper adherence. Indeed, several authors have recognized that maintaining links with coaches throughout injury is critical to rehabilitation (Bianco, 2001; 2002; Hardy, Burke, & Crace, 1999; Heil, 1993; Johnston & Carroll, 1998a ; Robbins & Rosenfeld, 2001; Rotella & Heyman, 1993; Shelley, 1999).

Coach Support—What Is It?

For the purposes of this chapter, coach support refers to social support activities that coaches engage in with the intention of helping their athletes. These activities are aimed at helping the athletes manage the uncertainty associated with stress and increase their sense of personal control over the environment (Albrecht & Adelman, 1987). There are a variety of ways a coach can extend social support to injured athletes, and these activities fall into three major categories:

- emotional support
- informational support
- tangible support

(Hardy et al., 1999). As shown in Table 2, emotional support includes behaviors such as listening without giving advice, showing empathy and concern, and challenging people to see things from a different perspective. Informational support includes behaviors aimed at validating one's experiences, recognizing and supporting coping

Table 2.

Social Support Types Grouped by Category

Category + Support Type	Definition
Emotional Support	
Listening support	Behaviors that indicate people listen to you without giving advice or being judgmental.
Emotional comfort	Behaviors that comfort you and indicate that people are on your side and care for you.
Emotional challenge	Behaviors that challenge you to evaluate your attitudes, values, and feelings.
Informational Support	
Reality confirmation	Behaviors that indicate that people are similar to you – see things the way you do – helps confirm your perceptions and perspectives of the world and helps you keep things in focus.
Task appreciation	Behaviors that acknowledge your efforts and express appreciation for the work you do.
Task challenge	Behaviors that challenge your way of thinking about your work in order to stretch you, motivate you, and lead you to greater creativity, excitement, and involvement in your work.
Tangible Support	
Material assistance	Behaviors that provide you with financial assistance, products, or gifts.
Personal assistance	Behaviors that indicate a giving of time, skills, knowledge, and/or expertise to help you accomplish your tasks.

Note: From Hardy et al. (1999).

efforts, and challenging people to keep up the good work. Finally, tangible support can be conceived of as material or personal assistance.

Discriminating among different forms of social support is important because it is likely that specific types of social support are needed under certain circumstances (Cohen & McKay, 1984; Cutrona & Russell, 1990). For example, Cutrona and Russell (1990) proposed that conditions of low controllability created a need for emotional support, while more controllable aspects of the stressor produced a need for informational and tangible support. Life domain affected by the stressor also influenced the nature of support needed. For instance, a financial loss would create a need for tangible support whereas the loss of a loved one would create a need for emotional support. In the case of the injured athlete worried about losing fitness, assistance with designing a fitness plan is likely to be more desirable than expressions of empathy.

How Does Coach Support Work?

In order to account for how coach support can be of assistance to injured athletes it is necessary to look to the social support literature. Two major perspectives have been put forth to explain how social support contributes to positive coping: the main effect theory and the buffering hypothesis. Both these perspectives view social support as a resource that protects individuals from the deleterious effects of stress. The main effect theory emphasizes how social support reduces the likelihood of experiencing stress (Pierce, Sarason, & Sarason, 1991; Sarason, Pierce, & Sarason, 1994), whereas the buffering hypothesis addresses how social support counteracts the impact of stress, once it is experienced (Cohen & Wills, 1985; Schwarzer & Leppin, 1991).

The main effect theory posits that through early social interactions, individuals come to develop perceptions about their ability to confront life challenges and whether social support will be available if needed. This "sense of support" can influence how situations are appraised (Pierce et al., 1991; Sarason et al., 1994). Recall that stress is experienced when it is perceived that the demands of a situation exceed one's coping resources (Lazarus & Folkman, 1991). It is believed that the sense that one is supported may foster more accurate and more positive appraisals of personal resources and enable individuals to develop more effective coping strategies. Compared to their low-sense-of-support counterparts, individuals high in sense of support are less likely to appraise life events as stressful because they believe they possess the necessary coping resources, and they are confident that help is available should the challenges posed by an event exceed these resources.

It is important to note that in spite of having a healthy sense of support, there will be times when individuals will feel overwhelmed by the challenges before them. As Hobfoll (1988) explained, coping with stress requires an investment of resources, but because resources are limited they can quickly become depleted and compromise coping. According to the buffering hypothesis, the social support received during times of stress can supplement, enhance, and actuate personal resources and thus increase a person's capacity to function (Cohen & Wills, 1985). In this case, social support serves to buffer or offset the negative effects of stress.

For social support to be effective, however, it must match the needs of the recipient (Cutrona, Cohen, & Ingram, 1990; Dunkel-Schetter & Bennett, 1990; Eckenrode & Wethington, 1990). A person whose house is on fire would much rather receive help in dousing the flames than expressions of sympathy for his predicament. The same holds true for the injured athlete; specific types of coach support will be required at given times throughout recovery.

Coach Support Needed

The injury and recovery process can be divided into three major phases:
(1) the occurrence of injury phase,
(2) the treatment and recovery phase, and
(3) the return to full training and competition phase.
Each of these phases presents its own unique set of challenges and thus engenders specific needs for coach support.

Phase 1: The Occurrence of Injury

This first stage is typically the shortest of the three. It begins with the occurrence of injury and includes the task of seeking and obtaining treatment. In this stage the athlete is likely to be in shock over what has just occurred and out of necessity will focus his or her energies on seeking and obtaining treatment. This preoccupation with practical matters will typically delay the processing of the event until the diagnosis and prognosis for recovery are received. It is at this point, when the reality of the situation sets in, that the emotional upheaval is likely to ensue (Heil, 1993). This is when the athlete may show mood changes and begin to worry about the implications of injury and a prolonged absence from sport.

During this stage, there is likely to be a high need for empathy and reassurance from coaches, and also advice and guidance on medical issues. Athletes have indicated that they were concerned about getting the best medical care possible and believed their coaches could help in directing them to suitably qualified medical professionals. The athletes with chronic injuries talked about needing advice on whether to have surgery. They explained that in addition to the medical opinion of their surgeons, input from coaches was desirable because their coaches knew best if the athletes could afford

Figure 3.
Coach support needed during injury and recovery.

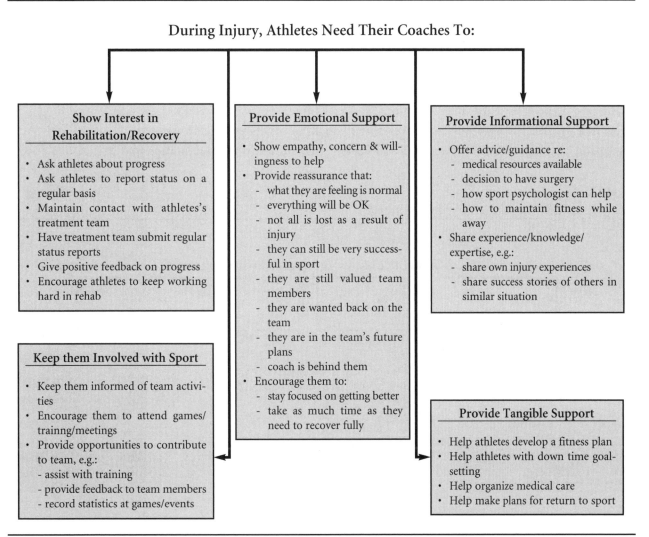

to take time off. It was felt that because of their expertise and experience in sport, coaches were well suited to offering guidance on such issues.

Phase 2: Treatment and Recovery

This next stage spans the beginning of treatment through recovery. This can be a very long stage marked by all sorts of ups and downs, depending on the extent of injury and the course of recovery. As mentioned earlier, injured athletes tend to worry a great deal about what their coaches think about them, about their positions on the team, and about the chance of regaining pre-injury form. To alleviate these concerns, athletes need reassurance that things will work out fine, that they are still a part of the team, and that their coaches believe in them and their ability to recover fully (Johnston & Carroll, 1998a; Robbins & Rosenfeld, 2000; Shelley, 1999). There is a range of support activities coaches can engage in to communicate such messages to their injured athletes. These activities are listed in Figure 3 and have been organized under five major categories: (a) monitoring of rehabilitation and recovery, (b) keeping athletes involved in sport, (c) provision of emotional support, (d) provision of informational support, and (e) provision of tangible support.

Monitoring of rehabilitation and recovery. It is important that injured athletes know that their coaches are interested in their rehabilitation and recovery. Not only does this interest signal concern but it also helps alleviate fears of being forgotten by the coach. Being monitored also creates a sense of accountability and can prove to be motivational for the athletes. By knowing that their rehabilitation efforts will not go unnoticed, athletes can use the opportunity to impress their coaches with their dedication and perseverance. As Susan, a national team swimmer, put it: "It was good to know that my coach knew I was doing everything I could to get better—that I wasn't just sitting around feeling sorry for myself and slacking off." Monitoring rehabilitation

Figure 4.
Benefits of continued involvement in sport.

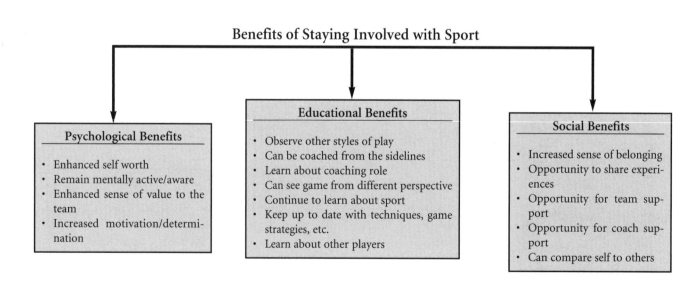

efforts also affords coaches the opportunity to offer feedback and encouragement to their athletes.

It must be noted, however, that while there may be motivational benefits associated with coach interest in rehabilitation, it can sometimes increase the athlete's distress rather than alleviate it. This is most likely to occur in situations in which athletes are experiencing rehabilitation setbacks or progress is slow. In times like these, athletes fear that the lack of progress may be misinterpreted as a lack of effort. Again, this is an opportunity for coaches to express their understanding of the rehabilitation process and to reassure athletes that eventually all will be well.

Keeping athletes involved in sport. Another way coaches can contribute to relieving their athletes' distress is by keeping them involved in sport, for instance, by inviting them to attend practices or team meetings or to watch games. Depending on the type of injury and the limitations imposed, injured athletes can still make a meaningful contribution to the sport. As Mary, a national team netballer, explained: "You are still an athlete. You still have something to offer. You can still have input and share ideas."

The benefits of continued involvement have been recognized in the literature and several authors have recommended this strategy as a tool for motivating injured athletes (Heil, 1993; Petrie, 1993; Udry et al., 1997; Wiese-Bjornstal, & Smith, 1999). As listed in Figure 4, continued involvement is beneficial on several levels. In terms of the psychological benefits, it can contribute to an enhanced sense of self-worth and value to the team. Being present and watching others can also serve to strengthen the athletes' resolve to work hard in rehabilitation and recover quickly.

With regards to the educational benefits associated with continued involvement, injured athletes can expand their knowledge of the game by observing different styles of play. They can also learn more about the coach's perspective by standing on the sidelines and listening to his or her comments. Furthermore, being present allows the athlete to keep up to date with techniques and strategies—a sure advantage when the athlete returns to full training and competition.

Depending on the type of injury and the stage of recovery, athletes may be able to run drills or even participate in some. Alternatively, they can use the opportunity to develop new skills not affected by the injury. Some athletes have suggested that coaches design specific drills for injured athletes so that they can use their downtime constructively. They explained that this would allow them to remain enthusiastic and motivated about their sport, especially if they could do the drills with some of their teammates.

On a social level, continued involvement can contribute to reducing feelings of isolation and loneliness. Injured athletes can share their experiences with others and benefit from the support and encouragement of their teammates and coaches. They can also use others as a basis of comparison for gauging their rate of progress. It's important to note that while continued involvement may be motivational for some, it can be distressing for others. Some athletes may find it difficult to watch their peers because it only serves to highlight their own deficiencies. Furthermore, it may contribute to a heightened fear of falling behind and not being able to catch up. Others may just find it difficult to watch the game and not be a part of it. Dean, a professional football player, offered this observation: "You're watching the game and you can't do anything about it. It's dangling there in front of you but you can't participate in it. It's very frustrating." The best thing to do is to let athletes know they are welcome to attend games and practices but to allow them the freedom to decide whether or not to do so.

One final caveat on the topic of continued involvement is that if coaches invite athletes to attend training sessions or games, they need to pay attention to them and give them something meaningful to do. Otherwise, the athletes will end up feeling worse. Paul, a national team basketball player, described his frustration at showing up to practice and being ignored by his coach: "I was totally and utterly frustrated because I was not asked to do anything. I just sat there and listened. It was so incredibly frustrating. It felt like I was invisible." Lara, a national team netballer, wasn't ignored by her coaches at training, instead she was treated like a gofer: "All you hear is, 'Do this, do that, get this, get that.' And sometimes you just want to tell them to get lost."

Provision of emotional support. Emotional support can play a significant role in relieving athletes' distress. Injured athletes need to know that their coaches care about them, that they understand what the athletes are going through, and that they are behind their athletes and willing to help however they can. Athletes also need reassurance from their coaches about treatment success, their position and value to the team, and their future in sport. Tina, a national team gymnast, described the need for emotional support in this manner: "Injured athletes have a lot of doubts about being able to come back and compete well. They need lots of reassurance. Coaches need to reassure them that they will be okay and that they're still a part of the team."

Concerns about the future are likely to be heightened by missing important events or experiencing rehabilitation setbacks. Encouragement and reassurance from coaches during such times can help the athletes put matters in perspective and redirect their efforts toward ensuring a successful rehabilitation. Coaches can also contribute to alleviating a lot of the pressure athletes feel by letting them know they can take the time necessary to recover fully.

It's important for coach contact to be present from the start, when athletes are likely to have the most doubts and concerns, and to be continued throughout rehabilitation. Otherwise, athletes may begin to worry about the motives behind the absence of contact. Recall that when in distress, individuals are prone to cognitive distortions. Athletes in this predicament may misinterpret the coach's silence as an indication that the coach doesn't care about them anymore or that something bad has happened (i.e., they've been replaced or dropped from the team).

Provision of informational support. Because of their involvement in sport and perhaps even as a result of their own past injury experiences, coaches have a wealth of relevant information they can share with injured athletes. Athletes have commented that it would be helpful for coaches to share their own experiences because it would show that they understood what the athletes were going through. Athletes offered another example of how coaches could provide informational support: sharing stories about athletes in similar predicaments who had recovered successfully and gone on to achieve great things in sport. Of course, it is important that these stories be relevant and intended to encourage the athlete rather than boast about one's own grit. As Sarah, a national team gymnast, expressed it: "They say stuff like when they broke their hand, they had to compete with a mangled hand, and you're thinking, yeah right! That is really annoying."

Positive feedback and encouragement on rehabilitation efforts is another way coaches can provide informational support to their athletes. Coaches can help keep athletes positive throughout rehabilitation and help them stay focused on the task. They can provide reassurance and use their knowledge of the athlete's personality to help them stay motivated. Mary, a national team netballer, explained: "No matter what was happening in rehabilitation, my coach always put a positive spin on it. That really helped me to stay focused and not worry so much."

Provision of tangible support. In terms of tangible support, athletes would like assistance from their coaches in developing a downtime fitness plan. Advice and guidance on how to maintain fitness while away from sport can help alleviate concerns about not being able to catch up to the rest of the field. Engaging in a downtime fitness plan can contribute to a heightened sense of control as it allows the athletes to feel they are doing something to facilitate the transition back to sport. Bianco and colleagues (1999) found that injured athletes sometimes worry that the training programs provided by physiotherapists are too general and not tailored to meet specific sport demands. Having a program designed by the coach can go along way in allaying such concerns. It also can help the athletes manage their downtime more efficiently because it provides them with a short-term goal-setting plan. However, coaches can also be of assistance in making long-term plans, thus helping the athletes stay positive and enthusiastic about the future.

Phase 3: The Return to Full Training and Competition

The third stage, which can also be quite long, begins with the return to full training and competition. As several authors (Bianco et al., 1999; Heil, 1993; Udry et al., 1997; Wiese-Bjornstal, & Smith, 1999) have noted, the injury experience does not end with getting the all-clear from one's doctor. There are still psychological hurdles for the athlete to confront upon the return to sport. The athlete may be physically healed, but psychologically, many challenges still lie ahead.

The return to full training and competition is a phase during which the athlete will be "testing" the recovered area. There is likely to be a significant amount of apprehension and holding back as athletes grapple with the fear of re-injury. This is a time when athletes will need their coaches to be very patient with them. They will have to allow the athletes the time and the space to become comfortable and confident with taking risks again. It's important to note that feeling psychologically ready can sometimes take a long time. One national team skier reported that it took him a full year before he was able to "let go and give 100%."

One way in which coaches can help returning athletes regain their self-confidence is by encouraging them to start slowly and build up gradually. To keep athletes motivated and focused during this time, coaches can assist in developing a goal-setting plan. They also can provide feedback and encouragement and focus on rewarding effort rather than outcome. A goal-setting plan can also be useful in those cases where rather than holding back, the returning athlete is overly eager to jump right in. In an effort to make up for lost time, the athlete may be inclined to take unnecessary chances and thus run the risk of re-injury. Again, this is an opportunity for coaches to impart their wisdom and play an instrumental role in protecting the athlete from further harm.

The Impact of Coach Support and Non-Support

In line with the propositions of the buffering hypothesis, research shows that coach support can play an important role in relieving athlete distress and encouraging adaptive coping behaviors (Bianco, 2001; Bianco et al., 1999; Heil, 1993; Johnston & Carroll, 1998a; Rees & Hardy, 2000; Robbins & Rosenfeld, 2001; Shelley, 1999; Udry et al., 1997). Specifically, the research shows that coach support can help restore confidence and feelings of self-worth by making athletes feel valued and important. As Lara, a national team netballer, recalled: "I was really depressed, but because my coach showed interest in me, it made me feel important, like I mattered." Coach support can also help increase confidence in the success of treatment and allay concerns about the future. Fred, a professional footballer, described the impact of his coach's support in the following manner: "My coach never had any doubts about my recovery. He believed I was going to come back and play and not have any problems. That was encouraging; it made me believe it as well."

It is clear that coach support can serve as an important motivational tool in rehabilitation and contribute to enhancing athlete commitment to recovery. It is also evident that lack of coach support, on the other hand, can have a detrimental effect on injured athletes (Bianco, 2001; Shelley 1999; Udry et al., 1997). Lack of support can contribute to decreases in self-confidence, motivation, and commitment to sport. Furthermore, a lack of coach interest can result in decreases in self-worth, making athletes feel like they are only valuable when healthy and playing. Bob, a professional soccer player, concluded: "We're people too. But the coach only sees the athlete, the machine. If you're not performing, then you don't count." Lack of coach support can also increase feelings of isolation and leave athletes feeling distanced from their team and their sport. Susan, a national team swimmer, described her experience this way: "I would have handled it a lot better if I knew I had the support of my coach—that he was there with me the whole time. But I didn't feel that. I felt distanced from everyone, from everything."

It is important to realize that coach support not only has an impact in the short-term with regards to coping with injury, but it also has an effect on the long-term working relationship between the coach and the athlete. Goldsmith and Parks (1990) suggested that social support activities serve as a vehicle for individuals to communicate their feelings about

(a) themselves,

(b) the recipient, and

(c) the relationship they share.

By telephoning an injured athlete in order to inquire about his or her progress, for example, a coach is ultimately communicating something about himself or herself (e.g., I am a caring person), the athlete (e.g., You are a valuable person), and their relationship (e.g., I care about you). These support messages are not stated explicitly; rather they are understood implicitly via the coach's expression of interest.

The messages conveyed through support interactions are important because they can alter one's sentiments and conduct toward the relationship partner (Barnes & Duck, 1994). Coach support activities that are seen as containing messages of caring and understanding, for example, can create feelings of warmth and gratitude and contribute to strengthening the coach-athlete relationship. Support activities that indicate a lack of caring and interest, on the other hand, can create feelings of estrangement and erode the coach-athlete relationship. The disappointment athletes feel from having been ignored, abandoned, or judged negatively by their coaches can lead to a strained working relationship upon the return to sport (Bianco, 2001; Shelley, 1999; Udry et al., 1997). John, a professional football player, said: "I felt betrayed and let down by my coaches. I no longer wanted to go out there and put everything on the line for my coaches." Thus, coach support during rehabilitation is not only important at the time of recovery but it is also integral to nurturing a positive working alliance long after recovery.

The Coach Support Process

Having established the multiple benefits of coach support in the recovery context, let us now examine the process of obtaining coach support. The process outlined in Figure 5 is an extension of the 4-stage social support model proposed by Pearlin and McCall (1990). Whereas these authors combined recognition of need and support-seeking, the present model presents them as separate processes. As shown in Figure 5, the coach support process comprises 5 stages, and each is influenced by coach and athlete characteristics, the quality of the relationship they share, and environmental factors. The process begins with the athlete acknowledging that coach support is needed

Figure 5.
The coach support process.

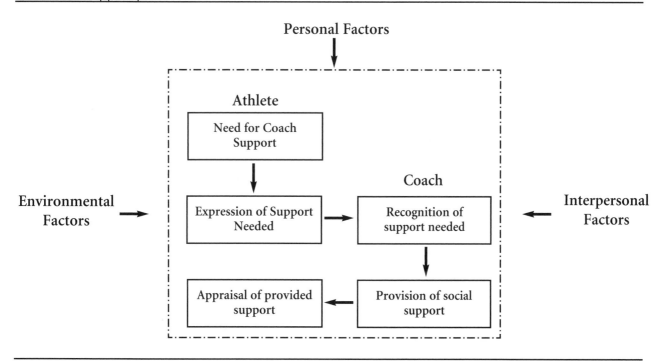

and then taking measures to communicate that need to the coach. This is followed by the coach recognizing the need for support and deciding whether he or she is able and willing to provide the support needed. Based on this decision, the coach offers social support to the athlete who, in turn, evaluates the support offered. This is a rather simplistic account of the process. In reality, the process of obtaining coach support can be rather complex and fraught with opportunities for breakdown. Let us consider each component separately in an effort to better understand the potential and pitfalls of the coach support process.

Step 1: Recognition of the need for support (athlete)

In order to ask for help, one needs to recognize that help is needed. The recognition that help is needed, however, can pose significant threats to self-esteem and thus may be resisted (Goldsmith & Parks, 1990). Instead, individuals may be more inclined to select other forms of coping that do not involve admitting a need for social support (Lazarus & Folkman, 1991). It is also possible that certain types of individuals need less support than others. As discussed earlier, people with a high sense of support tend to feel very capable of handling things on their own and therefore need less support than do their low-sense-of-support counterparts (Sarason et al., 1994). Affiliative need is another personality factor that may influence the need for support. According to Hill (1991), people can derive various types of rewards from social contact, and the value placed on these rewards will drive the need for social contact. Because they place a higher value on social rewards, individuals high in affiliative need are likely to have a greater need for social support compared to their low-affiliative-need counterparts.

The need for coach support is also influenced by environmental factors. As discussed previously, Cutrona and Russell (1990) proposed that the amount and type of support needed is determined, in part, by the nature of the stressor. The dimensions of a stressor that dictate support need are
(a) desirability,
(b) controllability,
(c) duration of consequences, and
(d) domain affected.
Thus, a career-ending injury that occurs during an Olympic event, for example, will create a greater need for support than a finger dislocation sustained during the off-season. The sociocultural context is also a consideration. In an environment that idealizes mental toughness, admitting a need for help can be particularly threatening to one's self-concept (Young & White, 1995; Young et al., 1994). As a result, there may be a tendency to downplay the need for support.

In terms of the influence of relationship quality, research shows people don't want support from those
(a) with whom they have a conflictive relationship,
(b) who have been unhelpful in the past, and
(c) who make them feel bad
(Hill, 1991; Sarason et al, 1994). It has been found that the support received under these circumstances often makes things worse rather than better (Rook, 1992). Evidence from sport injury studies (e.g., Bianco et al., 1999; Shelley, 1999) shows that coach support is

unwanted when the coach is ambivalent toward the relationship or the relationship is marked by a high degree of conflict. These findings serve to further highlight the importance of having established a good relationship with athletes beforehand.

Step 2: Expression of support need

As mentioned earlier, receiving coach support certainly has its benefits; however, the act of seeking support is fraught with personal costs (Eckenrode & Wethington, 1990). For example, asking for help can arouse feelings of embarrassment, vulnerability, and dependence on others. Moreover, it requires an open admission of one's own incompetence. This can be especially threatening in the sport environment. As Nixon (1994) observed, deeply embedded in athletic subcultures is the perception that needing or asking for help signifies weakness. Given that athletes are very concerned about what the coaches think of them, self-presentational concerns are paramount, particularly for those athletes who have not yet "proven themselves" to their coaches.

The nature of the coach-athlete relationship is another important determinant of support-seeking behavior. In an effort to minimize the personal costs inherent in support-seeking, individuals will express their support needs to those whom they believe will be

(a) responsive to their distress,

(b) motivated to help,

(c) accurate about the nature and degree of their difficulties, and

(d) willing to provide appropriate help

(Burleson, 1994).

Thus, it is important for coaches to establish an atmosphere that encourages safe disclosure. Athletes need to know that their requests for assistance will be well-received and not used against them at a later time. A relationship marked by conflict would certainly increase the risks associated with support-seeking.

Also at issue are gender differences. Asking for help may be especially difficult for male athletes. Evidence indicates that, with few exceptions, relative to men, women tend to

(a) engage in more self-disclosure,

(b) hold more positive attitudes toward seeking and receiving help, and

(c) seek help more and receive higher levels of help

(Hill, 1991). These tendencies are influenced by both gender and gender role prescriptions. Compared to women, men tend to be evaluated more negatively and viewed as less well adjusted when they disclose a personal problem because the masculine gender role holds that males are supposed to be strong and independent. Support-seeking on the part of females, however, is more acceptable because it is consistent with the feminine gender role that portrays females as weak and dependent

(Hobfoll & Vaux, 1993).

Overall, it seems that the decision to seek social support depends, in large part, on how vulnerable people feel to possible threats and whether they perceive that the costs of seeking social support outweigh the benefits. Substantial evidence indicates that people who might benefit from help often persist in their own failed problem-solving attempts rather than ask for help (Eckenrode & Wethington, 1990; Hill, 1991). The same is likely to hold true for the injured athlete who may feel there is too much risk involved in seeking coach support.

Step 3: Recognition of the need for support (coach)

Fortunately, it is not always necessary to ask for help in order to receive it. Research shows that individuals who are empathetic and socially aware are able to take the perspective of another and thus recognize the need for social support (Sheldon & Johnson, 1993). Because of their understanding of the importance of sport in the athlete's life, coaches are in a good position to appreciate the distressing nature of injury.

Figure 6.

Coach's role in athlete recovery.

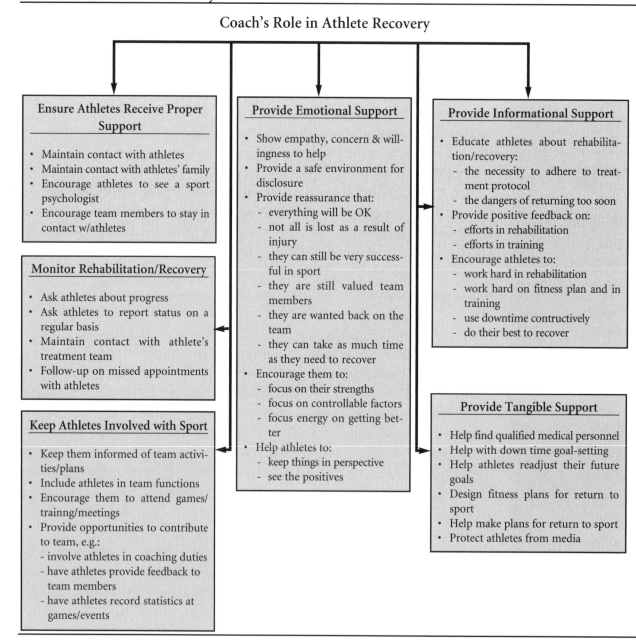

Moreover, if the coaches have had personal experience with injury (which is often the case), they are in an even better position to understand the upheaval and challenges engendered by injury.

Coaches who had had prior experience with injury explained that their understanding of the "psychological side" of injury was garnered from these experiences and not from any formal training they had received. These coaches had a good understanding of the stresses associated with injury and the need for social support. They also recognized that the support they provided played an important role in how athletes cope with injury. It was understood that coach support could contribute to stress relief, improved self-worth, increased self-confidence, and reduced isolation. It was also acknowledged that coach support could help foster adaptive coping behaviors, such as remaining positive about recovery and one's future in sport, focusing efforts on controllable aspects of recovery, and persevering in the face of rehabilitation.

As for the coach's understanding of the type of support needed, there seemed to be a good fit between what athletes need and what coaches think they need. The coaches felt their role was to

(a) ensure the athletes received adequate social support,

(b) monitor rehabilitation,

(c) keep injured athletes involved in sport,

(d) provide emotional support,

(e) provide informational support, and

(f) provide tangible support.

Examples coaches gave on how to fulfill this role are listed in Figure 6. Regarding the extent of involvement, this varied according to whether the coaches saw themselves as having a parental role versus a managerial role. Greater involvement occurred in the former case. In general, the coaches of younger athletes tended to see themselves in the parental role, while professional sport coaches saw themselves in the managerial role.

Although it may not be necessary to ask for help in order to get it, by not asking for what is needed, the right type (or, for that matter, any type) of support may not be forthcoming. If coaches draw mainly on their own injury experiences when deciding what type of support to offer, their efforts may be guided by what they personally needed and not necessarily what the injured athlete needs. Thus the support provided may not match the athletes' needs. The potential for a mismatch is likely to be reduced if the coach shares a good relationship with the athlete. As Pierce and colleagues (1991) pointed out, a healthy relationship paves the way to more accurate perceptions of support need.

Step 4: Provision of coach support

Just as there are costs and benefits to asking for support, there also are costs and benefits to providing support. Costs for helping can include experiencing extra demands on one's time, saying or doing the wrong thing, feeling discomfort with talking about feelings, becoming too involved in athletes' personal lives, and taking focus away from healthy athletes. On the other hand, the benefits for helping are being informed, being able to plan around the injury, and fostering a good relationship with the athlete.

Generally, the likelihood of extending help decreases as the costs for helping increase (Dovidio, Piliavin, Gaertner, Schroeder, & Clark, 1991). Dovidio and colleagues explained that to minimize their guilt for not helping in high-cost situations, people might resort to diffusing responsibility for helping or denigrating the person in need. In the case of the injured athlete, a coach could reason that it's not his job to babysit injured athletes or that the athlete got injured because she was careless and did not follow instructions.

Pearlin and McCall (1990) added that decisions to provide social support are also based on legitimacy judgments. They explained that support is likely to be withheld if the provider believes that

(a) the problem does not merit distress,

(b) the degree of distress shown is exaggerated, or

(c) the support provided in the past has not been used effectively.

The relational history between the provider and the recipient serves as the backdrop for making such decisions.

Legitimacy judgments are also based on implicit theories people hold about coping and the time course of adjustment following stressful life events (Coyne, Wortman, & Lehman, 1988). Social support is more likely to be extended to those who project they are actively problem solving and not overly depressed as opposed to those who use avoidant forms of coping or who become depressed (Silver, Wortman, & Crofton, 1990). Silver and colleagues noted that signs of distress might be tolerated in the early period following the event, but not for very long. Providers can become frustrated and upset when they do not see noticeable changes in a person's situation and may respond by withdrawing their support or avoiding the person in need.

Even though coaches may feel the need is legitimate, they also have to feel comfortable offering support. Knowing what to do and feeling capable of doing it do not necessarily go hand in hand. As Coyne et al. (1988) noted, people are not likely to involve themselves in situations that surpass their competencies. Even when a person feels capable, the gap between knowledge and skills can be substantial. Lehman and Hemphill (1990) claimed that although people often know in theory what support to provide, they are, for the most part, ineffective in translating this knowledge into action.

Step 5: Appraisal of support provided

In the last stage of the coach support process, the athlete makes a judgment about whether the provided support meets expected needs. The closer the perceived match, the greater the athlete's satisfaction with the coach support provided (Cutrona & Russell, 1990; Sarason et al., 1994). Satisfaction with support is important because it is believed to be the key determinant of the effectiveness of social support (Heller & Swindle, 1983; House, 1981). The perception of being supported creates a positive mental state that contributes to stress relief. The perception that support is lacking, on the other hand, creates an unpleasant mental state that further adds to one's psychological strain (House, 1981). Coach support, therefore, is most useful to injured athletes when the athletes believe it matches their needs. In line with this proposition, Bianco and colleagues (1999) reported that injured elite skiers who expected more coach support than was received reported low levels of satisfaction with coach support. Conversely, support attempts that met or exceeded skiers' expectations contributed to high levels of satisfaction with social support within the relationship concerned.

It's important to note that what matters is perceived support and not necessarily the actual support extended (Dunkel-Schetter & Bennett, 1990). People are affected by how they interpret their world (be it accurate or inaccurate) and not necessarily by how their world is (Heller & Swindle, 1983). What this implies is that even though a person may engage in behaviors that on the surface appear to be supportive, the actual supportiveness of those behaviors rests with how they are judged by the support recipient. Thus, a coach may do and say all the right things but if the athlete doesn't see it this way, the efforts will have been for naught.

A reasonable question to ask is why there would be a discrepancy in perceptions. One possible explanation has to do with relationship quality. Research indicates that the tone of a relationship greatly influences how support behaviors are interpreted (Pierce, 1994; Pierce et al., 1991). Support emanating from relationships marked by high levels of conflict, for example, can be viewed negatively by the recipient. Lucy, a downhill skier, explained her mistrust of her coach's interest in her rehabilitation: "He never cared about me when I was skiing—all of a sudden he was calling me to find out how I was doing? What did he want? To make sure I wasn't coming back?" As Hobfoll and Vaux (1993) noted, problems in a relationship are magnified under conditions of stress.

Barnes and Duck (1994) added that based on their daily interactions with one another, people come to develop expectations about each other's willingness and ability to provide social support. When a crisis arises, these expectations are set in motion, and the provider's actions are evaluated within the context of these expectations and against the backdrop of everyday interactions. Providers must thus be aware of these expectations if the support they provide is to be favorably evaluated. Hobfoll and Vaux (1993) explained that this is a difficult task because people tend to have unrealistic ideals about how others should react to their plight, particularly in terms of offering emotional support.

Also at issue is how the support message is conveyed. Scott, Furhman, and Wyer (1991) explained that messages have both a descriptive and an affective component and that the perception of another's communication is determined by the combined effect of both these features. Messages are interpreted in terms of their literal meaning (descriptive component) and what they imply (affective component). The implied message is inferred on the basis of the relationship history. The recipient's perception of the message will often elicit positive or negative emotions. Thus, the affective rather than the descriptive component of the message is often more important for understanding the effects of interpersonal communication. In evaluating coach support, it is likely that injured athletes are more concerned with the meaning behind the message rather than the choice of words. This is encouraging because it affords coaches more latitude in the provision of social support.

In terms of the types of messages that are likely to be evaluated more positively, sophisticated messages are best (Burleson, 1994). Sophisticated messages explicitly

- acknowledge,

- elaborate, and
- legitimize the feelings and perspectives of distressed others.

Unsophisticated messages, on the other hand, include

- unwanted or untimely advice,
- discouragement of open expression of feelings,
- minimization of feelings,
- pressure to make a more rapid recovery, and
- the use of automatic or scripted support.

Pearlin and McCall (1990) found that these types of messages tend to exacerbate rather than relieve distress. Compared to less sophisticated messages, sophisticated messages contribute to higher satisfaction with support interactions because they project a greater degree of involvement and are more accepting of the person in need. As a result, people who use sophisticated messages are better liked and evaluated more positively than those who use less sophisticated communication strategies (Burleson, 1994).

A final factor to consider with regard to support appraisal is that people tend to prefer support that is offered spontaneously over support that is solicited. Cutrona and colleagues (1990) explained that people often hold the perception that genuine support is entirely spontaneous and unsolicited. For this reason, support that is provided spontaneously might foster a greater feeling of being cared for.

Summary

It is clear that sport injury can be a devastating experience for athletes, especially those heavily invested in sport and whose injury is severe. Furthermore, the multitude of stressors associated with injury can overwhelm an athlete's coping resources and lead to a range of adjustment difficulties, including treatment non-adherence. Not complying with rehabilitation protocols is problematic because it can jeopardize the success of recovery and further exacerbate the athlete's distress. Coach support is an important coping resource that can contribute to relieving athlete distress and improving motivation for rehabilitation. However, in order for coach supportive to be effective, it must meet the athlete's needs. This requires that, at the very least, coaches have a good understanding of the experience of injury. Additionally, coaches need to have a good relationship with their athletes in order to have a better sense of what their specific needs might be. Both these factors will work toward facilitating the coach support process. The presence of coach support during recovery is beneficial not only to the athletes but the coaches as well. In the long term, athlete satisfaction with coach support will have a positive impact on the coach-athlete relationship and may contribute to better performance success.

Recommendations

Coach support is a complex process that involves efforts on the part of both the coach and the athlete for it to be successful. Listed below are some practical recommendations regarding what coaches and athletes can do to facilitate the process.

Athletes

- Make an effort to establish a good relationship with your coach prior to injury.
- When injured, be sure to ask for help if you need it.
- When asking for help, be reasonable and be specific about what you want.
- Make efforts to stay in contact your coach.
- Use your contact with your coach wisely. Don't whine and complain; instead, show that show that you are being proactive.
- Let your coach know how you are using your downtime, e.g., send weekly or bi-weekly updates.
- If your coach invites you to attend practices/games, be sure to show up.
- At games/practices, have a positive attitude and offer to help however you can.
- Use your downtime to learn as much as you can from your coach.
- Be appreciative of your coach's efforts.
- Don't complain to other athletes about your coach.

Coaches

- Develop a good on-field relationship with your athletes.
- Create an atmosphere that fosters open communication and disclosure.
- Let athletes know what the injury policy is and your position on the matter.
- Let athletes know how you see your role in the injury and rehabilitation process.
- Let athletes know what resources are available to them when they get injured, e.g., sport psychologist.
- Develop a database of medical professionals injured athletes can consult.
- Help guide athletes in their medical care decisions.
- Establish contact and consult regularly with the treatment team.
- Establish early contact with the injured athlete.
- Maintain contact throughout rehabilitation and recovery, e.g., weekly phone call.
- Ask about things other than progress.
- Keep athlete involved in the sport.
- Pay attention to athletes and give them something meaningful to do when they attend practices/games.
- Help athletes work on skills not affected by injury.
- Help athletes with short- and long-term goal setting.
- Encourage athletes to take the time necessary to recover fully.
- Recognize that returning athletes may be physically ready but not psychologically ready.
- Allow returning athletes to work at their own pace.
- With returning athletes, emphasize effort over performance.

References

Albrecht, T. L., & Adelman, M. B. (1987). Communicating social support. Newbury Park, CA: Sage.

Barnes, M. K., & Duck, S. (1994). Everyday communicative contexts for social support. In B. R. Burleson, T. L. Albrecht, & I. G. Sarason (Eds.), *Communication of social support: Messages, interactions, relationships, and community* (pp. 175-194). Thousand Oaks, CA: Sage.

Beck, A. T., Rush, A. J., Shaw, B. P., & Emery, G. (1979). *Cognitive therapy of depression.* New York: Guilford Press.

Bianco, T. (2001). Social support and recovery from sport injury: Elite skiers share their experiences. *Research Quarterly for Exercise & Sport, 72,* 376-388.

Bianco, T. (2002). *Coach support in the context of sport injury.* Unpublished doctoral dissertation, The University of Western Australia, Nedlands, Western Australia.

Bianco, T., Malo, S., & Orlick, T. (1999). Sport injury and illness: Elite skiers describe their experiences. *Research Quarterly for Exercise and Sport, 70,* 1-13.

Brewer, B. W. (1993). Self-identity and specific vulnerability to depressed mood. *Journal of Personality, 61,* 343-364.

Brewer, B. W. (1998). Adherence to sport injury rehabilitation programs. *Journal of Applied Sport Psychology, 10,* 70-82.

Brewer, B. W., Linder, D. E., & Phelps, C. M. (1995). Situational correlates of emotional adjustment to athletic injury. *Clinical Journal of Sport Medicine, 5,* 241-245.

Burleson, B. R. (1994). Comforting messages: Significance, approaches and effects, In Brant R. Burleson, Terrance L. Albrecht and Irwin G. Sarason (Eds.), *Communication of social support: Messages, interactions, relationships, and community* (pp. 3-28). Thousand Oaks, CA: Sage.

Cohen, S., & McKay, G. (1984). Social support, stress, and the buffering hypothesis: A theoretical analysis. In A. Baum, S. E. Taylor, & J. E. Singer (Eds.), *Handbook of psychology and health; Social psychological aspects of health* (Vol. 4). Hillsdale, NJ: Lawrence Erlbaum.

Cohen, S., & Wills, T. A. (1985). Stress, social support and the buffering hypothesis. *Psychological Bulletin, 98,* 310-357.

Coyne, J. C., Wortman, C. B., & Lehman, D. R. (1988). The other side of support: Emotional overinvolvement and miscarried helping. In. B. H. Gottlieb (Ed.), *Marshaling social support* (pp. 305- 330). Newbury Park, CA: Sage.

Crossman, J. (1997, May). Psychological rehabilitation from sports injuries. *Sports Medicine, 23,* 332-339.

Cutrona, C. E., Cohen, B. B., & Ingram, S. (1990). Contextual determinants of the perceived supportiveness of helping behaviors. *Journal of Social and Personal Relationships, 7,* 553-562.

Cutrona, C. E., & Russell, D. W. (1990). Type of social support and specific stress: Toward a theory of optimal matching. In B. R. Sarason, I. G. Sarason, & G. R. Pierce (Eds.), *Social support: An interactional view* (pp. 319-336). New York: Wiley.

Danish, S. (1986). Psychological aspects in the care and treatment of athletic injuries. In P. F. Vinger & E. F. Hoerner (Eds.), *Sports injuries: The unthwarted epidemic* (2nd ed., pp. 345-353). Littleton, MA: PSG Publishing.

Dovidio, J. F., Piliavin, J. A., Gaertner, S. L., Schroeder, D. A., & Clark, R. D. (1991). The Arousal: Cost-Reward model and the process of intervention: A review of the evidence. *Review of Personality & Social Psychology,* 86-118.

Doyle, J., Gleeson, N. P., & Rees, D. (1998). Psychobiology and the athlete with anterior cruciate ligament (ACL) injury. *Sports Medicine, 26*(6), 379-393.

Dunkel-Schetter, C., & Bennett, T. L. (1990). Differentiating the cognitive and behavioral aspects of social support. In B. R. Sarason, I. G. Sarason, & G. R. Pierce (Eds.), *Social support: An interactional view* (pp. 267-296). New York: Wiley.

Eckenrode, J. & Wethington, E. (1990). The process and outcome of mobilizing social support. In S. Duck (Ed., with R. C. Silver), *Personal relationships and social support* (pp. 83-103). London: Sage.

Fisher, A. C. (1990). Adherence to sports injury rehabilitation programmes. *Sports Medicine, 9,* 151-158.

Ford, I. W., Eklund, R. C., & Gordon, S. (2000). An examination of psychosocial variables moderating the relationship between life stress and injury time-loss among athletes of a high standard. *Journal of Sports Sciences, 5,* 301-312.

Goldsmith, D., & Parks, M. (1990). Communication strategies for managing the risks of seeking social support. In S. Duck (Ed., with R. Silver), *Personal relationships and social support* (pp. 104-121). London: Sage.

Gould, D., & Udry, E. (1995). The psychology of knee injuries and injury rehabilitation. In L. Y. Griffin (Ed.), *Rehabilitation of the injured knee* (2nd ed., pp. 86-98). St. Louis, MS: Mosby.

Gould, D., Udry, E., Bridges, D., & Beck, L. (1997). Stress sources encountered when rehabilitating from season-ending ski injuries. *The Sport Psychologist, 11,* 381-403.

Grove, J. R., & Gordon, A. M. D. (1995). The psychological aspects of injury in sport. In J. Bloomfield, P. A. Fricker, & K. D. Fitch (Eds.), *Textbook of science and medicine in sport* (2nd ed., pp. 194-205). Melbourne, Victoria: Blackwell.

Gutkind, S. M. (2004). Using solution-focused brief counselling to provide injury support. *Sport Psychologist, 18,* 75-88.

Hardy, C. J., Burke, K. L., & Crace, R. K. (1999). Social support and injury: A framework for support-based interventions with injured athletes. In D. Pargman (Ed.), *Psychological bases of sport injuries* (2nd ed., pp. 175-198). Morgantown, WV: Fitness Information Technology.

Heil, J. (1993). *Psychology of sport injury.* Champaign, IL: Human Kinetics Publishers.

Heller, K., & Swindle, R.W. (1983). Social networks, perceived support, and coping with stress. In R. D. Felner, L. A. Jason, J. N., Moritsugu, & S. S. Farber (Eds.), *Preventive psychology.* New York: Pergamon Press.

Hill, C. A. (1991). Seeking emotional support: The influence of affiliative need and partner warmth. *Journal of Personality & Social Psychology, 60,* 112-121.

Hobfoll, S. E. (1988). *The ecology of stress.* Washington, DC: Hemisphere.

Hobfoll, S. E., & Vaux, A. (1993). Social support: Social resources and social context. In L. Goldberger, & S. Breznitz (Eds.), *Handbook of Stress* (2nd ed., pp. 685-705). New York: The Free Press.

House, J. S. (1981). *Work stress and social support.* Reading, MA: Addison-Wesley.

Johnston, L. H. & D. Carroll (2000). Coping, social support, and injury: Changes over time and the effects of level of sports involvement. *Journal of Sport Rehabilitation, 9,* 290-303.

Johnston, L. H. and D. Carroll (1998a). The provision of social support to injured athletes. *Journal of Sport Rehabilitation, 7,* 267-284.

Johnston, L. H. and D. Carroll (1998b). The context of emotional responses to athletic injury: A qualitative analysis. *Journal of Sport Rehabilitation, 7,* 206-220.

Lazarus, R. S., Folkman, S. (1984). *Stress, appraisal and coping.* New York: Springer.

Lazarus, R. S., Folkman, S. (1991). The concept of coping. In A. Monat, R. S. Lazarus (Eds.), *Stress and coping: An anthology* (3rd ed., pp. 189-206). New York: Columbia University Press.

Leddy, M., Lambert, M., & Ogles, B. (1994). Psychological consequences of athletic injury among high-level competitors. *Research Quarterly for Exercise and Sport, 65,* 347-354.

Lehman, D. R., & Hemphill, K. J. (1990). Recipients' perceptions of support attempts and attributions for support attempts that fail. *Journal of Social and Personal Relationships, 7,* 563-574.

McDonald, S. A., & Hardy, C. J. (1990). Affective response patterns of the injured athlete: an exploratory analysis. *The Sport Psychologist, 4,* 261-274.

Nixon, H. L. II. (1994). Coaches' views of risk, pain, and injury in sport, with special reference to gender differences. *Sociology of Sport Journal, 11,* 79-87.

Pearlin, L. I., & McCall, M. E. (1990). Occupational stress and marital support: A description of micro-processes. In J. Eckenrode, & S. Gore (Eds.), *Stress between work and family* (pp. 39-60). New York: Plenum.

Pearson, L. & Jones, G. (1992). Emotional effects of sports injuries: Implications for physiotherapists. *Physiotherapy, 78,* 762-770.

Petrie, T. A. (1993). The moderating effects of social support and playing status on the life stress injury relationship. *Journal of Applied Sport Psychology, 5,* 1-16.

Pierce, G. R. (1994). The quality of relationships inventory: Assessing the interpersonal context of social support. In Brant R. Burleson, Terrance L. Albrecht and Irwin G. Sarason (Eds.), *Communication of social support* (pp. 247-266). Thousand Oaks, CA: Sage.

Pierce, G. R., Sarason, I. G., & Sarason, B. R. (1991). General and relationship-based perceptions of social support: Are two constructs better than one? *Journal of Personality & Social Psychology, 61,* 1028-1039.

Quackenbush, N., & Crossman, J. (1994). Injured athletes: A study of emotional responses. *Journal of Sport Behavior, 17,* 178-187.

Rees, T., & Hardy, L. (2000). An investigation of the social support experiences of high-level sport performers. *The Sport Psychologist, 14,* 327-347.

Robbins, J. E., & Rosenfeld, L. B. (2000). Athletes' perceptions of social support provided by their head coach, assistant coach, athletic trainer, pre-injury and during rehabilitation. *Journal of Sport Behavior, 24,* 277-297.

Rook, K. S. (1992). Detrimental aspects of social relationships: Taking stock of an emerging literature. In H. O. F. Veiel & U. Baumann (Eds.), *The meaning and measurement of social support* (pp. 157-169). New York: Hemisphere Publishing.

Rotella, R. J., & Heyman, S. R. (1993). Stress, injury, and the psychological rehabilitation of athletes. In J. M. Williams (Ed.), *Applied sport psychology: Personal growth to peak performance* (2nd ed., pp. 343-364). Palo Alto, CA: Mayfield.

Sarason, I. G., Pierce, G. R., & Sarason, B. R. (1994). General and specific perceptions of social support. In W. R. Avison, & I. H. Gotlib (Eds.), *Stress and mental health: Contemporary issues and prospects for the future* (pp. 151-177). New York, Plenum Press.

Schwarzer, R., & Leppin, A. (1991). Social support and health: A theoretical and empirical overview. *Journal of Social and Personal Relationships, 8,* 99-127.

Scott, C. K., Fuhrman, R. W., & Wyer, R. S., Jr. (1991). Information processing in close relationships. In G. J. O. Fletcher & F. D. Fincham (Eds.), *Cognition in close relationships* (pp. 37-68). Hillsdale, NJ: Lawrence Erlbaum.

Sheldon, K. M., & Johnson, J. T. (1993). Forms of social awareness: Their frequency and correlates. *Personality & Social Psychology Bulletin, 19*, 320-330.

Shelley, G. A. (1999). Using qualitative case analysis in the study of athletic injury: A model for implementation. In D. Pargman (Ed.), *Psychological bases of sport injuries* (2nd ed., pp. 305-331). Morgantown, WV: Fitness Information Technology.

Silver, R. C., Wortman, C. B., & Crofton, C. (1990). The role of coping in support provision: The self-presentational dilemma of victims of life crises. In B. R. Sarason, I. G. Sarason, & G. R. Pierce (Eds.), *Social support: An interactional view* (pp. 397-426). New York: Wiley.

Smith, A. M. & Milliner, D. K. (1994). Injured athletes and the risk of suicide. *Journal of Athletic Training, 29*, 337-341.

Smith, A. M., Scott, S. G., O'Fallon, W. M., & Young, M. L. (1990). Emotional responses of athletes to injury. *Mayo Clinic Proceedings, 65*, 38-50.

Smith, A. M., Stuart, M.J., Wiese-Bjornstal, D. M., Milliner, D. K., O'Fallon, W. M., & Crowson, C. S. (1993). Competitive athletes: Preinjury and postinjury mood state and self-esteem. *Mayo Clinic Proceedings, 68*, 939-947.

Sparkes, A. C. (1998). Athletic identity: An Achilles' heel to the survival of self. *Qualitative Health Research, 8*, 644-664.

Steadman, J. R. (1993). A physician's approach to the psychology of injury. In J. Heil (Ed.), *Psychology of sport injury* (pp. 25-31). Champaign, IL: Human Kinetics Publishers.

Taylor, A. H., & May, S. (1996). Threat and coping appraisal as determinants of compliance to sports injury rehabilitation: An application of protection motivation theory. *Journal of Sports Sciences, 14*, 471-482.

Taylor, J., & Taylor, S. (1997). *Psychological approaches to sports injury rehabilitation.* Gaithersburg, MD: Aspen Publishers.

Turner, R. J., & Roszell, P. (1994). Psychosocial resources and the stress process. In W. R. Avison & Gotlib, I. H. (Eds.), *Stress and mental health: Contemporary issues and prospects for the future* (pp. 179-210). New York: Plenum Press.

Udry, E., Gould, D., Bridges, D., & Tuffey, S. (1997). People helping people? Examining the social ties of athletes coping with burnout and injury stress. *Journal of Sport & Exercise Psychology, 19*, 368-395.

Wiese-Bjornstal, D. M., & Smith, A. M. (1999). Counseling strategies for enhanced recovery of injured athletes within a team approach. In D. Pargman (Ed.), *Psychological bases of sport injuries* (2nd ed., pp. 125-155). Morgantown, WV: Fitness Information Technology.

Young, K., & White, P. (1995). Sport, physical danger, and injury: The experiences of elite women athletes. *Journal of Sport & Social Issues, 19*, 45-61.

Young, K., White, P., & McTeer, W. (1994). Body talk: Male athletes reflect on sport, injury, and pain. *Sociology of Sport Journal, 11*, 174-194.

Chapter Fifteen | Suicide in Sport: Athletes at Risk

Jane C. Henderson
John Abbott College

If you are reading this then I guess I did the job. It is not anyone's fault, it was my decision nobody else's. I have been thinking about suicide since grade 7 I just never had the courage to just go ahead and do it. I'm just too tired of living just to damn lazy, and I do not feel like going on. I know I will never make it to Notre Dame sure I might be good on my team but to make it I would have to be the best in Canada, and I just don't have the talent. World Cup skiing is just something that is totally out of reach. I have never been the best at anything to make it big in this day en age it just isn't being in the right place at the right time. I want all my friends and family to just keep going on with there normal life with out me.

(Suicide note as written by a 15 year-old, captain of the football team and Most Valuable Player, killed himself by gunshot, (Corbella, 1996.)

Suicide is a conscious act of self-induced annihilation best understood as a multi-dimensional malaise in a needful individual who defines an issue for which suicide is perceived as the best solution (Shneidman, 1985, p. 203).

Statistics have shown that adolescent suicide is escalating. In fact, according to the Center for Disease Control and Prevention (2004), the incidence of suicide among teenagers and young adults has nearly tripled in the last 40 years. Suicide is now the second leading cause of death and the third leading cause of death among young people aged 15 to 24 (Anderson & Smith, 2003). Canada has the dubious distinction of having one of the highest teenage suicide rates in the industrialized world (Health Canada, 1994). However, completed suicides only partially reveal the extent of this phenomenon; suicide attempts are much more prevalent. It is estimated that an average of 500,000 teenage suicide attempts are made in the United States every year, or one per minute (Anthony, 1988). Most experts agree that the actual number of suicides in this age group is from 5 to 20 times higher after taking into consideration the suicides that are labelled accidental, such as drug overdoses or single-car accidents. Suicide then, especially among teenagers, is a virtually unrecognized public health problem.

Surprisingly, suicide experts are finding that more and more victims tend to be high achievers in school and sport as well as seemingly well balanced individuals. According to Lubell, Swahn, Crosby & Kegler (2004), all too many adolescents experience very high levels of stress that lead to depression that is exacerbated by difficulty coping with family, school, and community issues. Feelings of isolation often overwhelm teens and lead them to consider suicide as the only way out. Additionally, Lubell et al (2004) found that few schools have suicide prevention screening and crisis intervention programs for teens.

Media reports of recent suicides among Olympic level athletes in Canada, United States, and Greece suggest that athletes as a group are being overlooked as potential victims. Sport psychologists and others who deal with organized sport have often viewed athletes as more psychologically sound than their typical non-athlete peers, and therefore do not expect them to commit suicide. In fact, research focusing upon college students' attributions about suicide showed that athletes who committed suicide were viewed as more competent and in less distress than non-athletes who committed suicide (Lewis & Shepard, 1992). These young athletes were not regarded as having typical adolescent stressors and therefore suicide has rarely been a topic of significant research in sport. According to Swift (2006), "the suspected suicide of James Dungy, the 18-year-old son of Indianapolis Colts coach Tony Dungy, shocked the nation. But it was hardly an isolated case" (p. 60).

The suicides of five football athletes, all players of a Maine high school team, has drawn attention once again to the fact that athletes are not considered to be normal teens with typical teen troubles. Athletes are not expected to commit suicide and Swift (2006), maintains that "athletes are less likely to consider or attempt suicide than non-athletes but they are far more likely to either kill themselves or be seriously injured if they do attempt it. In short, an emotionally troubled athlete is more dangerous to himself than an emotionally troubled non-athlete" (p. 60). With virtually no statistics kept on the incidence of suicide in sport, according to status as either current participant or injured, cut, or dropped out, there is a paucity of information available to sport scientists. Typically, those at risk for suicidal behavior are believed to be suffering from severe psychopathology. However, recent research has revealed that sociodemographic variables such as parental loss, divorce, and disappointment are potent suicide risk factors (Holinger, 1989). Other studies have emphasized the role that stressful life events play in provoking suicide in youth (Pfeffer, 1986). A case in point: Sarah Devens, a captain of three sports teams at Dartmouth and probably the best woman athlete the school ever had. The stress of high expectations and her own competitive spirit may have contributed to her death by suicide (Callahan & Steptoe, 1995). Even Olympic world class athletes are driven to take their lives; Paul Thomson, a member of Canada's 1988 and 1992 Olympic Sailing team, died when he jumped off a bridge. It is thought that Thomson was grappling with what he felt were poor results at the 1992 Olympics (Ireland, 1994). The tragic deaths of Katrina Price, an all-star college basketball player who committed suicide after unsuccessfully trying out for a professional team, and Eleni Ioannou, a member of the Greek Olympic judo team who committed suicide prior to the Athens' Olympics, indicate that athletes are not by any means immune from the effects of disappointment (BBC Sport World Edition, 2004). The recent death of Italian cycling star, Marco Pantani, is viewed by some experts as being a suicide. There is much speculation about Pantani's death; however, he had been at the center of a legal probe into doping and, according to his mother, he died because of the constant persecution over drug charges (The Star, 2004).

According to Joiner (2006), suicide is very different from other forms of death. He suggests a link between depression and fearlessness, a common attribute among athletes. This combination becomes dangerous where suicide is concerned. Joiner points out that groups of people who are exposed repeatedly to pain and suffering, as are athletes, have higher suicide rates than other groups. A high tolerance for fear and pain, acquired most likely as a consequence of frequent exposure to these stimuli, may enable athletes to be highly adventurous. This tolerance, when combined with depression, may result in tragic outcomes. Especially vulnerable, then, would be athletes who are injured, cut from teams, or suffer great emotional losses, (i.e., performance decrement or personal losses). Joiner advocates the prevention of suicide through the strengthening of perceptions of belonging, as well as of personal and meaningful contributions to society. Brian Marston, father of one of the Maine football players, seems to support Joiner's notion that athletes have a tolerance or perhaps an affinity for fear. He says his son had a "streak of daredevil" in him: "Maybe he wanted to bring himself right next to suicide to see how it felt when he put that gun to his head, and something startled him" (Swift, 2006, p. 61).

Results from many studies expound upon the stress-reducing properties of exercise. Nevertheless, the relationship between exercise intensity and mood alteration remains unclear (Berger & Owen, 1992). The relationship between exercise and mood is not always a positive one. Berger & Owen (1992) concluded that although there is a need to clarify the relationship between exercise and mood, enough data exist to suggest that those wishing positive psychological benefits should avoid intense or prolonged exercise. Athletes vying for improved performance, however, often commit to gruelling and lengthy training sessions that are likely to result in extreme fatigue and negative emotion. Along with other existing stressors, and interacting with certain personality traits, intense training may be detrimental to the psychological well-being of teenagers. For some athletes then, strenuous exercise may increase the risk of suicidal behavior. In a study of 5,000 college students classified according to whether or not they participated in physical activity, surprisingly, women who reported frequently engaging in vigorous physical activity on six or seven days a week had twice the risk of suicidal behavior as the inactive women in the study (Brown & Blanton, 2002). This association between physical activity and suicidal behavior in women was independent of distorted weight perception. The researchers suggest that collegiate women may be using exercise to cope with stress.

Psychopathology may not be the only reason teenagers in general, or athletes in particular, take their own lives. In light of the recent occurrence of suicide in sport, it appears crucial for sport psychologists to reexamine their perceptions and assumptions about the risk of suicide among athletes. One longitudinal study has determined that 69 major league baseball players have committed suicide. Most of these occurred during the off-season or after retirement (Coleman & Lester, 1989). Because sport represents a microcosm of society (Eitzen & Sage, 1982), and since suicide rates are increasing, especially among young adults, athletes will be at least as vulnerable to suicidal behavior as the general population. The rigors of an athletic lifestyle may even place athletes at greater risk for suicide under some circumstances but actually lessen the risk under others.

Why Are Athletes at Risk?

Many theories attempt to explain suicide; however, experts agree that suicide among the young has a number of distinguishing features. According to the Center for Disease Control and Prevention (Auchmutey, 1998), teenagers who try to kill themselves do not fit the stereotype that characterizes older people attempting to extinguish their pain—many are not depressed, but rather angry and overwhelmed by some sort of rejection. A number of factors may precipitate suicidal behavior in athletes. Among these are the following:

- age group (15–24 years) (Anderson & Smith, 2003)
- biochemical fluctuations due to diet and weight loss and intense training (Wurtman & Wurtman, 1986; Young, 1986)
- concussion (Bailes & Jordan, 2000)
- personal loss: relationships, injury, retirement, performance, cuts from sport teams (Coleman & Lester, 1989; Gore, Aseltine & Colton, 1992; Pfeffer, 1986; Smith & Millener, 1984)
- narcissistic and perfectionist personalities (Miller, 1990)
- coaching behaviors, sexual identity issues, and alcohol and drug use (Anthony, 1987a, 1987b)

Age and Developmental Considerations

Most high school, college, and professional athletes are part of a high-risk age group for suicide. Coincidentally, the prevalence of suicidal thoughts peaks among young people in the 15-to 24-year age group, which is twice the rate for other age groups (Emond et al., 1988). In the United States, suicide is the second leading cause of death for persons 15 to 24 years of age. More than 1 in every 1,000 children will attempt to commit suicide before reaching the age of 25 (Center for Disease Control, 1986). What makes this age group especially vulnerable is the tendency for "all-or-nothing" thinking. In the course of normal developmental process, adolescents do not think abstractly. Unlike adults, they have neither the experience nor the ability to see that every defeat does not result in permanent consequences. In a study of 13,257 Kansas State University students in the years 1989 to 2001, mental health issues were shown to be increasingly more prevalent, more complex, and of increasing severity (Putukian and Wilfert, 2004). During this period, the number of students seen for depression doubled and the number of students having suicidal ideation tripled. It is suggested that college-age students do not seem to have the skills to deal with ever increasing pressures of a complex world (Putukian & Wilfert, 2004) and that student athletes are certainly not immune to these pressures. Putukian and Wilfert (2004) further note

(a) that the assumption that student athletes might be better adjusted and at lower risk for mental health issues than the general population of college-age students is false, and

(b) that student athletes may be, in fact, at higher risk.

Furthermore, team dynamics restrict athletes from taking their problems outside the team, and professional mental health counseling often is not sought. Mental health problems facing athletes may be an embarrassment to athletic departments who would rather they not exist.

Adolescence is a period of rapid and profound physical and cognitive emotional changes or, as Petersen and Hamburg (1986) suggest, a "critical transition period." Most adolescents "successfully navigate through adolescence learning to use developing skills to solve problems" (Berman & Jobes, 1994, p. 55). However, a minority of adolescents experience great difficulty in achieving the challenging and difficult transition to adulthood. For some, suicide appears to be the only solution. Experts agree that suicidal individuals tend to view suicide as impermanent and deny its reality (Allen, 1987); rather, they view it as a continuation of pain-free life and fail to understand that suicide results in a permanent state—death. A study by Tousignant, Hamel, and Bastien (1988) of 2,327 secondary school students in the province of Québec, Canada, (average age 16.3) revealed that 6.7% of young people have already attempted suicide. In addition, three times as many girls as boys attempt suicide; however, more boys succeed, as they tend to choose more lethal means (Garfinkle, Froese, and Hood, 1982).

Concussion

Recent research points out that head injuries in sport are doubly dangerous for teens whose brains are at a critical developmental stage (Kontos, Collins, & Russo, 2004). Kontos et al. (2004) point out that concussions affecting nearly 300,000 athletes in the United States each year are responsible for causing biochemical disturbances in the brain. Larsen, Starkey, and Zaichkowsky (1999) have documented the many emotional symptoms due to concussion including

- depression,
- anxiety,
- anger, and
- confusion.

According to Bailes and Jordan (2000) in a study of 1,800 retired National Football League players, a highly significant association exists between concussion and clinical depression. Researchers have thus hypothesized that at least one high school star football player, Corey Bischof, died by suicide as a result of the biochemical and neurological problems associated with the effects of a concussion (Caruso, 2003).

Dietary Factors

Dietary practices and associated biochemical changes related to weight loss in athletes may be involved causally in psychological depression, which in turn may be a factor in suicide. Athletes trying to lose weight might be under considerable stress that may be associated with depressive episodes. Nutritional deficiency may also affect mood (Wurtman & Wurtman, 1986; Young, 1986). For instance, folate deficiency has been shown to cause a decrease in the level of the brain chemical serotonin (Botez, Botez & Maag, 1984), which in turn has been speculated to be linked with depression (Young, 1986).

A variety of violent impulsive behaviors have also been linked with lower than normal levels of serotonin. According to Waters (1994), The National Institute of Mental Health reports that based upon 22 autopsies of the brain and body fluids of suicide victims, there appears to be a connection between low levels of serotonin (a neurotransmitter) and suicide. The precursor of serotonin is L-tryptophan, normally produced by the body but dietarily contained in many carbohydrate foods. Animal studies have confirmed that altering dietary L-tryptophan can influence serotonin levels (Wurtman & Wurtman, 1984). Sufficient levels of brain serotonin are known to be important in the regulation of eating, mood, and impulse control (Garfinkle & Kaplan, 1985). It is conceivable that athletes restricting their diets in an attempt to make weight may be placing themselves at greater risk for depression and impulsive behavior. A negative relationship has been found between platelet 5HT (the precursor to serotonin) concentration and suicidal behavior (Muck-Seler, Jakouljevic & Pivac, 1996). 5HT is involved in the regulation of mood, where its action is inhibitory. It also tends to depress the central nervous system's activity in regulation of sleep, pain, arousal, dreaming, and impulse control. For some individuals with a genetic 5HT abnormality, sport may be a suicide mediator. Sport may be causally related in predisposed individuals by exposing them to intense training and dieting, thus resulting in low levels of 5HT. Some athletes may have genetically determined 5HT abnormality that may be exacerbated by diet and intense training. Research that examined women of normal weight who diet shows a significant relationship between dieting and depressed mood. Further study of the influence of high or low carbohydrate intake during weight loss on high-intensity physical performance in college wrestlers demonstrates that rapid weight loss is associated with low carbohydrate intake, which adversely affects the wrestlers' physiology and psychology. Their physical performance is impaired, and tension, depression, anger, fatigue, and confusion scores on the Profile of Mood States (POMS) are significantly elevated (Horswill, Craig, Hickner, Scott & Costill, 1990).

The fact that suicidal tendencies may have a strong neurochemical basis must be emphasized so that athletes should not feel shame when seeking professional assistance in dealing with them. None of the risk factors independently is likely to be the cause of suicide, but it is the manner in which they interact that determines who will and who will not commit suicide.

The following model delineates the relationship of a 5HT abnormality with associated behaviors and a predisposition to suicide.

Predisposition to Suicide:	Coping Mechanism:	Maladaptive Coping	Create 5HT Abnormality?	Athlete with 5HT Abnormality:	Increased Potential to Suicide
- Family History - Personality - Life Events - Concussion	- Narcissism - Intense Training - Compulsive Exercise - Eating Disorder			- Impulsivity - Aggression - Depression	

Although eating disorders have been linked with depression, a causal relationship has not been established. Herpertz and Remschmidt (1989) have shown that adolescent patients suffering from major depression disorder have significantly lower body weight than do those without a current episode. In addition, the researchers reported a highly significant negative correlation between body weight and depressive symptoms. Highly restrained eaters of normal body weight demonstrate impaired cognitive functioning which, Green, Rogers, Elliman, and Gatensy (1994) explain in terms of anxiety resulting from the stressful effects of imposing and maintaining dietary restraint. Recent suicides and attempted suicides of successful female athletes focus attention on the problem of diet and eating disorders in sport. Gymnastics, figure skating, running, wrestling, diving, and swimming are among the sports wherein weight problems and eating disorders appear to be developing at an alarming frequency (Rosen, McKeag, Hough & Curley, 1986).

A case in point concerns a nationally ranked distance runner who thought being thin would make her run faster. She attempted suicide by jumping into a river near her home. The runner survived, suffering paralysis, and wrote her experiences of disordered eating in a book entitled *Dark Marathon* (Wazeter & Lewis, 1989). Wazeter chronicles a life of extreme dieting and the associated irrational and obsessional thinking that followed. Although researchers are uncertain what comes first, the biochemical imbalance in the brain that causes athletes to lose weight or behavior leading to the weight loss, the argument is probably moot. There is a growing body of literature that has investigated eating disorders, especially among female athletes. Less is known about the relatively small number of males who develop eating discords and have been seen by doctors. However, the research of Garfinkle, Garner, and Goldbloom (1987) suggests that many of these males are competitive athletes. More research is required to clarify this issue, and the relationship between disordered eating and striving for enhanced performance deserves closer attention. A high proportion of competitive female athletes resort to dangerous weight control behavior to maintain an edge over their opponents and to satisfy expectations of coaches and judges (Black & Burckes-Miller, 1988). Even seemingly casual comments by coaches who are overly concerned with their athlete's weight may prompt young athletes to resort to dangerous weight control behaviors to deal with the perceived criticism (Rosen & Hough, 1988). While many coaches express concern about this issue, very few seem to be aware of the extent of the problem and how their actions might influence athletes' thinking and behavior (Jaffee, 1988).

A list of hypothesised risk factors for the development of eating disorders includes

- cultural,
- familial, and
- individual categories.

These factors are believed to interact and thereby result in dieting that enhances an individual's sense of self-control and consequent self-worth (Garfinkle & Garner, 1982). Among those who may be at high risk for developing eating disorders are "women who, by career choice, must be thin to achieve." This category includes athletes (Garfinkle, Garner, & Goldbloom, 1987, p. 625). Coaches should approach the matter of weight control in relation to sport performance with care and insight. A negative, critical approach by the coach can have a devastating effect on the athlete's self-esteem, general behavior, and sport performance, which may lead to a cycle of disordered eating, depressed mood, and impulsive behavior.

Personal Loss

Most people show only a temporary lowering of mood after a loss or disappointment. Familial interactions and other life stressors involving loss have been identified as important sources of risk for suicide in youths (Gore, Aseltine, & Colton, 1992).

Many difficulties are involved in collecting empirical data about suicide, including the deaths of its victims. "The people who are most important to understand are by definition unavailable to the suicide researcher" (Berman & Jobes, 1994, p. 68). Therefore, researchers rely upon retrospective study of suicide attempters or ideators, although these derived data may not be generalizable to suicide completers. However, stressful events have been found to be involved in suicidal behavior in young people, including

- divorce or separation in the family, disciplinary problems at home or at school (Shaffer, 1974);
- unsupportive and disinterested fathers, stress in early years resulting in parent-child difficulties (Tousignant, 1993);
- physical illness or injury (Tousignant, Hanigan & Bergeron, 1984); and
- various psychological disorders.

Events that have been shown to trigger suicide attempts in youth include the loss of something or someone that is important to the victim and resultant humiliation (Pfeffer, 1986). Particularly relevant is the loss of a supportive person, that is, the loss of someone with whom the subject has a steady relationship. The importance of loss of social support as a contributor to suicidal risk is therefore underscored. Depression is difficult to assess and thus diagnose in adolescents because they express it in a great variety of ways (Davidson & Choquet, 1981). Thus the perceived loss these young people experience is even more important.

Many suicide theories exist that emphasize different underpinning factors, but no single understanding of the nature of suicide prevails. Therefore no definite checklist of **risk factors** has emerged from the literature that will describe any one suicidal adolescent. One may "read between the lines" in order to identify common themes that may operate synergistically. Nonetheless, the following are frequently cited as being causally related to suicide attempts in youth (Berman & Jobes, 1994):

1. Negative personal history including early life events, narcissistic injury, inadequate or negative models for coping, and biochemical vulnerabilities.

2. Psychopathology: Severe psychopathology such as schizophrenia and paranoia would generally contraindicate participation in sport. Narcissism, compulsivity, aggression, and low frustration and disruptions tolerance are personality characteristics that could be related to suicide in sport.

3. Humiliation: anticipated or real, loss of self-esteem or punishment.

4. Rigidity.

5. Social isolation.

6. Hopelessness.

Again, none of the above risk factors is independently likely to be the cause of suicide; it is the manner in which they interact that determines who will and who will not commit suicide. These stressors, in and of themselves, do not pose a risk for most adolescents; however, those with weak stress management skills are vulnerable to suicide. Those who are coping with a social loss or a blow to their self-esteem seem to be especially vulnerable (Shaffer, 1974).

Athletes who have committed suicide have tended to be good students and well-known within their community of peers. Two groups of people who are most at risk for suicide clusters are overachievers and underachievers (Swift, 2006). There may be, of course, the problem of recording bias and publicizing only the most sensational stories; nevertheless, very talented athletes are taking their lives. Shaffer, Garland, Gould, Fisher, and Trautman (1988) note a subgroup of suicide completers who show evidence of anxiety, perfectionism, and distress at times of change and dislocation. Berman and Jobes (1994, p. 93) describe these individuals as the "high achieving star." Following are a few recent sport suicides and speculative suicides that have drawn public attention:

- Marco Pantani (2004). Cycling star, after being accused of doping. His mother regards his death as suicide due to humiliation (The Star, 2004).
- Eleni Ioannou (2004). Greek Judo Olympic athlete, during the Olympics, after an argument with her boyfriend (BBC Sport, 2004).
- Robert Howard (2004). Former U.S. Olympian, after failing third attempt at making the U.S. Olympic Track Team (NBC Sports, 2004).
- Corey Bischof. (2004) Star U.S. High School Quarterback, after sustaining a serious concussion while playing football (Caruso, 2003).
- Justin Strzelczyk (2004). Offensive lineman for the Pittsburgh Steelers, after being released in 2000, died in a single-car accident (Jenkins, 2004). There is speculation this accident may have been a suicide. Single-car accidents are viewed by experts as likely being suicides, especially among young males (Leadbeater, Blatt & Quinlan, 1995).

Accounts from coaches, teammates, and parents depict most of the young athlete suicide victims as "normal teenagers," although perfectionistic, and typically the "last one expected to commit suicide." The victims tended to live with one parent or step-parent and had a confrontational or aloof relationship with the other parent. Many indications point toward a perfectionist attitude: "[The suicide victim] was the big hockey star in lower grades, but at the regional school there were a lot of other hockey players. He was used to being the best and then he went to the middle; he wasn't used to that and he didn't think people liked him anymore" (Fine, Globe, & Mail, 1990). This statement is congruent with research showing that suicide is often preceded by an event or events viewed by the victim as humiliating or contributing to a loss of self-esteem. High-performance athletes are under immense amounts of stress, according to Mark Tewksbury, who described his circumstances after winning a gold medal in swimming at the Barcelona Olympics:

> Finally I stopped beating myself up for being depressed and realized I was human. There wasn't anything wrong with me; I just didn't have any sense of balance. In less than three months, everything in my life had changed. I went from being unknown to being a celebrity, a commodity and a role model; from swimming six hours a day to never swimming at all. Instead of being with a team most of the time, I was always alone. I travelled by myself; I worked out by myself; I spent 90 percent of my time away from home. I felt completely out of control and depressed because I was lost. I did not have a sense of who I was any more. (Tewksbury, 1993, p. 214)

Injury

Another common stressor in the lives of athletes is injury. Studies investigating athletes' emotional response to injury show that more seriously injured athletes experience the most depressed mood (Smith, Scott, & Wiese, 1990), and depressed mood associated with long-lasting injury was found to be causally related to attempted suicides (Smith & Millener, 1994). Smith and Millener (1994) identified factors common to suicidal athletes in their study:

(a) surgery,

(b) a 6-week to 1-year rehabilitation process,

(c) depleted athletic skill,

(d) lack of perceived athletic competence, and

(e) being replaced by another athlete in their sport positions.

Injury results in many life changes for an athlete. The psychological stress brought about by injury is well documented in the sport psychology literature. It is thought that the primary stressor is loss of affiliation, or the social support system, which is an important part of much athletic life.

> After stressful events people turn to those closest to them as a source of strength. It is those closest to us who carry our burdens when we are incapable, who offer a shoulder on which to cry, shelter from adversity, and solace from grief. Significant others share their resources to help those for whom they care through these most difficult periods of life. (Hobfall, & Stephens, 1990, p. 459)

An injury may bring to an abrupt end feelings of belonging, so important to all humans but particularly for athletes. For some, issues of self-validity and esteem routinely addressed on the playing field are difficult to deal with elsewhere. Many athletes are limited in personal coping resources to deal with such a change in social status. As many adolescent suicides occur impulsively (Shaffer et al., 1988), coping strategies for dealing with loss of affiliation and the associated changes brought about by injury should be taught to athletes.

Retirement

Retirement may also be a time of increased stress for athletes. A study of suicides in major league baseball reveals that the 69 players who committed suicide did so mostly after career termination (Coleman & Lester, 1989). Retirement, like injury, is often viewed as a loss of athletic identity and value. Social support mechanisms may break down and athletes may be insecure about their purpose in life. Hopelessness or powerlessness is well documented as an important precursor and indication of increased suicide risk (Berman & Jobes, 1994). In writing about football players' difficulties after retirement, Le Batard (2005) noted that although athletes are expected to be well prepared for life and balanced after a life in sport that does not always seem to be the case. Furthermore, Le Batard (2005) noted the following:

> [Many players] limped through retirement, depressed and drunk and lost as they staggered through the streets in search of the next party. There is nothing that replaces the gladiator rush of Sundays, not children, not religion, not anything. . . . [I]n a lot of cases, they were successful specifically because they weren't balanced before football. It takes a certain maniacal zeal to climb atop sports, to outwork all the other competition addicts, and that zeal can cripple the development of other parts of your personality. The more lopsided you are, the more your world revolves around nothing but that football, the more you ignore other parts of your personality, sculpting and sculpting and sculpting at that one thing until you've made it excellent. And then you reach adulthood with arrested development. (Le Batard, 2005, p. C3)

Being Cut or Dropped

In furthering the discussion of loss or disappointment as a potential precipitator of athletic suicide, reactions associated with being cut or dropped from a team also deserve attention. Such responses may be similar to those for injury, in both the element of humiliation and diminished self-esteem. As the majority of suicide victims are male, it is interesting to note that they are much more likely than females to have experienced a specific trauma or loss of status directly before suicide. Relationship breakups are likely to be involved (Thompson, 1987). Teams are similar to families in structure and social function. "Sometimes emotionally disturbed and alienated youngsters seek a sense of belonging in new families" (Berman & Jobes, 1994, p. 94).

Loss of this new "family or relationship" could be a heartbreaking occurrence for some youngsters, especially those whose home life is lacking in nurturing qualities.

Injury, retirement, and being cut may result in loss of attachment to the team, to teammates, to social prestige, to social relationships. Many researchers (Berman & Jobes, 1994; Ramsay, Tanney, Tierney & Lang, 1994) have documented **attachment loss** as an important precipitator of suicide that cannot be underestimated. Studies of suicide notes verify self-harm behavior can result from problems with attachments (Ramsay et al., 1994). Thus, attachment loss may be a very important issue when considering the vulnerability of athletes to suicide.

Again, the multidimensional aspect of suicide causality, particularly among athletes, must be emphasized. No single factor fully clarifies this phenomenon.

Narcissism

As previously indicated, affiliation and attachment to a team provide many athletes with strengths and security that may enhance their invulnerability to suicidal behaviour. Garmezy (1985), Rubenstein, Heeran, Housman, Rubin, & Stechler (1989), have identified stress-resistant children as those who perceive their families to be cohesive and adaptable and who belong, as valued members, to a peer group. These children are seen as having fewer suicidal tendencies. Affiliation, then, serves as a protector, but what happens when the attachments to the peer group break down, as in the case of injury, retirement, cuts, or performance decrement? What occurs depends on the psychological resources of the athlete. High-achieving athletes are by necessity narcissistic and egocentric and thereby motivated to spend many hours and years in gruelling training. Narcissism is defined as an unconscious lack of self-esteem, where the locus of self-control is external and the need for attention is never satiated. A certain amount of narcissism is healthy and necessary. Unhealthy narcissism develops in a child, for instance, when parents are unable to separate themselves from the child and thus live vicariously through the child's achievements. Through the child's performance (sport) the parent strives to satisfy his or her needs and thus the child is unable to develop a healthy sense of self. Miller (1990), a psychotherapist writing about narcissism and the gifted child, speaks of these children who have been praised and admired for their talents and achievements and who have been a source of parental pride. She notes that instead of having a strong and stable self-assurance, the opposite is the case.

> In everything they undertake, they do well and often excellently, they are admired and envied; they are successful whenever they care to be—but all to no avail. Behind all this lurks depression, the feeling of emptiness and self-alienation and a sense that their life has no meaning. Additionally, as soon as "the drug of grandiosity" fails, as soon as they are not on top, not definitely the superstar or whenever they suddenly get the feeling they failed to live up to some ideal image and measure they feel they must adhere to, they are plagued by deep feelings of guilt and shame. (Miller, 1991, p. 6)

There is much dispute as to the cause of these narcissistic disturbances in highly gifted people (Kohut, 1971; Mahler, 1968). However, it appears that as young children, their sense of self was poorly or inadequately developed apart from their need for achievement and admiration.

Young people with low self-esteem may be attracted to sport because it provides an opportunity for attention and satisfies their narcissistic needs. According to Dielens (1984), participation in physical activity is linked to narcissistic tendencies because of the overemphasis on self. Sport provides a forum for displaying the great self, to be seen and to be admired. But as athletic ability improves, deep self-doubt may not be alleviated for some. These athletes increase their training in an effort to cope with the feelings of "not being good enough." Sometimes such training becomes overtraining and is counter-productive to performance. Injury may be the result. In addition, eating disorders may be prompted by feelings of low self-esteem. A cycle of food deprivation, dieting, and ensuing performance decreases due to overtraining and lack of proper nutrition results in a depressed mood. If the athlete suffers an injury to self-esteem, perhaps through an ostensibly innocent remark about performance given by the coach and negatively perceived by the athlete, a sense of "being no good" may be triggered. Tragically, some self-destructive act could be the result.

Role of the Coach

Few would question that coaches have a very important impact on the behavior of their athletes. Coaches, therefore, must then be willing to ask themselves serious and self-reflective questions about their own behavior, tactics, and communication skills. Most will acknowledge that youth sport has become more and more competitive in recent years. Ideally, sport participation should prepare children for the team play that will some day be a part of their professional and personal lives. Unfortunately, this is not always the case. Anthony (1988a) suggested that some suicides occur as a direct result of a devastating experience within the competitive realm. A tragic example is the case of the small-town football coach who, on the day of cuts, walked into the locker room to find that one of the rejected players had hanged himself (Anthony, 1988). The competitive environment should be an emotionally healthy one that promotes the values that young people need to succeed in life. As one coach commented, "I think the ideal of wholesale rejection of aspiring competitors through cuts is an unhealthy practice. If creative minds got together, we could come up with another way of handling cuts that would leave no one feeling totally worthless" (Anthony, 1988a, p. 5). This is just one issue that needs to be addressed by all who are in positions of youth coaching. Anthony (1988 b) also suggested that coaches must be willing to assess themselves on certain coaching practices. The essential point is that coaches must be fair, constructive, and sensitive in criticizing the performances of their athletes and, in doing so, help preserve their self-worth. Moreover, coaches must be open and non-judgmental and demonstrate moral and personal commitment to excellence rather than only to a winning record.

Coaches are essentially role models. If team leaders do not promote caring and concern among those whose lives are in their trust, their athletes will not develop as profoundly as possible. Thus, sport, rather than being a positive experience, becomes a deleterious and potentially harmful one.

Many believe the drive for excellence is fueled essentially by narcissism (Miller, 1990). Athletes who need and desire admiration and respect may be traumatized by the unproductive criticism of their coaches. Often coaches do not understand the emotional fragility of the athletes in their charge. Very few coaches know much about the lives of their athletes outside of sport. Does the athlete live with both parents? Is the parental relationship a healthy one? What coping mechanisms has the athlete developed to deal with disappointment? How well does the athlete deal with rejection? How will he or she cope if cut or injured? How important is sport in determining his or her identity? These are essential issues that require the coach's understanding in order that he or she may enhance the relationship with the athlete. Athletes have more than an athletic identity, and sadly, this fact is sometimes overlooked by their coaches.

The majority of teenagers who kill themselves provide an array of clues about their imminent suicidal behavior to those in a position to notice. According to Brent, Perper, and Allman (1987), 85% of adolescent completers in their study had made noticeable suicidal threats in the week prior to their deaths. Tragically, such threats are not usually taken seriously or are totally missed by those in a position to respond. Prevention of an adolescent suicide often fundamentally depends on the awareness and sensitivity of key people in the young person's life who seriously respond to obvious or veiled suicidal cues and make referrals to those who can help (Berman & Jobes, 1994).

Often coaches know so little about the "other" lives of their athletes that they are not cognizant of any of these signs. Talking about feelings and emotions has not been an integral part of the athletic milieu. In fact, athletes sometimes fear that their coaches will discover that they have confided in a sport psychologist, because it might show weakness. Parker and Price (1996), in a study of sport psychology issues in college athletics, stated that "athletes do not want their coaches to know they are engaging in mental skills training. Confidentiality is paramount." Additionally, Parker and Price pointed out that many coaches who have problems communicating effectively with their athletes tend toward an autocratic leadership style and feel that the athlete, not the coach, is the problem when the athlete has performance decrements. It follows, then, that coaches can miss clues indicating that their athletes may be having serious difficulties.

Teammates may also miss important signs and symptoms. An attitude that feelings are not to be discussed may prevail among team members, and thus an athlete exhibiting perceived signs of weakness is not taken seriously. Consequently, tell-tale signals are often dismissed by teammates and coaches. Only after suicide and death have occurred are those who have been close to the athlete able to perceive the cries for help that had been given. Even then, these signs are too often dismissed as having been irrelevant.

Prevention of Suicide in Athletes: Understanding Vital Signs

An understanding of why talented athletes may take their own lives ultimately leads to a discussion of what one can do to prevent these untimely deaths. Sport can be a positive influence in the lives of young people, in which they are taught life skills that are difficult to learn in other environments. However, for some, sport can have a negative harmful effect. Children whose whole identity is reflected through sport performance may be at risk for an ego-shattering experience through sport. The lessons these children learn about themselves through sport may be self-destructive and reinforce low self-esteem.

As has been discussed previously, those involved in the development of sport, especially coaches and teammates, must be more aware of the fragile balance of an athlete's life. Too much importance placed upon performance at an early age may lead to an imbalance in the athlete's perception of the role of sport performance in determining identity. Coaches must be alert to the signs that an athlete is struggling with serious self-esteem issues, and show empathy and sensitivity when relating to the athlete, especially when critiquing sport performance.

Additionally, coaches, parents and team officials must be aware of the indicators of suicidal ideation or impending suicide. These include verbal, behavioral, and situational factors. Recognition of an impending suicide may not surface on the competitive field, but may be hinted at in locker room or inter-team talk. It is not true that athletes who talk about suicide will not do it; if anything, the reverse is true.

Verbal behaviors may include, but are not limited to the following:

- blatant statements or jokes about suicide or death
- preoccupation with dying or death

The behavioral indicators of suicidal thought are very broad and diverse and include any noticeable change in behavior from the normal for that person. Of note might be the following:

- changes in eating, sleeping and grooming habits
- changes in energy level
- changes in school and/or sport practice habits
- sudden personality changes
- self-destructive behavior
- difficulty in concentration

Situational factors in the lives of athletes that might be related to suicidal behavior have been discussed earlier in this text. They include the following:

- broken home
- perfectionist attitude
- recent significant loss—in performance, of a family member, break-up of a significant relationship, injury, termination from sport
- alcoholism in family; other problems at home
- suicide history in family or previous suicide attempt
- striving for weight loss to enhance performance
- psychological or emotional problems
- recent concussion

Suicide may be prevented by parents, coaches, teammates, sport psychologists, athletic trainers and physical therapists when they are aware of the danger signals and prepared to respond to them. Rosenberg, Eddy, Wolpert, and Broumas (1989) estimated that training of gatekeepers in the signs and symptoms of suicidal ideation could potentially reduce youth suicide by approximately 13%. Such professionals may be able to refer vulnerable athletes to well-trained experts. Many opportunities to divert suicide are missed because those in a position to notice cries for help have missed important cues. Experts believe that those who commit suicide have not decided to take their own lives until they actually do it. Suicidal individuals seek those whom they trust and feel connected to in some way, such as friends, family members, or coaches (Ramsay, Tanner, Tierney, & Lang, 1994). One of the most important factors in preventing suicide is the presence of a supportive resource. Many suicidal episodes are short-lived, and a supportive person's talking and listening may draw the suicidal individual away from self-destructive thoughts and at the same time provide the necessary hiatus to mobilize professional assistance, if required. School counselors or other community resources could be asked to provide this training to all sport personnel, including athletes. Often coaches do not want to discuss suicide, or human failings in general, because they are apprehensive about directing their athletes' thoughts in a negative manner. However, experts agree that talking about suicide does not create or increase the risk (Ramsay et al., 1994). Open discussion and genuine concern about suicidal thoughts can be a source of relief and often are among the key elements in its prevention. In fact, the avoidance of these subjects can be a contributing factor in suicide, leaving a person at risk to feel more isolated, helpless, and hopeless (Ramsay et al, 1994). The sporting environment should be a safe place where participants feel at ease to discuss and cope with emotional needs. Sadly, it is often not the case.

A questionnaire attached to the athlete's medical information could be used to explore an athlete's coping resources. Some sample questions might include the following:

1. If I were cut from the team, I would
2. If the coach berated me, I would
3. Five people I could talk to if I needed to:
4. After a loss I generally feel
5. After my playing career is over, I am going to
6. If I should be seriously injured, I would
7. My concerns about my weight are
8. After my concussion, I felt

The coaching staff should be alert to athletes who are not able to name people to whom they could talk to in an emergency. Additionally, by prompting athletes to think about how they might cope in various situations, the groundwork is being laid for athletes to be more prepared should these scenarios actually arise. Stress-coping resources are learned responses that must be taught to athletes. Attention to those athletes who have had concussions, either recently or sometime in the past, is vitally important. As already noted, a concussion can precipitate an extreme emotional reaction in some people. Additionally, it is important to take into consideration those athletes in the process of losing weight. The associated biochemical change could serve as a precursor to an emotional and physical upheaval.

The key to success in preventing suicide is early intervention. Every suicide threat must be taken seriously. Adults often tend to minimize the importance and intensity of adolescent feelings and respond to a young person's crisis without an appreciation of his or her feelings (Ramsay et al., 1994). The threat of suicidal behavior is usually an act of desperation, a cry for help rather than a manipulation. Any statement or action about suicide must be taken as a serious invitation to respond. It is a normal response to feel anger or frustration in dealing with such a situation; however, the underlying reason for these feelings is often one of inadequacy. Teammates, coaches, and trainers feel they do not have the training to effectively deal with a suicidal person. The feeling may be justifiable, but it should not deter one from providing empathy or referring the person to an available, competent expert who is able to offer help. On high school, college, and university campuses, as well as in non-school settings, athletic administrators and coaches must be in tune with athletes' mental as well as physical health. Athletes should be screened accordingly. A referral system to accommodate the special needs of a student athlete must deal with the athlete's resistance to seeking help and their feelings of inadequacy in having to seek mental health assistance. Efforts should be made to remove all too prevalent stigmas about seeking help for mental/emotional problems that prevent athletes from availing themselves of accessible services.

Summary

There are a number of practical things that the coach, trainer or sport psychologist can do when help is needed. Ramsay et al. (1994) likened the initial intervention of non-specialist suicidal help to a "lifeguard," that is, an intermediary between a suicidal person and professional care. Every situation is different, but it is important for the helper to know that providing any demonstration of support for the suicidal person could potentially decrease the suicidal feelings.

Involving oneself with young people in sport demands a responsibility beyond the norm because these individuals have not yet fully fashioned their feelings, their ability to express themselves, and in sum, their lives. The vulnerability of their youth makes it incumbent upon responsible adults to be trained to listen to the "music behind the words." By doing so, they will not only assist their young athletes in attaining prowess but also greatly enhance the total of their lives and preclude one of the great tragedies in the human experience, the loss of human potential, the death of a child.

References

Allen, B. (1987). Youth suicide. *Adolescence, 22,* 271-290.

Anderson, R., & Smith, B. (2003). Deaths: Leading causes for 2001. *National Vital Statistical Report, 52*(9), 1-86.

Anthony, M. (1988a). Teenage suicide: Coaches can play important role as counselors for athletes. *Interscholastic Athletic Administration, 14*(3), 20-23.

Anthony, M. (1988b). Teenage suicide: Spreading a network of caring over field of athletic competition. *Interscholastic Athletic Administration, 14*(2), 4-6.

Auchmutey, J. (1998, October 12). Gone too soon, growing problem of teen suicide haunts America. *Atlanta Journal Constitution,* p. C1.

Bailes, J., & Jordan, B. (2000, May). Concussion history and current neurological symptoms among retired professional football players. Paper presented at annual meeting of American Academy of Neurology, San Diego, CA.

BBC Sport. World Edition (2004, August 24). Tragic judo star dies. Retrieved November 19, 2004, from http://news.bbc,co.uk/sport2/hi/Olympics-2004/3544542.stm

Berger, B., & Owen, D. (1992). Preliminary analysis of a causal relationship between swimming and stress reduction: Intense exercise may negate the effects. *International Journal of Sport Psychology, 23,* 70-85.

Berman, A. K., & Jobes, D. A. (1994). *Adolescent suicide assessment and intervention.* Washington, DC: American Psychological Association.

Black, D., & Burckes-Miller, M. (1988). Male and female college athletes: Use of anorexia nervosa and bulimia nervosa weight loss methods. *Research Quarterly, 59*(3), 252-256.

Botez, M., Botez, T., & Maag, U. (1984). The Wechsler subtests in mild organic brain damage associated with folate deficiency. *Psychological Medicine, 14,* 431-437.

Brent, D., Pepper, J., & Allman, C. (1987). Alcohol, firearms and suicide among youth. *Journal of the American Medical Association, 257,* 3369-3372.

Brown, D., & Blanton, C. (2002, July). Physical activity, sports participation, and suicidal behavior among college students. *Medicine & Science in Sports and Exercise, 34*(7), 1087-1096.

Callahan, G., & Steptoe, S. (1995, July 24). An end too soon. *Sports Illustrated, 83,* 32-36.

Caruso, K. (2003). Concussions can lead to suicide. *Prevent Suicide Now*. Retrieved November 19, 2004, from www.preventsuicidenow/concussions-can-lead-to-suicide.html

Center for Disease Control and Prevention, National Center for Injury Prevention and Control (producer). (2004). Web-based Injury Statistics Query and Reporting System (WISQARS) [Online]. Retrieved June 21, 2004, from http://www.cdc.gov/ncipc/wisqars/default.htm

Coleman, L., & Lester, D. (1989, April). *Boys of summer, suicides of winter*. Paper presented at the annual meeting of the American Association of Suicidology, San Diego.

Corbella, L. (1996, March 16). Recalling a life too short. *The Calgary Sun*.

Davidson, F., & Choquet, M. (1981). *Le suicide de l'adolescent: étude épidémiologique* (Adolescent Suicide: Epidemiology Study). Paris: Les Éditions ESF

Dielens, S. (1984). Narcissisme et activités physiques à la mode: Profil psychologique des pratiquants d'aérobie, de jogging et de bodybuilding. (Narcissism and physical activities: Psychological profile of aerobics, jogging and bodybuilding participants). *Revue de l'Éducation physique, 241*, 21-24

Eitzen, D., & Sage, G. (1982). *Sociology of American sport*. Dubuque, IA: William C. Brown.

Emond, A., Guyon, L., Camirand, T., Shenard, L., Pineault, R., & Robitaille, Y. (1988). *Et la santé ça va? Rapport de l'enquête Santé Québec*. (How's your health? Inquiry report of Health Quebec). Québec: Les Publications du Québec.

Fine, S. (1990, April 2). Student gave few hints of plan to end his life, acquaintances say. *Globe and Mail*.

Garkinkel, B., Froese, A., & Hood, J. (1982). Suicide attempts in children and adolescents. *American Journal of Psychiatry, 138*, 35-40.

Garfinkel, P., & Garner, D. (1982). *Anorexia nervosa: A multidimensional perspective*. New York: Brunner/Mazel.

Garfinkel, P., Garner, D., & Goldbloom, D. (1987). Eating disorders: Implications for the 1990s. *Canadian Journal of Psychiatry, 32*, 624-630.

Garfinkel, P., & Kaplan, A. (1985). Starvation based perpetuating mechanisms in anorexia nervosa and bulimia. *International Journal of Eating Disorders, 4*, 651-655.

Garmezy, N. (1985). Stress-resistant children: The search for protective factors. In J.E. Stevenson (Ed.), *Recent research in developmental psychopathology, Journal of Child Psychology and Psychiatry Book*, (Suppl. 4), 213-233. Oxford: Permagon Press.

Gore, S., Aseltine, R., Colton, M. (1992). Social structure, life stress and depressive symptoms in a high-school aged population. *Journal of Health and Social Behaviour, 33*, 97-113

Green, M., Rogers, P., Elliman, N., & Gatenby, S. (1994). Impairment of cognitive performance associated with dieting and high levels of dietary restraint. *Physiological Behavior, 55*, 447-452.

Health Canada. (1994). *Suicide in Canada: Update of the report of the task force on suicide in Canada*. Ottawa, ON: Author.

Herpertz-Dahlmann, B., & Remschidmt, H. (1989). Anorexia nervosa and depression. On the relation of body weight and depressive symptoms. *Nervenartz, 60*(8), 490-495.

Hobfall, S. E., & Stephens, M. A. P. (1990). Social support during extreme stress: Consequences and intervention. In B. R. Sarason, I. G. Sarason, & G. R. Pierce (Eds.), *Social support: An interactional view* (pp. 454-481). New York: John Wiley and Sons.

Holinger, P. (1989). Epidemiologic issues in youth suicide. In Pfeffer, C., *Suicide among youth*. Washington, DC: American Psychiatric Press.

Horswill, C., Hickner, R., Scott, J., & Costill, D. (1990). Weight loss, dietary carbohydrate modifications and high intensity, physical performance. *Medicine and Science in Sports and Exercise, 22*(4), 470-476.

Ireland, J. (1994, May 30). When the spotlight fades, Olympic athletes fall victim to depression. *Calgary Herald*, p. A1, A2.

Jaffee, L. (1988). Eating disorders and coach-athlete relationships. *Melpomene Report, 7*(1), 12-13.

Jenkins, B. (2004, October 1) Update, *USA Today*, 21C.

Joiner, T. (2006). *Why people die by suicide*. Boston: Harvard.

Kohut, H. (1971). *The analysis of self*. New York: International Universities Press.

Kontos, A., Collins, M., & Russo, S. (2004). An introduction to sports concussion for the sport psychology consultant. *Journal of Applied Sport Psychology, 16*(3), 220-235.

Larson, J., Starkey, C., & Zaichokowski, L. (1996). Psychological aspects of athletic injuries as perceived by athletic trainers. *The Sport Psychologist, 10*, 37-47.

Leadbeater, B., Blatt, S. & Quinlan, D., (1995). Gender-linked vulnerabilities to depressive symptoms, stress, and problem behaviours in adolescents. *Journal of Research on Adolescence*. 5, 1-29.

Le Batard, D. (2005, February 9). Life after NFL tough to tackle. *Montreal Gazette*, p. C3.

Lewis, R., & Sheppard, G. (1992). Inferred characteristics of successful suicides as a function of gender and context. *Suicide and Life-threatening Behavior, 22*(2), 187-196.

Lubell, K., Swahn, M., Crosby, A., & Kegler, S. (2004) *Methods of suicide among persons aged 10-19 years — United States, 1992-2001*. Retrieved March 4, 2006, from http://www.cdc.gov./mmwr/PDF/wk\mm5322.pdf

Mahler, M. (1968). *On human symbiosis and the vicissitudes of individuation*. New York: International Universities Press.

Miller, A. (1990). *The drama of the gifted child*. New York: Basic Books.

Muck-Seler, D., Jakovljevic, M., & Pivac, N. (1996). Platelet 5-HT concentrations and suicidal behavior in recurrent major depression. *Journal of Affective Disorders, 39*, 73-80.

NBC Sports (2004, September 29). *Olympian haunted by failures, suicide note says*. Retrieved November 19, 2004, from www.msnbc.msn.com/id/6135796

Parker, K., & Price, F. (1996, October). *In the trenches, applied sport psychology issues at the NCAA division 1 level*. Paper presented at the annual meeting of the Association for the Advancement of Applied Sport Psychology, Williamsburg, VA.

Peterson, A., & Hamburg, B. (1986). Adolescence: A developmental approach to problems and pathology. *Behavior Therapy, 17*, 480-499.

Pfeffer, C. (1986). *The suicidal child*. New York: Guilford.

Putukian, M., & Wilfert, M. (2004) *Student athletes also face dangers from depression*. Retrieved March 1, 2006, from http://www.suicidereferencelibrary.com/test4~id~1374.php

Ramsay, R., Tanney, B., Tierney, R., & Lang, W. (1994). *Suicide intervention handbook*. Calgary, AB: Living Works Education.

Rosen, L., & Hough, D. (1988). Pathogenic weight control behaviors of female college gymnasts. *The Physician and Sportsmedicine, 16*(9), 140-143.

Rosen, L., McKeag, D., Hough, D., & Curley, V. (1986). Pathogenic weight control behavior in female athletes. *The Physician and Sportsmedicine, 14*(1), 79-86.

Rosenberg, M., Eddy, D., Wolpert, R., & Broumas, E., (1989). Developing strategies to prevent youth suicide. In Pfeffer, C., *Suicide among youth*, (pp. 203-225). Washington, DC: American Psychiatric Press.

Rubenstein, J. L., Heeren, T., Housman, D., Rubin, C., & Stechler, G. (1989). Suicidal behavior in "normal" adolescents: Risks and protective factors. *American Journal of Orthopsychiatry, 59*, 59-71.

Shaffer, D. (1974). Suicide in childhood and early adolescence. *Journal of Psychology Psychiatry, 15*, 275-291.

Shaffer, D., Garland, A., Gould, M., Fisher, P., & Trautman, P. (1988). Preventing teenage suicide: A critical review. *Journal of the American Academy of Child and Adolescent Psychiatry, 27*, 675-687.

Shneidman, E. S. (1985). *Definition of suicide*. New York: John Wiley & Sons.

Smith, A., & Millener, E. (1994). Injured athletes and the risk of suicide. *Journal of Athletic Training, 29*(4), 337-341.

Smith, A., Scott, S., & Wiese, D. (1990). The psychological effects of sports injuries: Coping. *Journal of Sportsmedicine, 9*, 352-369.

Suicide among children, adolescents, and young adults – United States. (1995). *Journal of School Health, 65*(7), 272-274.

Swift, E. (2006, Jan 9). What went wrong in Winthrop? *Sports Illustrated*, 60-65.

Tewksbury, M. (1993). *Visions of excellence*. Toronto: Penguin.

The Star (2004, February 18). Doping allegations lead to Pantani's death, cyclist's mother insists. Retrieved November 19, 2004, from www.thestar.co.za/index.php?/fSectionId=132&fArticleId=351706.

Thompson, T. (1987). Childhood and adolescent suicide in Manitoba: Demographic study. *Canadian Journal, 32*, 264-269.

Tousignant, M. (1993). La santé mentale dans l'enquête de la Défense Nationale. (National defense mental health inquiry.) *Rapport final de recherche*. Montréal, mai 1990.

Tousignant, M., Hamel, S, & Bastien, M.F. (1988). Structure familiale, relations parents-enfants et conduites suicidaires à l'école secondaire. (Family structures, parent-child relationships and suicidal conduct in high school.) *Santé mentale Québec, 13*, 79-93.

Tousignant, M., Hanigan, D., & Bergeron, L. (1984). *Le mal de vivre: Comportements et idéations suicidaires chez les cégepiens de Montréal*. (The Pain of Living : Behaviors and Suicidal Ideations in Montreal Cegep Students). *Santé mentale Québec, 9*, 122-123.

Tragedy in Texas. (1999, February 1). *Sports Illustrated*, 30.

Waters, H. (1994, April 18). Teenage suicide: One act not to follow. *Newsweek, 123*, 49.

Wazeter, M., & Lewis, G. (1989). *Dark marathon*. Grand Rapids: Zondervan Publishing.

Wurtman, R., & Wurtman, J. (1984). Nutrients; neurotransmitter synthesis and the control of food intake. In Stunkard, J. & Stellar, E., (Eds.), *Eating and its disorders* (pp. 77-86). New York: Raven Press.

Young, S. (1986). The clinical psychopharmacology of tryptophan. In Wurtman, R. & Wurtman J. (Eds.), *Nutrition and the brain: Vol. 7. Food constituents affecting normal and abnormal behaviours* (pp. 49-88). New York: Raven Press.

Section Five | Special Considerations and Case Studies

Section 5, the book's last, has five chapters. The first, (chapter 16), prepared by Louis M. Makarowski, is concerned with ethical and legal issues of which those working professionally with injured athletes should be cognizant.

The second chapter (17) by Wendy Sternberg, describes a significant sensory experience that typically accompanies sport injury—pain. Its neural bases are explained in detail to the extent that readers derive a helpful understanding of this phenomenon.

Frances A. Flint has written the next chapter (18) in this section, which emphasizes the need to match psychological oriented rehabilitative interventions with injury characteristics for optimal rehabilitative results (e.g., type of sport, re-injury or not, stage of athlete's rehabilitation, etc.)

Renee Newcomer Appaneal and Megan D. Granquist are the authors of the next chapter (19). Here, as well as in the book's very last chapter (20) by Barbara B. Meyer and Kyle T. Ebersole, detailed accounts of therapeutic interventions done with injured athletes are described in case study format.

Chapter Sixteen

Ethical and Legal Issues for Sports Professionals Counseling Injured Athletes

Lou M. Makarowski
Pensacola, Florida

The renowned basketball personality Magic Johnson tested positive for HIV before retiring from the Los Angeles Lakers of the National Basketball Association. The surprising disclosure undoubtedly prompted many counselors and psychologists to consider the following question: "What would I have done, or what should I have done, with such information were Mr. Johnson a client of mine?"

Answers to this question have important implications for the well-being and competitive achievement of Johnson's teammates, as well as the ethical stress level and liability exposure of professional helpers. This chapter examines some of the ethical and legal issues relevant to those who provide service to athletes who are injured, ill, or in some way psychologically or physically compromised. Some of those helpers, although well-intentioned, have only modest training or professional preparation for the difficult responsibilities they undertake. This chapter is designed to be of assistance to such readers

Introduction

Trainers and team physicians are in the forefront in sport health care, while others attend to the physical and mental deficits of athletes. Healthcare providers of all kinds should abide by professional, moral, ethical, and legal principles and directives (Board of Certification [BOC] Role Delineation Study Fifth Edition, 2004, p. 19)

Sport psychologists, athletic trainers, counselors, and physical therapists are expected to follow a code of ethical conduct. "The BOC defines and enforces ethical behavior on the part of the practicing AT by requiring compliance with the Standards of Professional Practice. Non-compliance with or violation of

BOC requirements can result in revocation of the credential." Athletic trainers are expected to adhere to the dictates of the National Athletic Trainers Association (NATA) Board of Professional Association (NATA, 1990).

An employee of an organization, however, may find that his or her job description conflicts with ethical professional requirements (Ungerleider & Golding, 1992; Voy, 1991), and sport counselors may be held legally accountable for the ways in which they discharge their responsibilities.

The American Medical Association now recognizes athletic trainers as allied health providers. Forty-three states license athletic trainers, at the A.T.C. level (NATA Fact sheet, 2006, Fact 5). The scope of the supporting legislation varies from state to state, but the trend toward licensure is very likely to continue. With increasing professional status comes increased vulnerability to lawsuits. Tortuous activity of all types will increase as trainers and counselors are held legally accountable for ever-increasing levels of knowledge.

The fact that licensed athletic trainers may now open free-standing clinics is an indication of their presumed skill, knowledge, and ability. Malpractice insurance for trainers has therefore become significantly more costly, because insurers project that monetary awards paid to plaintiffs who sue trainers for damages will continue to increase. As public knowledge of sports' inner workings grows, so will the creativity of lawyers who seek to protect athletes from exploitation and to protect the public from incompetent or unethical sport professionals (Voy, 1991).

Professional helpers may assume roles as trainers, assistant coaches, psychological counselors, or representatives of organizations that employ them. Ethical conflicts are a major source of stress and anxiety and are likely to be different for a psychologist than they are for a coach, university professor, health club employee, or professional boxing promoter.

Ethical stress occurs when a trainer's personal interpretation of right and wrong differs from that of the client, employer, or employing organization. Such dissonance may produce anxiety or worry that resides at a low level of awareness until trainers find themselves confronted with some ethical challenge or legal proceeding. Counselors, psychologists, and trainers deal with ethical stressors regularly and minimize their potential adverse reactions by developing a strong ethical philosophy as well as a system that guides their personal decision-making.

Derivation of Ethical Codes

Ethical imperatives define who and what we are, and value conflict among them may engender stress. Ethical conflict may provide inspiration and impetus for changing ethical and legal codes. The philosophical basis of codes originates with the principle of justice. Ethical conflict is a result of our perception of injustice.

Each of us is defined by the interaction of nature, learning, experience, and opportunity. Our individual behavioral responses in specific circumstances are determined by nature, learning, and volition.

Volition is the exercise of will, and it guides the choices we make. Will may be defined as the total conscious process involved in effecting a decision. Decisions may involve action or the absence of action. Will is influenced by conscious and subconscious energy, images, emotions, and thoughts. Concepts are composed of images and values. Values are priority assignments that greatly influence choices.

The choices we make are the external signs from which the nature of our character is defined and inferred by us and by others. Conscience is a reflection (approval or disapproval) or rational faculty that discerns the moral characteristic of actions (Butler, 1873). Consideration of right and wrong are the subject matter of morality. Morality represents ideal forms of right and proper conduct. Kant concluded that reason is not intended to produce happiness, but to produce good will. Good will is one that acts for the sake of duty (Solomon, 1982).

The science of ethics informs individuals what should be, in principle. Organizations also specify what should be in the ideal sense. Ethics is the science of moral values and duties or the study of ideal human character, actions, and ends.

Freedom of will is a fundamental, theological principle, with respect to the notion of blame. Someone who is forced to make decisions cannot be held responsible or blamed for the end result of a forced choice. Freedom to choose is a fundamental principle of morality as well. Freedom to choose is a right implied by the Constitution of the United States, but it by no means implies that choice is absent of consequences.

Rather, the freedom is one of choice. When people exercise free will and choose a course of action, they are then accountable for the rightness or wrongness of the choice. The concept of freedom is central to the discussion of ethics and legality as well. Obviously, the concept of free will is of paramount importance in considering the principle of justice.

Justice is one of the primary principles of civilization and democracy. The perception of justice is also a primary influence on motivation in sport and life. Sport professionals sometimes engage in questionable practices in an attempt to provide a just, or equal, playing environment for their athletes, team, or organization.

Virtually all of society's guidelines, rules, regulations, codes, and laws are intended to maintain that which is just, right, and fair. The reflective nature of ethical decision making helps bring objectivity to ones' personal definition of justice.

Value-Based Decision-Making Tools

Value-based decision-making includes ethics in a behavioral value system composed of attitudes and beliefs, as well as values. A behavioral value is something one likes to do. A behavioral attitude consists of physical, intellectual, emotional, social, and spiritual habits. A behavioral belief is simply a value plus an attitude that grows with time. All this leads to one's behavioral potential. The potential to behave, with opportunity, leads to actual behavior.

Behavior is the basis of a moral action that leads one to act morally and ethically, and it is vital that actions are accompanied by behavioral value systems. When this is not the case, unethical and immoral action transpires. We all have a value system and behave according to its dictates. Our system may be a hedonistic one, where the Pleasure Principle rules. One extreme of this principle is: "If it feels good or gives us advantage, regardless of the consequences, do it." Values emphasizing altruism and service exemplify the other extreme. Most of us fall somewhere between these two endpoints of the continuum. The most efficient value system leads to behavior that produces a healthy lifestyle. A healthy lifestyle incorporates physical, emotional, intellectual, social, and spiritual health. It is a lifestyle that usually results in high performance, minimal amounts of stress, and low levels of risk of injury.

In order to make decisions based on your value system, an accurate knowledge of yourself is necessary. To serve others ethically, a clear understanding of your personal value system is crucial. Knowledge of your personal value system will help in gaining

Figure 1.
Value Decision-Making Flow Chart

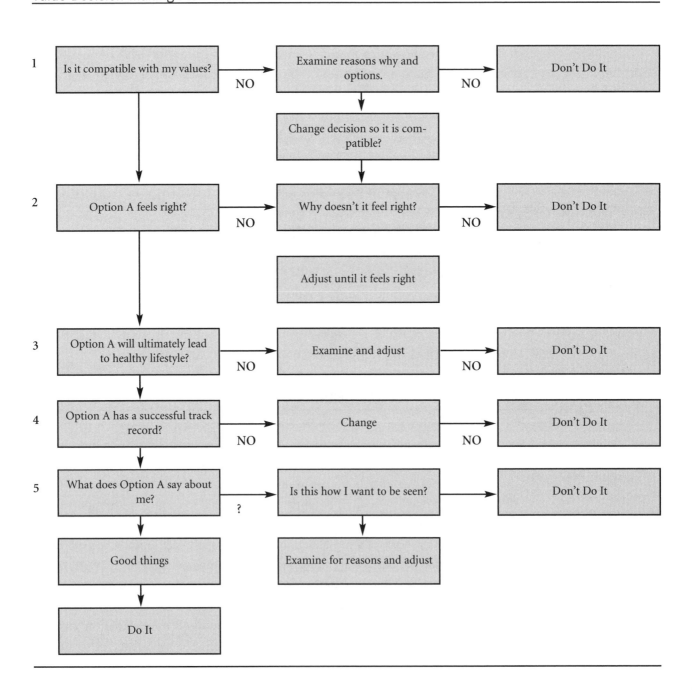

an understanding of yourself as well as others. You will also be in a better position to communicate value-laden information in a way that athletes and clients will accept.

Your personal value system can create ethical stressor if it is in conflict with the decisions you make. Your value system may also provide emotional blind spots that account for inordinately unrealistic and demanding behaviors from athletes.

Value Decision-Making Guidelines

Self-administered questions that may provide helpful insights to counselors, athletic trainers, sport psychologists, and physical therapists are:

1. Is my decision/action compatible with my goals, values, and expectations?
2. Does it feel right?
3. Where does the act ultimately lead?
4. What is the track record of others when making a similar decision? What is my track record when making a similar decision?
5. By doing this, what am I saying about myself?

Value decision making is a dynamic process. The flow chart in Figure 1 illustrates one method to assist in decision making.

In the struggle to evaluate the decision-making process, a matrix for examining decisions may also prove helpful. These guidelines and systems based on the work of Sid Simon (1974) and Louis Raths (1966) can be helpful in maintaining consistency and clarity in thinking when counseling athletes.

For example, if you are struggling with a decision of whether or not to work for a prominent coach who insists that steroids be a part of the training regimen, "steroids" should be listed on the first line of the matrix. If you are troubled by the method chosen to help junior athletes "make weight," list "weight loss" in the matrix. If sex is being exchanged for playing time, and you are struggling to decide just how badly you want to play, include "sexual barter" in the matrix.

Other areas of value concern complete the matrix.

Decision-Making Matrix

Decisions/Situations	1	2	3	4	5	6	7
Steroids	7	6	5	6	7	7	5
Weight Loss							
Sexual Barter							
Blood Doping							
Abusive Relationships							
Cheat or Not to Cheat							
Painkillers							

For each decision/situation included in the matrix above, select the number that best describes *you* in the decision process, and enter the number on the horizontal axis of the box. The answering scale is a continuum numbered 1 through 7, with 1 indicating a definite yes and 7 indicating a definite no. Other responses indicate varying degrees of agreement.

Answering Scale

1–4, decision is consistent with your values

5–7, decision is inconsistent with your values

1. Freely made the decision?
   Yes 1 - 2 - 3 - 4 - 5 - 6 – 7 No

2. Like the position taken?
   Yes 1 - 2 - 3 - 4 - 5 - 6 - 7 No

3. Looked at the pros & cons?
   Yes 1 - 2 - 3 - 4 - 5 - 6 - 7 No

4. Examined outcomes?
   Yes 1 - 2 - 3 - 4 - 5 - 6 - 7 No

5. In accordance with my values, attitudes, and beliefs?
   Yes 1 - 2 - 3 - 4 - 5 - 6 - 7 No

6. Stand up for my actions?
   Yes 1 - 2 - 3 - 4 - 5 - 6 - 7 No

7. Made a personal commitment?
   Yes 1 - 2 - 3 - 4 - 5 - 6 - 7 No

Interpretation

If the decision you are considering produces values that mostly lie between 1 and 4, your decision will likely promote a healthy lifestyle with low levels of stress and injury potential. If values mostly lie between 5and 7, as in the first one (Steroids), your decision likely will promote an unhealthy lifestyle, involve substantial stress levels, and increase the risk of injury.

Ethical/Legal Issues

Professional helpers who attempt to function as the "Morals Police" may unnecessarily limit their contribution to the athlete/patient and to the employing organization. When interacting with athletes, counselors and trainers must make every effort to work within the value system of the client. If for some reason they are unable to listen empathically and nonjudgmentally, they are ethically obligated to assist the athlete in locating a more impartial confidant. The professional helpers must not breech the client's right to confidential, competent treatment in the referral process or in the transition to a more appropriate counselor.

The penalty for a psychologist who violates the client's right to confidentiality could be extreme. The results of breaching such rights might include being found guilty of malpractice by the legal system with penalties that could include substantial monetary damages. Loss of license may result from conviction of violation of professional statutory proscriptions. For lesser ethical breaches, which do not involve civil or criminal misconduct, the penalties for psychologists or trainers might range from censure to expulsion from professional organizations.

Ethical decision making greatly reduces the likelihood of any form of criminal, civil, or malpractice violation. Codes for counselors routinely define ethicality as practicing within the limits of the law. Conduct that violates legal mandates will almost always be unethical. Personal value decision-making tools guide decision making that complies with legal codes as well as contributes to a healthy lifestyle.

A trainer or counselor who serves athletes in areas that provoke ethical concerns should consider referring them to a colleague who does not have such conflict. Risks of all sorts prevail in the sport environment. Athletes at all levels are often attracted to risk. They see it as a challenge. Mastery of risk is a thrill that makes sport exciting (Tricker & Cook, 1990). In a highly competitive environment, it is easy for athletes and support staff to get caught up in a "win at any cost" mentality. When ends justify means, risks associated with cheating may be emotionally denied. They may also be considered part of the excitement, a necessary evil, or even a demonstration of willingness to pay the price of success.

Sport professionals working with elite athletes will regularly be confronted with evidence of illegal or unethical practices designed to enhance performance (Ungerleider & Golding, 1992; Voy, 1991). An athlete quoted by Ungerleider and Golding (1992) reported anonymously:

> My belief is that if I had to take an estimate, about sixty-five percent of the top five, let's say top ten in the world in every event, are doing something illegal. That basically is the growth hormones in the ballistic events and blood doping for the distance events. I think all of the major distance runners that have run really incredible times are blood doping. I think middle distance runners are using a combination of blood doping and steroids. (p. 119)

If such claims are true, the ethics of some sport physicians and administrators may be called into question. In fact, some coaches have been known to refuse to train athletes who wanted to compete clean (Voy, 1991).

Other areas of unethical behavior are also to be found in sports. Manipulating academic eligibility requirements is unethical. Unethical behavior may also include overt child abuse, unethical weight loss practices, or sexual barter (Rotella & Connelly, 1984). In the case of moral issues, boundary violations, illegal activity, or abusive relationships, the motivation for condoning such practices may also be justified by the belief that everyone is doing it.

Recognizing abuse can be difficult in the competitive environment. Personal criteria of abuse are culture laden and highly subjective. Legal criteria are clear. In the sport environment, abusive behavior is disguised, tolerated, and, at times, celebrated. The need for aggression in sport may even encourage acceptance of abusive coaching or parenting activities that are designed to increase aggressive behavior at game time. Abusive behavior may be publicly abhorred but privately condoned when it leads to success.

Without a well-developed value-based decision system to guide their counsel, professional helpers may ultimately compromise their integrity. Risk may entail experiencing censure by professional or employing organizations even if the ethical violation is not criminal in nature. Criminal penalties or civil suits may follow ethical breeches that violate statute law as well.

Ethical Standards

The National Athletic Trainers Association (NATA) completed a role-delineation validation study for the entry-level athletic trainers' certification examination (2004). Its Board of Certification (BOC) works to protect the public by identifying individuals who are competent to practice the profession of athletic training. Consistent with this mission, the primary function of the athletic training examination is "to assess competence in the discipline of athletic training and the role of the athletic trainer." (BOC Role Delineation Study Fifth Edition, 2004, p. 1)

NATA considered six major domains as essential components for competent functioning at the entry level (NATA, 2004):
1. Prevention
2. Clinical Evaluation and Diagnosis
3. Immediate Care
4. Treatment, Rehabilitation, and Reconditioning
5. Organization and Administration
6. Professional Responsibility

(p. 3)

"The variety of patients with whom an AT must communicate regarding risk and prevention has expanded. These patients, termed 'appropriate' in the domain, are associated with (1) the sports medicine team, (2) the clinical setting, and (3) fitness facilities. ATs also communicate risk because of legal considerations" (NATA, 2004, p. 4). Education and counseling skills are viewed as critically important competencies for entry-level certified athletic trainers. The advising of athletes and coaches, as well as others interested in athletic endeavors, is clearly within the purview of the work of a trainer. The NATA Board of Certification emphasizes the importance of education and communication across all domains.

Some sport professionals are all too well aware of the limitations their academic training provides for the challenges they face in counseling athletes. Others express a willingness to counsel on virtually any topic. In recent years NATA has stressed the importance of the trainers' need to maintain the highest ethical and professional standards. NATA has recently created the Domain of Professional Responsibility to underscore the significance of maintaining the highest ethical and professional standards. For these reasons it might be useful to review some of the ethical guidelines that have been imposed upon psychologists by The American Psychological Association. The ethical guidelines discussed in this chapter are drawn from The Ethical Principles of Psychologists and Code of Conduct of The American Psychological Association, 2002.

Five general principles state the aspirational norms that guide psychologists toward the highest ideals of psychology:
1. Beneficence and Nonmaleficence
2. Fidelity and Responsibility
3. Integrity

4. Justice
5. Respect for People's Rights and Dignity

This code represents a dynamic set of ethical standards for work-related conduct which requires "a personal commitment and lifelong effort to act ethically; to encourage ethical behavior by students, supervisees, employees, and colleagues; and to consult with others concerning ethical problems" (American Psychological Association [APA], 2002, p. 3).

The NATA Code of Ethics (2005) reflects similar aspiration goals. It emphasizes the need for trainers to

- respect confidentiality,
- avoid discriminations,
- comply with pertinent laws and regulations,
- report illegal activity,
- restrict their scope of practice to those areas in which they have received formal training, and
- avoid "conduct that could be constructed as a conflict of interest"

(NATA, 2005, p. 6). Because counseling is clearly a primary job function of psychologists it seems reasonable to extend the counseling and educational ethics of psychology to other healthcare providers who counsel. Psychologists are expected to supplement, but not violate, the ethical code values and rules based on guidance drawn from personal values, culture and experience. This ethic has implications for other sport professionals as well.

Counselor's Role

Boundary and role delineation aspects of the sports consultant's job are other issues inherent in the nature of the job itself. A sport consultant may spend a great deal of time with a team or with an individual athlete during conditioning, practice, travel, and competition. When athletes and professional helpers eat, sleep, sweat, mourn, and celebrate together, it is easy for boundaries to become blurred, particularly in matters of a personal nature. The sport professional should keep the athlete informed, at all times, of the nature of the relationship, and of shifts in the relationship that may occur as a result of changes in the trainer's responsibility. As the athlete confides more and more in the professional helper, value blind spots and guiding ethical codes need to be well defined.

Another issue of ethical significance when counseling athletes pertains to the dangers of developing an overly dependent relationship as opposed to encouraging independent behavior. Van Hoose & Kottler (1980) warned that failure to set and hold to time guidelines when counseling may reinforce dependent behavior on the part of clients and encourage them to renege on their responsibility for self-direction. The authors point out that fostering excessive dependency in response to intervention would not only be destructive to the client, but could also be ethically questionable.

Contractual obligations pose ethical dilemmas for the sport consultant who provides ongoing personal counseling. Sport psychologists or trainers with a counseling degree should be aware of their contractual obligation to the client. A client may quit the counseling at any time for any reason; however, a psychologist or sports professional who terminates a counseling relationship without sufficient notice may be liable for malpractice if the client sustains damages of a type recognized by law. In other words, when functioning in the role of a counselor, trainers might be held legally accountable if they depart from the standard of care that a jury might consider appropriate for that particular relationship. Obviously, individuals who misrepresent themselves as psychologists are subject to sanction by the state for such misconduct. All professionals, in and outside of sport, counsel in a variety of ways. Coaches frequently consider molding young people's values as the most important and rewarding part of their job. Certainly, they do not consider themselves as providers of psychotherapy (Zeigler, 1987).

Consider the case of the athlete who may deliberately injure himself as a face-saving way to avoid competitive stress (Kane, 1984). NATA would emphasize the importance of recognizing the problem and referring such an athlete to an appropriate professional therapist. When the sports professional uses referral and informal counseling techniques, athletes may leave competition or compete at a reduced level and still maintain their dignity. This type of intervention is not only ethically appropriate, but is also consistent with NATA recommendations for competent functioning in virtually all domains. The transfer process should entail follow-up, if harm to an athlete or another person is suspected.

Sport professionals who find themselves questioning their competency to deal with serious psychological situations should be applauded. Being scrupulous may be the best liability insurance. The athlete should be informed of the seriousness of the matter and told that a high level of training is ordinarily required to provide help with this type of problem. Athletes should be made to understand that psychologists, psychiatrists, and other therapists who are more qualified are readily available. To direct the athlete to such services is consistent with NATA and APA guidelines.

Knowledge of referral procedures and community resources are specifically referenced as minimum competencies for Certified Athletic Trainers by NATA. In fact, knowledge of "professional resources for stress management and behavior modification" is specifically referenced under NATA's Prevention Domain. The Domains of Treatment, Rehabilitation, and Reconditioning direct the trainer to have knowledge of available psychosocial, community, family, and healthcare support systems (NATA, 2004). NATA further delineates the knowledge required:

1. Knowledge of psychological effects related to rehabilitation, recovery, and performance.
2. Knowledge of referral resources.
3. Knowledge of psychosocial dysfunction.

NATA's panel of experts identified specific skills necessary in order to implement the Domain IV Knowledges:

1. Skill in identifying appropriate patients for guidance and counseling.
2. Skill in using appropriate psychosocial techniques (e.g., goal setting and stress management) in rehabilitation.
3. Skill in referring to appropriate healthcare professionals.

4. Skill in using effective communication.
5. Skill in providing guidance/counseling for the patient during the treatment, rehabilitation, and reconditioning process. (NATA, 2004, pp. 23, 24)

Athletic trainers who engage in counseling athletes with social and/or personal problems would be considered incompetent by the standards of NATA 2004 were they to exceed the boundaries of their competence to counsel.

Trainers are expected to have knowledge in the areas of psychology, sport psychology, and developmental psychology, as well as of psychological readiness for the return to activity. They should have skill in evaluating the athletes' present physical and psychological status as it pertains to sports participation. The trainer is also expected to have knowledge of implications of unhealthy personal situations (e.g., substance abuse, eating disorders, victims of assault, abuse, etc.). Lastly, the trainer is expected to have skill in recognizing the athletes' need for information regarding personal and/or community health topics. Trainers should also be skilled with instructional methods as well as information dissemination procedures regarding personal and/or community health topics (NATA, 2004, p. 21). While the counseling mission of the Certified Athletic Trainer is important, there appears to be a shift in emphasis. In 1991 trainers were clearly encouraged to refer counseling to mental health professionals. In the 2004 BOC document, those knowledges and skills have been deemphasized. In fact, the entire Domain of Education and Counseling has been deleted. This de-emphasis on referral to mental health professionals may increase the liability exposure of trainers who are encouraged to do more counseling yet lack formal training in counseling theory and practice. Now more than ever it is incumbent upon the trainer to be mindful of the standard of care to which professional counselors are required to adhere.

Conflicting Interests

Sport consultants who also function as coaches may risk the appearance of conflict of interest. This appearance can be problematic, imposing unnecessary hardship on the athlete and the counselor. The APA Ethical Standard 3.07 offers sound guidance in this area:

> When psychologists agree to provide services to a person or entity at the request of a third party, psychologists attempt to clarify at the outset of the service the nature of the relationship with all individuals or organizations involved. This clarification includes the role of the psychologist (e.g., therapist, consultant, diagnostician, or expert witness), an identification of who is the client, the probable use of the services provided or the information obtained, and the fact that there may be limits to confidentiality. (APA, 2002, p. 6)

Adherence to such ethical guidelines clarifies for whom the professional helper is actually working. Consultants and helpers have an obligation to their employers, but they also have a responsibility to the athletes whom they counsel. In performance-enhancement settings, it is possible to maintain a very positive relationship with both management and athlete.

Athletes should be made to understand that what they share will remain in confidence unless it is a matter of life and death to them or someone else. For psychologists working in a counseling role, this is a standard guideline. There are times, however, when this requirement is not the rule, such as in the case of military psychologists, or in certain organizational or forensic settings. Military psychologists must inform their clients of their duty to follow the chain of command. Information is therefore not confidential.

Begin every new personal counseling relationship by reviewing the limits to which information discussed can ethically be kept confidential. It is important that neither the athlete or professional helper be misled. A psychotherapist's records may be subpoenaed and admitted into evidence in some jurisdictions even where the psychologist/patient privilege is recognized. Most, if not all jurisdictions recognize, at a minimum, the priest/penitent and psychologist/patient relationship as confidentially protected.

Too Much, Too Soon

Communication is good. Confession may be good for the soul, as catharsis can alleviate energy-sapping stress. But, too much self-disclosure, too soon, can be harmful (Derlega & Chaikin, 1975). Some clients will begin talking about stressful situations and express thoughts and feelings that have been on their minds for some time. Beware of clients who seem to say too much, too soon, particularly if they are new clients. Be mindful that sometimes a client who tells too much too soon may feel violated later.

Even self-reliant, emotionally stable, independent people with a streak of cynicism can become overwhelmed, highly stressed, and depressed. Many times, having the opportunity to "unload" will be good medicine. Athletes will appreciate your willingness to listen, as well as the liberty to seek assistance as they feel the need.

Occasionally, an athlete who is obviously agitated and under pressure will visit a trainer or counselor volitionally. If the athlete is highly emotional or anxious, reassure him or her of your availability. The athlete does not need to reveal all issues in one meeting. On occasion, you may deem it appropriate to discourage too much self-disclosure. Inform the athlete that confidential revelations are not legally exempt from discovery by the legal system in the jurisdiction in which you work.

Athletes raised with an aggressive, competitive, racist, or "macho" mentality may feel compromised if they are encouraged to reveal too much of themselves in a moment of weakness. Later, they may feel uncomfortable. They may even resent the counselor, feeling that they have been robbed of their dignity or taken advantage of in their moment of weakness. This reaction is not typical, but it does occur. A confident manner will project a reassuring sense of optimism that a solution will be found.

It is a counselor's responsibility to have a clearly established protocol when counseling. With internal consistency among personal morality, ethical principles, and legal responsibilities, making ethically and legally correct decisions will be more comfortable.

Potential Traps

In a situation where the athlete says, "I have to share something, but you must promise not to tell," counselor/trainer may respond with, "It is my role to listen. I will be happy to listen to what you have to say, if you trust me to use what you tell me in your best interests."

By telling the client, "I'd like you to tell me anything you trust me to use in your best interest," counselors offer the opportunity to be of professional assistance without having their hands tied. This approach is likely to be appropriate when dealing with children, but adults may press for higher levels of secrecy. At that point, an explanation of the limits of confidentiality would be in order.

Triangles

Triangles can be particularly challenging for many helping professionals. In such a situation a client will share some information about a second party. You are put in a position of trying to help someone solve a problem involving someone else without permission to involve that third party. Here again, the best course of action is to be a reflective listener. Avoid the temptation to rescue the athlete from the problem. In such a situation it is best to do nothing, unless, of course, the athlete is psychotic, suicidal, or homicidal.

Triangle situations require problem-solving without the power or authority to do so. Keep in mind that the counselor is a facilitator who assists athletes in solving their own problems. An exception to the facilitator role occurs when an athlete is clearly in danger and lacks access to a power base adequate to cope with the danger. Children and teenagers who are abused are cases in point. Adult victims of crime are also in this category.

Victims of abuse require immediate response from the counselor, who is, moreover obliged to report the abuse. In doing so, the professional helper provides the best chance of halting it.

Cultural Values and Ethical Counseling

Racial bias can prove ethically challenging for those who are counseling athletes. Racial, or for that matter, any values that would conflict with your ability to provide unbiased consultation are considered reasons to refer the client to someone else. If referral is not practical, the client should be made aware of any of the counselor's values that may influence his or her counsel.

Gender identity issues have ethical implications for personal counseling. Ethical conflicts sometimes arise when sexual preference differs for counselor and client. Counselors have an ethical duty to refer clients to another healthcare professional when the counselors experience anxiety or discomfort with the clients' sexual orientation. Sexual nepotism, or favoring individuals of one's sexual preference, is increasingly discussed as a problem among psychologists who counsel and offer services to female sport teams. The ethical warning to avoid misuse of power when counseling holds true for homosexual as well as heterosexual coaches, trainers, and sport psychologists (York, 2006.)

Sexual harassment, discrimination, and lack of respect for the values and human differences among those the professional counsels are clearly unethical and to be avoided. Exploitative relationships are unethical. Sexual relations between counselor and client are considered exploitative, unethical, and are the leading reason for malpractice awards against professional counselors.

Documentation of Work

Ethical and legal considerations require that records be kept about services performed. This is particularly important in the private sector, although institutional and organizational policies may be similar. If policy doesn't require record-keeping, prudence does.

When dealing with sensitive personal information, it is critical to have minimum entries in the confidential file for each session or meeting. The notes do not need to be exhaustive, but should include a minimum of information, such as

- the date,
- who was present,
- problem addressed,
- recommendations made,
- estimates of progress, and
- plans for the future.

This makes it possible for counselors to document positions taken in the event that they are ordered to appear in court. This is particularly true in cases where athletes are in crises with significant areas of abuse or emotional disturbance, such as depression or suicidal ideation.

It is also important to document things that were said and done during rehabilitation of sport injuries. Such documentation may help protect counselors, trainers, or psychologists from litigation. If sued, deposed, or brought into court as expert witnesses, professional helpers will be able to present their professional responses emphatically when citing records that support their contentions. Appropriately kept records will also enable the athlete to receive an important message. The athlete client is likely to be more reasonable, knowing that a record of previous encounters is available. Malpractice situations are unpleasant for both plaintiff and defendant. When professionals are sued for malpractice, it is easier to defend their conduct when documentation is available. Lawsuits are sometimes brought in revenge for real or imagined slights or offenses.

When counseling or referring, be sure to note the problem or issue, your estimate of the client's mental state at time of consultation (e.g., lucid, clear or desperate, despondent). Note your recommendation or action, especially if referral was made. The notes need to provide sufficient information so that another professional might evaluate the scope of the problem and the appropriateness of documented recommendations. This may be enough to convince an adversarial party's attorney and expert that there is no likelihood of deviation from the standard of care.

It is important to recognize that the burden of a plaintiff's proof is not always easy. A tort is a civil wrong. The requirements of proof for a plaintiff in tort are four in number:

- The first is duty. This means that there must have been a duty of the defendant to the plaintiff, that duty arising from the professional relationship.
- Second, there must have been a breach of that duty by either an overt act or the failure to act by the person who owes the duty.
- Third, there must be damages proven that are recognized by law.

- Last, there must be proof that the act or non-act must have resulted proximately in the damages accrued (J.D. Williams, personal communication, January, 2006).

Summary

Ethical guidelines of The American Psychological Association and virtually all human relations ethics codes affirm the dignity of the client. Virtually all codes ban discrimination, sexual harassment, or other types of harassment and encourage respect for the rights and diverse values and opinions of the people served. It is helpful to realize that counselors, trainers, and psychologists are privileged in that clients share information with them. The act of sharing, particularly sensitive personal information, involves considerable risk on the part of the athlete. By increasing awareness of personal values, the professional helper's work with athletes will be enhanced.

References

American Psychological Association. (October 8, 2002). *Ethical Principles of Psychology and Code of Conduct.* Washington, DC: Author.

Derlega, V., & Chaikin, A. (1975). *Sharing intimacy.* Englewood Cliffs, NJ: Prentice-Hall.

Kane, B. (1984). Trainer counseling to avoid three face-saving maneuvers. *Athletic Training, 19(3),*171-174.

Makarowski, L (1996). *How To Keep Your C.O.O.L With Your Kids.* (p. 126) New York, NY: A Perigee Book.

McGuire, R. (1990). History and evolution of drugs in sport. In R. Tricker & D. L. Cook (Eds.), *Athletes at risk: Drugs and sport (p.* 10). Dubuque, IA: Wm. C. Brown.

National Athletic Trainers' Association. (2005). *The FACTS about Certified Athletic Trainers and The National Athletic Trainers' Association* [Data file]. Texas: NATA.

National Athletic Trainers' Association Board of Certification, Inc. (2004). *Certainty in the Professional Practice of Athletic Trainers (5th ed.).*Omaha, NE: Board of Certification, Inc.

National Athletic Trainers' Association. (2005). *NATA Code of Ethics* [Data file]. Texas: NATA.

Raths, L., Merrill, H., & Simon, S. (1966). *Values and teaching.* Columbus, OH: Charles E. Merrill.

Rotella, R. J., & Connelly, D. (1984). Individual ethics in the application of cognitive sport psychology. In W. F. Straub & J. M. Williams (Eds.), *Cognitive sport psychology* (pp. 102-112). Lansing, NY: Sport Science Associates.

Shake racial stereotypes. (1991, December 19). *USA Today,* p. 12A.

Simon, S. B., Howe, L. W., & Kirschenbaum, H. (1974). *Value clarification.* New York: Hart.

Thompson, A. (1983). *Ethical concerns in psychotherapy and their legal ramifications.* Lanham, MID: University Press of America.

Tricker, R., & Cook, D. L. (Eds.). (1990). *Athletes at risk: Drugs and sport.* Dubuque, IA:Wm. C. Brown.

Ungerleider, S., & Golding, J. M. (1992). *Beyond strength.* Dubuque, IA: Wm. C. Brown.

Van Hoose, W. H., & Kottler, J. A. (1985). *Ethical and legal issues in counseling and psychotherapy* (2nd ed). San Francisco: Jossey-Bass

Voy, R. (1991). *Drugs, sport, and politics.* Champaign, IL: Leisure Press.

York, Frank.(2006). *The National Psychologist,15(22),* 15,19.

Zeigler, E. F. (1987). Rationale and suggested dimensions for a code of ethics for sport psychologists. *The Sport Psychologist, 1,* 138-150.

Chapter Seventeen | Pain: Basic Concepts

Wendy F. Sternberg
Haverford College

Introduction

Pain is unlike other sensory experiences. Although all of our sensory capacities are evolved adaptations designed to help us locate food, mates, and other resources and to avoid predation or potentially harmful substances, pain sensation is arguably the most important for survival. Individuals who are deaf, blind, or anosmic (unable to smell) are able to negotiate the world on their remaining senses, (although they would likely have been unfit in the ancestral environment); those who cannot feel pain live injury-filled lives, unable to recognize or avoid harmful stimuli in the environment (Melzack & Wall, 1996).

Pain can be distinguished from other sensory modalities on a number of other characteristics. For example, in most sensory systems, habituation occurs in response to constant stimuli such that the perceptual experience of these unchanging stimuli diminishes over time. No such habituation occurs in pain sensation—indeed, the opposite often occurs; sensitization is the process whereby the perceptual response to noxious (tissue damaging) stimuli may become heightened in the face of repeated stimulation. Furthermore, pain is understood in terms of its emotional as well as its sensory aspects. Like all sensory experiences, pain can be described on a "sensory-discriminative" dimension, on which the location, quality, and intensity of the experience are characterized. But unlike other sensations, pain can be characterized by its unpleasantness (the affective, or emotional dimension)—indeed, if the sensation is not unpleasant, it is not pain. In no other sensory modality is emotion a defining component of the perceptual experience.

It is useful at this point to distinguish between the terms "sensation" and "perception." "Sensation" describes the general process by which stimulus energy (e.g., photons of light, sound waves traveling through the air, or high-intensity pressure, temperature, or mechanical stimuli) contacts the sensory receptors (usually specialized neurons or structures associated with neurons located at the periphery of the body) and causes a change in neural activity that is transmitted to the central nervous system (brain and spinal cord) through afferent (incoming) neural pathways. Thus, sensation is the process by which stimulus energy is received, transduced into the electrochemical energy of the nervous system, and represented as a unique pattern of neural activity in the brain. In contrast, "perception" refers to the conscious, subjective experience, one that involves higher order processing of those incoming sensory signals that arise in the periphery. In a very real sense, perception is *in the brain*, although our conscious experience incorporates a sense of location in the world (including the body, e.g., "where it hurts"). It is the activity of cortical circuitry in the regions of the brain that receive input from afferent neurons, specifically those responding to tissue damage (or impending damage) in the periphery, that gives rise to pain perception.

In this chapter, the neural basis of pain sensation and perception will be described, in terms that are useful to the athlete wishing to learn more about the physiological basis of injury-induced pain. Special attention will be given to the brain's modulatory influence over afferent stimulation, because the experience of many individuals, athletes and non-athletes alike, clearly illustrates the tenuous link that exists between injury and pain. Injury occurs in the absence of pain, and in many cases of persistent pain, great suffering occurs in the absence of injury. Far from being a passive recipient of messages received and transmitted from the periphery, the brain is capable of generating the neural experience of pain in the absence of input. Furthermore, the brain actively modulates its own input, and is capable of diminishing the information that eventually reaches its processing centers. It is this descending inhibition that may allow athletes to continue to compete despite injury (in some cases, being blissfully unaware of the injury).

The organizational scheme that will be utilized to describe the underlying neural basis of pain involves the four stages of pain described by Fields (1987):

Nociception is activity in peripheral neurons designed to detect the presence of noxious (tissue-damaging) stimuli that impinges on the body. These peripheral neurons are called *nociceptors*; they are embedded in the skin, joints, and muscles, and their function is to alert the central nervous system that tissue damage is occurring or will occur if the stimulus continues.

Transmission is communication of nociceptive information from the periphery (where the nociceptors interface with the outside world) to the central nervous system (brain and spinal cord).

Modulation is the process by which the brain can exert its influence over the incoming nociceptive information.

Perception is conscious interpretation of the nociceptive stimulus as *pain* (see Figure 1).

Figure 1.

Information flow in the nervous system.

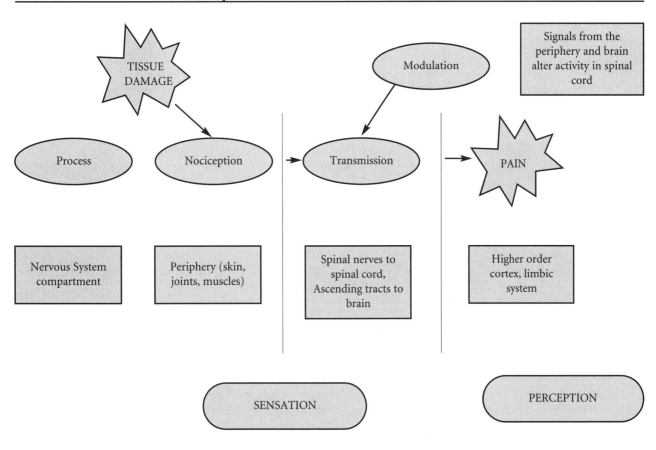

Nociception starts in the periphery in response to tissue damage. These signals are transmitted through spinal nerves to the dorsal horn of the spinal cord. Output from the spinal cord to the brain is ultimately interpreted by the brain as pain. However, modulatory influences from the brain and the periphery alter activity in the spinal cord.

Pain Pathways: From Nociception to Perception

Under normal conditions, pain perception is the outcome of neural activity in the peripheral and central nervous system pathways designed to respond to noxious (tissue damaging) stimuli. A specialized class of peripheral neurons called **nociceptors** detects the presence of high-intensity temperature, mechanical, or chemical stimuli impinging on the body and responds when such stimuli reach tissue-damaging (or potentially tissue-damaging) range. These cells have their cell bodies (including the nucleus, genetic material, and cellular machinery) located just outside the dorsal (toward the back) aspect of the spinal cord in the dorsal root ganglion (DRG). In addition to the long projection fiber from the periphery (where information about tissue damage is gathered), DRG cells extend a short fiber into the spinal cord dorsal horn (Figure 2). The peripheral end of the DRG cells are highly concentrated in the skin, joints, connective tissue, skeletal muscles, and blood vessel walls, whereas few such receptors are located in the visceral organs (those that are located in visceral organs respond exclusively to distention, or stretch, in those organs). Nociceptors extend

Figure 2.

Schematic diagram of pain input pathway.

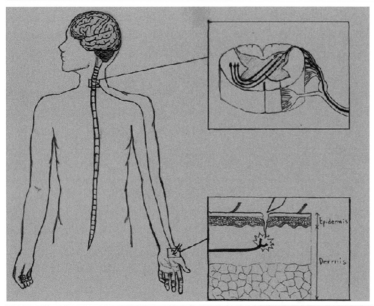

A noxious stimulus impinging on the skin (inset, bottom) activates nociceptors in the periphery, sending signals along primary afferent fibers into the relevant spinal cord segment (inset, top). The swelling outside the dorsal surface of the spinal cord contains the cell bodies of these primary afferent fibers (cell bodies not shown). The second order cells arise in the spinal cord dorsal horn and send their output up the anterolateral quadrant of the spinal cord white matter to the brain. (Illustration by Ashley G. Kim.)

from the periphery into the spinal cord via the spinal nerves. Thus, intermingled with the nociceptive projections into the spinal cord are those sensory neurons that respond to innocuous temperature and touch stimuli (e.g., light pressure, tickle, vibration, warmth, cooling, etc.). The nociceptors can be distinguished from the non-nociceptive afferent projections anatomically and physiologically.

Nociceptive afferents are characterized by their small diameter and relative lack of myelination (the fatty covering that insulates most projection fibers in the nervous system). The condition of congenital insensitivity to pain described earlier results from a genetic mutation that prevents the growth of small diameter peripheral axons (Mardy et al., 1999). The smallest of these are the unmyelinated C-fibers that in mammalian nervous systems are almost exclusively nociceptive, responding to high-intensity thermal, mechanical, and chemical stimuli (and are thus termed "polymodal" nociceptors). Their peripheral termini are described as free nerve endings, whereby noxious stimuli impinge directly on the peripheral extension to produce an excitatory signal (Cesare et al., 1999) that is then transmitted to the central nervous system. Neurologically intact subjects report a subjective shift from warmth to pain when peripherally applied thermal stimuli reach the 43–45°C range (Magerl & Treede, 1996). This psychophysical function is detectable in the increased activity of C-fibers isolated in vitro when the skin is exposed to temperatures above 42°C, and has been associated with ion conductance through a particular type of TRP cation channel (known as TRPV channels) gated by the vanilloid receptor VR-1 (Cesare et al., 1999).

Stimulation of the vanilloid receptor by capsaicin, the active ingredient in chili peppers, also opens TRPV cation channels, explaining the heat and pain that often arise from contact with the substance. Thus, when a thermal stimulus reaches "nociceptive threshold," positively charged ions enter peripheral terminals of nociceptive afferents in that region, causing electrical signals to be transmitted through their axonal extensions as they course through the spinal nerve into the spinal cord. All nociceptive afferent projection fibers are small in diameter and either unmyelinated (as in C-fibers) or thinly myelinated (Aδ fibers), making them among the slowest conducting neurons in the nervous system (axon diameter and myelination are positively associated with speed of conduction).

Other subtypes of TRP cation channels (TRPA, TRPC, and alternate types of TRPV, (see Lin & Corey, 2005, for review) open in response to other forms of noxious stimuli, such as cold, (stimulated by menthol, Reid, 2005), mechanical pressure, and a variety of noxious chemical irritants. Mutant mice that lack TRPA channels fail to respond to mustard oil (the irritant found in the condiment wasabi), garlic extracts, and the volatile irritant acrolein (Bautista et al., 2006), suggesting a common underlying mechanism activated in response to a wide range of potentially noxious insults impinging on the skin, joints, and muscles.

The output ends of the nociceptive afferents (those that communicate with cells in the spinal cord) form synapses in the dorsal gray matter of the spinal cord, particularly in the superficial layers (those closest to the entry point at the back of the spinal cord). Spinal cord segments consist of a central region of gray matter (axon terminals,

Figure 3.

Light microscopic image of a section of mouse thoracic spinal cord, removed 1 hour after exposure to a noxious stimulus (dilute acetic acid administered into the gut cavity, which causes mild abdominal pain).

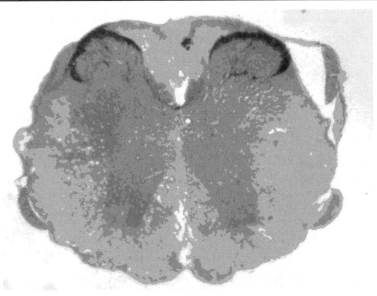

The darkly stained regions at the top of the figure (dorsal horn of the spinal cord gray matter; arrows) indicates presence of fos protein, a neural activity marker.

dendrites, cell bodies) surrounded by an outer region of white matter (myelinated axons projecting to and from the brain), forming the characteristic butterfly shape (Figure 3). The dorsal horns of spinal cord gray matter contain the second order neurons in the somatosensory (i.e., touch, temperature, pain) system that receive input from primary afferent fibers, and send their output through the white matter to supraspinal targets, in a number of ascending tracts (including the spinothalamic, spinoreticular, and dorsal column pathways). The darkly stained regions of the spinal cord dorsal horn in Figure 3 illustrate activity in the superficial dorsal horns following exposure to a mild chemical irritant injected into the gut cavity in the mouse. The staining reflects cells that contain the protein c-fos, a product of gene expression whose production is a reflection of underlying neural activity (Morgan & Curran, 1991; Curran & Morgan, 1995).

These second order cells extend projections up the spinal cord toward the brain. When these ascending projections enter the brainstem, they form synaptic contact with neurons located in brainstem nuclei, including the thalamus. The thalamus then redirects this information to the appropriate area of the primary somatosensory cortex in the parietal lobe. A somatotopic map of the body surface is represented in the cortex (particular locations in the cortex correspond to particular locations on the body surface), providing a neural substrate for the localization of painful experience. From the primary somatosensory cortex, information regarding tissue damage is transmitted to higher order cortex, located both in the parietal lobe and to diffuse locations in the cerebral cortex, including the frontal lobes and limbic systems. It is this higher order processing that produces the quality, intensity, and meaning of the subjective experience. The somatosensory cortex is not the only target of nociceptive information. Brain areas associated with arousal (e.g., the reticular formation) and emotion (the limbic system) also receive direct input from the ascending nociceptive tracts, in addition to receiving information by way of the somatosensory cortex.

Functional brain-imaging studies in humans illustrate the role of multiple brain areas in producing pain experience; distinct regions of the cortex and brainstem are differentially associated with certain aspects of pain experience, such as detection threshold, pain unpleasantness, and pain intensity (Tolle et al., 1999). Thus, the multifaceted perceptual experience of pain reflects the underlying neural activity of brain areas processing sensory and emotional information that arises from tissue damage (real and impending) in the periphery, in order to organize appropriate behavioral responses and to provide a powerful motivation to avoid similar stimuli in the future.

The key step in the ascending nociceptive process is the output from the spinal cord to the brain (in the case of noxious stimuli that impinge on the body above the neck, the trigeminal nerve system plays an important analogous role to the spinal nerve/spinal cord system). Neurons with cell bodies in the superficial layers of the spinal cord dorsal horn, whose axons extend up the spinal cord into the brain, are termed *pain transmission neurons* (PTNs). As was first proposed by Melzack and Wall (1965), the superficial dorsal horn of the spinal cord also contains local neurons that can alter the firing rate of the PTNs by virtue of forming modulatory synapses. Such modulatory inputs to the PTNs can be activated by descending projections from the brain (often inhibitory in nature) or by nociceptive and non-nociceptive afferents. The effectiveness of non-nociceptive afferents in dampening pain sensation is illustrated in the common phenomenon of pain relief induced by rubbing or massaging an affected area. Descending pain control circuitry, on the other hand, originates in the brain and descends via the midbrain and lower brain stem to the spinal cord where inhibitory synapses with ascending pain transmission neurons prevent or diminish the upward flow of nociceptive information.

Experimental evidence for such descending pain modulation was first provided by the observation of analgesia (pain relief) resulting from electrical stimulation of midbrain sites (Reynolds, 1969; Mayer et al., 1971) and its subsequent elimination by the lesioning of downstream nuclei in the medulla or descending spinal cord pathways (Prieto et al., 1983). Thus, the brain is capable of limiting its own input by preventing the upward flow of nociceptive information from the spinal cord. Modulation in the spinal cord can also produce heightened responses from the PTN, as will be discussed in a later section.

The observation of stimulation-produced analgesia preceded the discovery of the brain's own pain-killing compounds, the endogenous (occurring within) opioid peptides, chemicals similar in structure to narcotic drugs like morphine (Goldberg, 1988). In the early 1970s scientists isolated the receptor that was responsible for the powerful effects of opiate compounds (e.g., opium, heroin, and morphine) and later discovered the endogenous ligands that acted on these receptors: enkephalins, endorphins, and dynorphins (Pert and Snyder, 1973; Hughes et al., 1975). Opioids (both endogenous and exogenous) achieve their analgesic effects by binding to opiate receptors in the nervous system, particularly in loci distributed throughout the pain modulatory pathway (other mechanisms of opiate analgesia also exist; see Corbett et al., 2006, for review). The opiate receptor blocker, naloxone, has been shown to eliminate or reduce the analgesia arising from electrical stimulation of the midbrain (Akil et al., 1976; Cannon et al., 1982). These observations suggest that electrical stimulation and opiate administration achieve their analgesic effects via the same underlying neural substrates—by activating descending analgesic mechanisms that send inhibitory output to the PTNs in the dorsal horn of the spinal cord.

The observation of stimulation-produced analgesia, and the subsequent discovery of an entire system devoted to pain inhibition, presented researchers with two puzzles:

- First, electrical stimulation and administration of poppy plant extracts (i.e., opium, morphine, etc.) could not be the natural triggers for endogenous pain inhibitory circuitry. The first major question to be solved, then, was what was the natural trigger for endogenous pain inhibition?
- A second, related question was why did the nervous system evolve such circuitry?

As discussed at the outset of this chapter, intact pain perception is essential for survival, thus, the very existence of endogenous pain inhibition posed a problem for the formulation of pain perception as a protective property of the nervous system. Both questions were answered by the observation in the laboratory of an ecologically valid environmental manipulation that could activate endogenous pain inhibitory mechanisms. The key environmental factor is stress. Under conditions of extreme stress, when organisms must mobilize all available resources to meet the demands of challenges in the environment, the "fight-or-flight" mechanisms include a temporary pain inhibitory effect. Analgesia resulting from acutely stressful events in laboratory animals can be readily elicited in response to a variety of environmental stressors. The significance of such stress-induced analgesia (SIA) for the competitive athlete will be discussed later.

The descending pain inhibitory pathways originate in the hypothalamus, the brain structure that governs the hormonal and neural response to stressful situations. From the hypothalamus, axons project downstream to the periaqueductal gray matter in the midbrain, to various nuclei in the rostroventral medulla, then down the spinal cord to form inhibitory synapses in the dorsal horn, where local inhibitory mechanisms are activated that dampen the output of the PTNs (Basbaum & Fields, 1984). These brain and spinal cord regions are rich in opiate receptors, and electrical stimulation in any of the brainstem regions mentioned above produces analgesia. Thus, pain perception at any moment in time is a reflection of the balance of activity in both the ascending, afferent nociceptive pathways, and the activity of descending, efferent (outgoing from the brain) antinociceptive pathways that modulate the afferent input.

Pain Pathways in Action: Response to Injury

The pathways and processes described above are activated under non-pathological conditions in the presence of real or impending tissue damage. (Note that many pathological pains are due to the activation of these mechanisms in the absence of injury.) Noxious stimuli that produce tissue damage directly activate nociceptors, but that is only the first step in the nociceptive process. A variety of chemical mediators appear in damaged tissue (released from dead and dying cells, and synthesized by local inflammatory mechanisms), which then stimulate nociceptors in the area of damage and reduce the threshold of nociceptors located in the primary region of the injury. Because nociceptors are more sensitive (rather than less) in the presence of ongoing stimulation, nociceptors are said to exhibit sensitization. The perceptual manifestation of this sensitization is termed *hyperalgesia*—that is, a heightened response to a noxious stimulus. For example, the pain ratings of a low-intensity heat stimulus (41°C) in injured tissue are comparable to that previously produced by a much higher stimulus intensity (49°C) (Meyer and Campbell 1981). Stimuli applied to injured tissue need not be noxious to produce a pain response—*allodynia* is pain produced from an innocuous stimulus, another form of sensitization. The pain resulting from light touch on sunburned skin is a common example of allodynia. Also occurring at the site of damaged tissue is spontaneous pain. That is, in the absence of direct or ongoing mechanical, thermal, or chemical stimulation, subjects with injury report pain arising from the injured area.

Pain, hyperalgesia, and allodynia that occur at the site of injury are due to the activation of nociceptors by the tissue damaging stimulus and by chemical stimulation of nociceptors by intracellular contents spilled from dead or dying cells (e.g., ATP, K+ ions) that, when applied to peripheral afferents, produce strong levels of neural excitation. In addition, chemical mediators are synthesized in damaged tissue during the inflammatory process. In response to injury, capillaries in the affected area dilate (producing redness) to allow the increased flow of blood to the area to promote healing. Contained within the region of inflammation are several enzymes that synthesize pain-producing chemicals in the injured area. Prostaglandin is a product of an enzymatic cascade that is produced in damaged tissue by the enzyme cyclooxygenase (COX) that modifies metabolic products of arachadonic acid (an intracellular chemical that is spilled into the extracellular space upon tissue injury). Prostaglandin is capable of activating nociceptive afferents in a dose-dependent manner (Moncada et al., 1975). Peripherally acting analgesics (such as aspirin and ibuprofen) work by inhibiting COX, thereby preventing prostaglandin synthesis. All of these chemical mediators, synthesized at the site of tissue injury and inflammation, are capable of producing activity and lowering the threshold for activation in nociceptors, thereby producing the perceptual phenomena of primary (at the site of injury) hyperalgesia.

In addition to the changes that occur in the periphery that result in sensitization, changes also take place in the central nervous system that can heighten pain sensitivity following injury. So-called central sensitization is a result of synaptic strengthening, such that the connections between nociceptive inputs and their dorsal horn PTN targets are more efficient, allowing lower intensity stimuli to produce a larger response. Similar forms of synaptic plasticity occur with non-nociceptive inputs. Normally, non-nociceptive inputs do not trigger activity in PTNs, but following injury, low-threshold primary afferents (i.e., those that normally respond to innocuous stimuli) become capable of causing activity in PTNs through a strengthening of interneuronal connections. Spinal cord neurons also exhibit an expansion of their receptive fields following injury, such that PTNs in the spinal cord are abnormally activated by non-nociceptive afferents from the regions surrounding the injury, resulting in secondary (surrounding the area of injury) hyperalgesia. The perceptual experience of heightened pain sensitivity in regions surrounding an injured area can be elicited only by mechanical (i.e., pressure) stimuli—surrounding regions do not become overly sensitive to heat, but palpating or stroking an area surrounding an injury can produce a heightened pain perception (see Raja et al.,1 1999).

The mechanisms in place in the spinal cord that produce central sensitization represent a kind of cellular learning, whereby synapses are strengthened in response to use. The key factor in producing long-lasting changes in the spinal cord is the afferent barrage—that is, a high-intensity burst of incoming stimulation (as would be experienced during a severe injury) necessarily causes a large degree of activity in its targets in the spinal cord. Later on, though, that high-intensity stimulation is seen to have caused changes in the spinal cord such that a low level of stimulation is capable of reactivating the targets in the spinal cord in a more efficient, robust manner. Similar kinds of cellular learning occur throughout the nervous system in brain areas involved in behavioral learning, and although there are some differences, it is largely believed that the mechanisms underlying both forms of synaptic strengthening depend on similar underlying mechanisms (Ji et al., 2003). One mechanism relies on the neurotransmitter glutamate released from nociceptive afferents binding to the NMDA subtype of glutamate receptor in spinal cord dorsal horn neurons. Certain specializations of the NMDA receptor allow synaptic strengthening to occur in response to high-intensity activity across a synapse. Although such synaptic plasticity generally serves organisms well, in the context of pathological pain, the efficiency of spinal cord circuitry in strengthening synaptic connections contributes to its insidious nature. Therefore, a great deal of promise lies in the treatment of long-lasting post-injury pain by preventing its onset, by interfering with the process of cellular learning in the spinal cord at the time of peripheral injury. Recent laboratory evidence suggests that an NMDA antagonist infused into the spinal cord at the time of peripheral nerve injury reduced the cellular manifestations of sensitization in rats (Wilson et al., 2005). Whether such treatments are similarly effective for peripheral nerve injury in clinical populations has not yet been determined.

Pain Inhibition: Activation by Stress

Stress-induced analgesia, the reduction in pain sensitivity that has been observed under conditions of stress, has been studied extensively in laboratory animals. Rats and mice exposed to a variety of laboratory stressors exhibit profound reductions in pain sensitivity. Stressors that have been employed include

- restraint,
- cold,
- predator exposure,
- swim,
- forced exercise,
- footshock, and
- metabolic stressors

(Kelly, 1986). The advantage to studying stress-induced analgesia in laboratory settings is that with precisely controlled stress exposure, it is feasible to understand the temporal characteristics of endogenous analgesia and the neurochemical and neuroanatomical substrates of the brain's own capacity for pain inhibition.

It is well known that opiate drugs cause analgesia, and that descending pain inhibition in the form of electrical stimulation produces analgesia through an opiate-mediated mechanism. Therefore, an obvious hypothesis regarding the neurochemical quality of stress-induced analgesia is that endogenous opioid released during stress is the underlying neurochemical mechanism producing analgesia in the spinal cord. Indeed, SIA can be blocked by the opiate blocker, naloxone, and tolerance and cross-tolerance develop, suggesting that endogenous opiate neurotransmitters released during stress are responsible for the pain-inhibitory effects of stress (Girardot & Holloway, 1984; Terman et al., 1984; Girardot & Holloway, 1985).

However, SIA is not always naloxone-reversible, suggesting that alternate forms of SIA exist (Watkins & Mayer, 1982; Terman et al., 1984). Similarly, not all brain stimulation analgesia can be eliminated by naloxone, indicating a multiplicity of analgesia systems present in the nervous system (and implying the adaptive importance of endogenous pain inhibition). It is generally accepted that stress-induced analgesia has multiple neurochemically and anatomically distinct mechanisms, and that qualities of the stressor are capable of eliciting different forms of analgesia. Stressor severity appears to be the key quality that determines the neurochemical quality of the subsequent SIA. More severe stressors produce naloxone-insensitive SIA; less severe stressors produce naloxone-reversible (and by definition, opioid) SIA (Mogil et al., 1996). There have been several neurotransmitter systems implicated in naloxone-insensitive forms of analgesia, such as histamine, excitatory amino acids, and noradrenergic mechanisms. There is also some evidence that naloxone-insensitive SIA can be reversed by concurrent administration of a combination of opiate receptor subtype antagonists, suggesting that even naloxone-insensitive SIA may be opioid mediated (Watkins et al., 1992). Whatever the distinct neurochemical profile, it is clear that a redundancy of neurochemical systems is built in to mammalian nervous systems.

The "fight-or-flight" response is well preserved across mammalian species, so it is reasonable to expect that acutely stressful situations would also result in a reduction in pain sensitivity in humans. Indeed, humans possess pain inhibitory circuitry that can be activated by deep-brain electrical stimulation (Richardson, 1983; Richardson, 1995), and non-pharmacological mechanisms of pain inhibition commonly used in humans (such as acupuncture, hypnosis, and relaxation) are likely to achieve their effects, at least in part, through activation of descending analgesia mechanisms. The role of endogenous opioids, however, in producing non-pharmacological analgesia against pain of clinical and experimental origin in humans is not well established (Spiegel & Albert 1983; Moret et al., 1991).

But what are the naturally occurring circumstances that give rise to endogenous pain inhibition in humans? Anecdotal evidence of athletes continuing to compete despite painful injury, or even being unaware of injury until after competition is over, suggests that pain perception is inhibited during athletic competition. It has been well established that athletic competition produces elevations in the stress hormone, cortisol (Suay et al., 1999; Bateup et al., 2002; Salvador et al., 2003; Edwards et al., 2006), and can therefore be construed as a "stressor." In an explicit test of the hypothesis that athletic competition activates SIA responses, experimental pain sensitivity was assessed in male and female intercollegiate athletes (basketball players, fencers, track athletes) immediately following a game, race, or bout, and was compared to subjects' own pain responses two days prior to and two days following the competition. Athletes' pain sensitivity was lower when tested at the athletic competition compared to their own responses at either baseline session (Sternberg et al., 1998), suggesting an analgesic effect of competition.

The effects of competition on pain sensitivity may not be limited to athletic contests; similar reductions in pain sensitivity were observed in male (but not female) subjects engaged in a videogame competition (Sternberg et al., 2001). Conversely, exercise without competition can also produce an analgesic response (see Koltyn, 2000, for review); however, the threshold for activation of exercise analgesia may vary by sex (Sternberg et al., 2001). Thus, it is conceivable that athletic competition (and other kinds of competition-related activity) inhibits pain through a stress-induced analgesia mechanism.

Summary

Pain is a normal, adaptive consequence to tissue-damaging stimuli. Pain encourages recuperative behaviors so that proper healing may take place, and its negative emotional component discourages repeated contact with pain-producing stimuli. The experience of pain in the context of sport, however, is complicated by the rewarding and motivating aspects of participation, as well as the modulatory effects of exercise and competition. Furthermore, the meaning of pain to an individual is an important determinant of the distress that it produces. This review has primarily been concerned with the physiological factors underlying pain perception in the nervous system. There are myriad psychological factors that intervene between nociception and perception that have their effects by operating on the modulatory circuitry that exists within the central nervous system. The brain is capable of both generating and inhibiting the perceptual experience of pain, regardless of the presence of noxious stimuli.

References

Akil, H., Mayer, D. J., & Liebeskind, J. C. (1976). Antagonism of stimulation-produced analgesia by naloxone, a narcotic antagonist. *Science, 191,* 961-962.

Basbaum, A. I., & Fields, H. L. (1984). Endogenous pain control systems: brainstem spinal pathways and endorphin circuitry. *Annual Review of Neuroscience, 7,* 309-338.

Bateup, H. S., Booth, A., Shirtcliff, E. A., & Granger, D.A. (2002). Testosterone, cortisol, and women's competition. *Evolution and Human Behavior, 23,* 181-192.

Cannon, J. T., Prieto, G. J., Lee, A., & Liebeskind, J. C. (1982). Evidence for opioid and non-opioid forms of stimulation-produced analgesia in the rat. *Brain Research, 243,* 315-321.

Cesare, P., Moriondo, A., Vellani, V., & McNaughton, P.A. (1999). Ion channels gated by heat. *Proceedings of the National Academy of Sciences USA, 96*(14), 7658-7663.

Corbett, A. D., Henderson, G., McKnight, A. T., & Paterson, S. J. (2006). 75 years of opioid research: the exciting but vain quest for the Holy Grail. *British Journal of Pharmacology, 147* (Suppl. 1) S153-162.

Curran, T. & Morgan, J. I. (1995). Fos: an immediate-early transcription factor in neurons. *Journal of Neurobiology, 26*(3), 403-412.

Edwards, D. A., K. Wetzel & Wyner, D. R. (2006). Intercollegiate soccer: saliva cortisol and testosterone are elevated during competition, and testosterone is related to status and social connectedness with team mates. *Physiology & Behavior, 87*(1), 135-143.

Fields, H. L. (1987). *Pain.* New York: McGraw-Hill.

Girardot, M. N. & Holloway, F. A. (1984). Intermittent cold water stress-analgesia in rats: cross tolerance to morphine. *Pharmacology Biochemistry & Behavior, 20,* 631-633.

Girardot, M. N. & Holloway, F. A. (1985). Naltrexone antagonizes the biobehavioral adaptation to cold water stress in rats. *Pharmacology Biochemistry & Behavior, 22,* 769-779.

Goldberg, J. (1988). *Anatomy of a Scientific Discovery.* New York: Bantam Books.

Hughes, J., Smith, T. W., Kosterlitz, H. W., Fothergill, L. A., Morgan, B. A., & Morris, H. R. (1975). Identification of two related pentapeptides from the brain with potent opiate agonist activity. *Nature, 258*(5536), 577-80.

Ji, R. R., Kohno, T., Moore, K. A., & Woolf, C. J. (2003). Central sensitization and LTP: Do pain and memory share similar mechanisms? *Trends in Neurosciences, 26,*(12), 696-705.

Kelly, D. D. (Ed.). (1986). *Stress-induced analgesia.* Annals of the New York Academy of Sciences. New York: New York Academy of Sciences.

Koltyn, K. F. (2000). Analgesia following exercise: A review. *Sports Medicine, 29*(2), 85-98.

Lin, S. Y. & Corey, D. P. (2005). TRP channels in mechanosensation. *Current Opinion in Neurobiology, 15*(3), 350-357.

Magerl, W. & Treede, R. D. (1996). Heat-evoked vasodilatation in human hairy skin: axon reflexes due to low-level activity of nociceptive afferents. *Journal of Physiology, 497*(Pt 3), 837-848.

Mardy, S., Miura, Y., Endo, F., Matsuda, I., Sztriha, L., Frossard, P., et al. (1999). Congenital insensitivity to pain with anhidrosis: novel mutations in the TRKA (NTRK1) gene encoding a high-affinity receptor for nerve growth factor. *American Journal of Human Genetics, 64*(6), 1570-1579.

Mayer, D. J., Wolfle, T. L., Akil, H., Carder, B., & Liebeskind, J. C. (1971). Analgesia from electrical stimulation in the brainstem of the rat. *Science,174,* 1351-1354.

Melzack, R. & Wall, P. D. (1965). Pain mechanisms: A new theory. *Science, 158*(8699), 971-979.

Melzack, R. & Wall, P. D. (1996). *The challenge of pain (updated 2nd ed.).* New York: Penguin Books.

Meyer, R. A. & Campbell, J. N. (1981). Myelinated nociceptive afferents account for the hyperalgesia that follows a burn to the hand. *Science, 213*(4515), 1527-1529.

Mogil, J. S., Sternberg, W. F., Balian, H., Marek, P., Sadowski, B., & Liebeskind, J. C. (1996). Opioid and nonopioid swim stress-induced analgesia: a parametric analysis in mice. *Physiology and Behavior, 59*(1), 123-132.

Moncada, S., Ferreira, S. H., & Vane, J. R. (1975). Inhibition of prostaglandin biosynthesis as the mechanism of analgesia of aspirin-like drugs in the dog knee joint. *European Journal of Pharmacology, 31*(2), 250-260.

Moret, V., Forster, A., Laverriere, M. C., Lambert, H., Gaillard, R. C., Bourgeois, P., et al. (1991). Mechanism of analgesia induced by hypnosis and acupuncture: Is there a difference? *Pain, 45*(2), 135-140.

Morgan, J. I. & Curran, T. (1991). Stimulus-transcription coupling in the nervous system: involvement of the inducible proto-oncogenes fos and jun. *Annual Review of Neuroscience, 14,* 421-51.

Pert, C. B. & Snyder, S. H. (1973). Opiate receptor: demonstration in nervous tissue. *Science, 179*(77), 1011-1014.

Prieto, G. J., Cannon, J. T., & Liebeskind, J. C. (1983). N. Raphe magnus lesions disrupt stimulation produced analgesia from ventral but not dorsal midbrain areas in the rat. *Brain Research, 261,* 53-57.

Raja, S. N., Meyer, R. A., Ringkamp, M., & Campbell, J. N. (1999). Peripheral neural mechanisms of nociception. In P. D. Wall & R. Melzack (Eds.), *Textbook of pain* (4th ed., pp. 11-58). Edinburgh, Scotland: Churchill Livingston.

Reid, G. (2005). ThermoTRP channels and cold sensing: what are they really up to? *Pflugers Archiv, 451*(1), 250-263.

Reynolds, D. V. (1969). Surgery in the rat during electrical analgesia induced by focal brain stimulation. *Science, 164,* 444-445.

Richardson, D. E. (1983). Intracranial stimulation for the control of chronic pain. *Clinical Neurosurgery, 31,* 316-322.

Richardson, D. E. (1995). Deep brain stimulation for the relief of chronic pain. *Neurosurgery Clinics of North America, 6*(1), 135-144.

Salvador, A., Suay, F., Gonzalez-Bono, E., & Serrano, M. A. (2003). Anticipatory cortisol, testosterone and psychological responses to judo competition in young men. *Psychoneuroendocrinology, 28*(3), 364-375.

Spiegel, D. & Albert, L. H. (1983). Naloxone fails to reverse hypnotic alleviation of chronic pain. *Psychopharmacology (Berl), 81*(2), 140-143.

Sternberg, W., Bokat, C., Kass, L., Alboyadjian, A., & Gracely, R. (2001). Sex-dependent components of the analgesia induced by athletic competition. *Journal of Pain 2*(1), 65-74.

Sternberg, W. F., Bailin, D., Grant, M., & Gracely, R. H. (1998). Competition alters the perception of noxious stimuli in male and female athletes. *Pain, 76,* 231-238.

Suay, F., Salvador, A., Gonzalez-Bono, E., Sanchis, C., Martinez, M., Martinez-Sanchis, S., Simon, et al. (1999). Effects of competition and its outcome on serum testosterone, cortisol and prolactin. *Psychoneuroendocrinology, 24*(5), 551-566.

Terman, G. W., Lewis, J. W., & Liebeskind, J. C. (1984). Endogenous pain inhibitory substrates and mechanisms. *Advances in Pain Research, 7,* 43-56.

Terman, G. W., Shavit, Y., Lewis, J. W., Cannon, J. T., & Liebeskind, J. C. (1984). Intrinsic mechanisms of pain inhibition: Activation by stress. *Science, 226,* 1270-1277.

Tolle, T. R., Kaufmann, T., Siessmeier, T., Lautenbacher, S., Berthele, A., Munz, F., et al. (1999). Region-specific encoding of sensory and affective components of pain in the human brain: a positron emission tomography correlation analysis. *Annals of Neurology, 45*(1), 40-7.

Watkins, L. R. & Mayer, D. J. (1982). Multiple endogenous opiate and non-opiate analgesia systems: evidence of their existence and clinical implications. *Annals New York Academy of Sciences,* 273-299.

Watkins, L. R., Wiertelak, E. P., Grisel, J. E., Silbert, L. H., & Maier, S. F. (1992). Parallel activation of multiple spinal opiate systems appears to mediate 'non-opiate' stress-induced analgesias. *Brain Research, 594,* 99-108.

Wilson, J. A., Garry, E. M., Anderson, H. A., Rosie, R., Colvin, L. A., Mitchell, R. & Fleetwood-Walker, S. M. (2005). NMDA receptor antagonist treatment at the time of nerve injury prevents injury-induced changes in spinal NR1 and NR2B subunit expression and increases the sensitivity of residual pain behaviours to subsequently administered NMDA receptor antagonists. *Pain, 117*(3), 421-432.

Chapter Eighteen

Matching Psychological Strategies with Physical Rehabilitation: Integrated Rehabilitation

Frances A. Flint
York University

Psychological interventions are consistently used to assist athletes during the period of recovery after sport injury. Traditionally, the timing of the use of these psychological strategies and skills has been based primarily on feedback from injured athletes, from experience of sports medicine professionals, or as a response to rehabilitation-disruptive behavior from athletes. To date, athletic therapists/trainers have not had a framework upon which to integrate psychological or sport-related interventions. Anchoring psychological and sport aspects of rehabilitation to the physical healing process provides such a framework. Proactive psychological interventions can now be employed in order to enhance the recovery process and provide total body rehabilitation for injured athletes.

For many years there has been a consensus that psychological intervention has a role to play in sport injury rehabilitation (Evans & Hardy, 2002; Flint, 1998b; Udry, 2001). Most of the discussion regarding the use of psychological strategies or skills in injury recovery relates to which skills can be most effective and when these interventions should be utilized. While we do not have a significant body of evidence-based practice on which to establish guidelines for psychological skills and strategies to assist in injury rehabilitation, we do have feedback from athletes through anecdotal reports and qualitative research (Podlog & Eklund, 2006, Vergeer, 2006). Injured athletes struggle with the experiences of removal from their normal sport routine and with the associated difficulties of rehabilitation. Having open lines of communication with them while they encounter rehabilitation and through after-recovery reflections helps sports medicine professionals understand their needs and wants.

Integrated Rehabilitation

What is integrated rehabilitation? It is a recognition that we cannot treat just the physical injuries of the athlete—that the complete person must be considered within a rehabilitation design that accommodates for not only the physical/physiological injury, but also psychological and sport aspects. The approach to treating the whole person and not just the injury has been called a "biopsychosocial" approach (Brewer et al., 2005) and was initially described for sport injury rehabilitation by Weiss and Troxel (1986). By utilizing the Integrated Rehabilitation Model (Flint, 1998a), the needs of the whole person are addressed during the recovery process.

Physical Recovery from Injury

What physical/physiological implications are there for each phase of rehabilitation? We know that the body follows an orderly process of healing so that anatomic continuity can be regained (Leadbetter, 1978). Throughout each phase of the healing process, the body releases specific hormones and chemicals to remove dead tissue, limit swelling, create new arteries, and bring in collagen for tissue regeneration. This process takes time, and appropriate sequencing and is not something that can easily or appropriately be accelerated. What we do not know at this time is what influence physiological factors have on psychological well being or vice versa:

- Do the severity of an injury and the amount of tissue damage influence the psychological response?
- Does the psychological outlook of the athlete positively or negatively influence the physiological process of healing?

To date, the majority of research has investigated these two factors independently without considering the impact each has on the other (Flint, 1998c). It is easy to understand, however, that we must attempt to marry all of the areas that influence the healing process and the athlete so that a complete recovery is achieved (Flint, 1998b). There is no point in encouraging physical healing without promoting psychological and sport-related factors simultaneously. All too often athletes are declared physically fit to play without the issues of psychological and sport readiness being considered. In order to assist in simultaneously addressing all the issues of physical/physiological and psychological responses and sport factors, we can use the healing process for the appropriate timelines for various strategies and skills applications.

Healing Process

Typically, we use a classification of mechanism of injury to identify the two basic etiologies of injury: macrotrauma and microtrauma (see Figure 1).

- In macrotrauma, we see a single, traumatic event as the mechanism of injury. In this case, the athlete sustains a fracture, strain (muscle), sprain (ligament), contusion, laceration, dislocation, or neurological injury usually caused by an external impact on the body. The episode is sudden and could be self-inflicted or from an opponent or sport implement.
- Microtraumatic injury, on the other hand, is caused by multiple, small impacts that gradually break down tissue. These injuries are usually classified as stress fractures, tendonopathies, or "overuse." This kind of injury may take weeks or months to become symptomatic as the athlete continues to work the body part. There is a distinctly different psychological impact in microtraumatic

injury because the situation develops over many weeks and the athlete's performance gradually decreases without apparent cause (Flint, 1998b). As the athlete works even harder to improve performance, the tissue experiences more trauma, resulting in a final breakdown. Sports medicine professionals working with athletes who have overuse injuries must note that the level of frustration can be much higher with microtrauma because there isn't a single event or any one causative incident that the athlete can point to as the beginning of the injury.

Figure 1.

The onset and progression of macrotraumatic injury

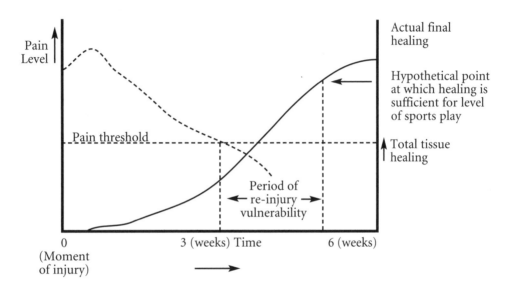

Reprinted by permission from W.B. Leadbetter, 1992. Cell-matrix response in tendon injury. *Clinics in Sports Medicine, 11,* 561-562

The difference between macro and microtrauma with respect to the process of healing relates mainly to the acute phase where we typically see all the signs of inflammation with macrotrauma, but not with microtrauma (Leadbetter, 1992). Microtraumatic injuries generally do not show the signs of inflammation because the repeated damage to the tissue is just below clinical levels until the yield or "breaking" point in the tissue is reached. When the yield point is reached, pain is generally the primary symptom experienced by the athlete. Since the primary cause of microtrauma is repeated, minor level damage, most often athletes attempt to work through the pain in order to keep training and competing. It is only when the pain becomes unbearable or a diagnosis of overuse injury is made that an athlete will be restricted in workouts. It is easy to see, therefore, why this kind of injury creates high levels of frustration and potentially long periods of rehabilitation.

Figure 2.

The onset and progression of microtraumatic injury

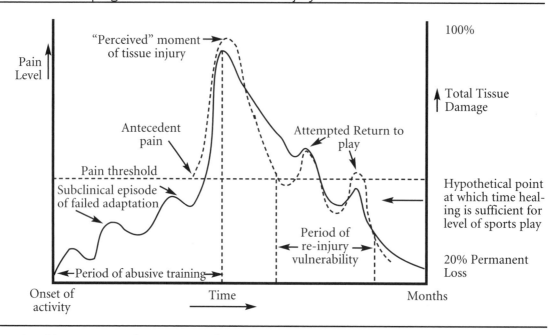

Reprinted by permission from W.B. Leadbetter, 1992. Cell-matrix response in tendon injury. *Clinics in Sports Medicine, 11,* 561-562

Figure 3.

Integrated Rehabilitation Model

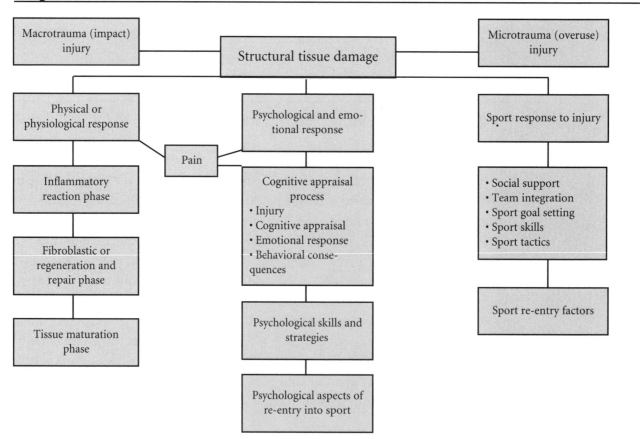

The healing process is divided into three phases based on the body's reaction to the injury and to the kinds of biological functions that occur in order to heal the damaged tissue. Initially, we have an acute or inflammatory phase, followed by the fibroblastic or proliferative (sometimes called repair and regeneration) phase, and culminating with the tissue maturation or remodelling (sometimes called functional) phase. It is a distinguishing feature in a microtraumatic injury situation that the acute or inflammatory phase may not be evident since the tissue damage gradually accumulates over time staying just below noticeable signs of trauma.

Acute or Inflammatory Phase

During this phase, the body typically reacts to the trauma with vascular, chemical, and cellular mediators in an attempt to control the damage. The cardinal signs of inflammatory were described by Celsus nearly 2000 years ago as dolar (pain), tumor (swelling), calor (heat), rubor (redness) and, added later, functio laesa (loss of function)(Cameron, 2003). These signs are typically seen with macrotraumatic injuries, but not as commonly with microtraumatically caused injuries. This inflammatory phase lasts 2–4 days but may be influenced somewhat by the kinds of therapy received. This is not to say that sports medicine professionals attempt to speed up healing, but rather that they try to prevent the lingering effects of inflammation, which can delay the overall healing process.

Fibroblastic Phase

Other than a reduction in swelling, redness, heat, and pain, there aren't any overt signals that the body is now moving on in the healing process. Within the fibroblastic phase, there are several overlapping functions that begin about 5 days after the injury and continue for about 3–4 weeks (Starkey & Johnson, 2006). Once the inflammation has abated, the rebuilding of tissue begins with an influx of fibroblasts, a matrix of new tissue is laid down, and new blood vessels (angiogenesis) are formed. If an athlete returns to competition during this phase, there may be a healing setback as the matrix of tissue (collagen) is not mature and is unable to withstand forces placed upon it. Unfortunately, because the obvious signs of inflammation have abated and pain is greatly reduced, athletes may feel that they can return to competition. Depending on the extent of the initial injury, the mind may not be in congruence with the body and the athlete may be frustrated in being held back from returning to sport. Obviously, this is not the case with severe injury where the athlete is still experiencing physical restrictions, but it is a common occurrence with less trauma.

Maturation Phase

This is a critical phase in healing because the weak and unruly matrix of new collagen experiences mechanical stressors that help to align the matrix fibers along these lines of stress. This realignment of collagen may take up to 18 months to be completed, but is critical to the regaining of strength. This is why the phase is called maturation or remodelling. It is also the phase where the majority of sport-specific functional rehabilitation takes place as the athlete is prepared to return to competition. Athletes often return to competition before this phase has been finalized with ongoing rehabilitation while competing.

Matching Psychological Skills and Strategies with the Healing Process

Although we have little evidence-based clinical research to support the premise that psychological skills and strategies should be matched to the healing process, it seems intuitive and logical that this approach be utilized. The injured athlete is experiencing various physiological/physical reactions to the trauma and specific therapeutic treatments, so at least we have a framework with which to match other interventions (see Table 1). As the rehabilitation progresses and new treatments or therapies are used, adjustments to the skills or strategies can be made and there can be some anticipation of events to come (i.e., setbacks or plateaus).

The keys to the initiation of various psychological skills and strategies within the rehabilitation program are open lines of communication among the athletes, sports medicine professionals, coaches, and any sport psychology consultants working with the athletes. Injured athletes appreciate a collaborative approach to the recovery process and since it is a "process" with relatively established phases, there can be open discussion about the days, weeks, or months ahead. Beginner injured athletes who do not have any experiences on which to base their behavioral response to the injury and rehabilitation effort will need considerable guidance from the therapy staff and previously injured athletes. If the injured athlete can be encouraged to make the same commitment to the rehabilitation program as was made to the sport, then the recovery process can be more successful.

At the outset, immediately after the injury has occurred, there may be a period of time when the athlete may not want to address the issues of rehabilitation. Still having the injury scenario in mind, the athlete may be going through a cognitive appraisal of what effects the injury is going to have on current and future endeavors. For example, the interaction of the injury scenario and the environment in which the athlete competes creates a matrix of influences. These influences can come from family, coaches, teammates, medical personnel, or the athlete himself or herself. Keeping this in mind, sports medicine professionals should be patient and wait until the athlete is ready to open up to discussion and information. Providing counseling at this phase has much to do with listening and being empathetic.

A. Acute Phase

Acute phase psychological skills and strategies are needed to deal with a number of matters:
(a) emotions related to the injury situation,
(b) understanding the current injury situation (diagnosis) and future situation (prognosis),
(c) understanding the healing process,
(d) understanding the realities of pain,
(e) understanding the change in status from athlete to injured athlete,

Table 1.

Rehabilitation Goal-Setting Chart (Adapted from Flint, 1998b)

Physical or Physiological Goals	Psychological Goals	Sport Goals
Inflammatory Reaction Phase (Clinical Goals)	**Cognitive Appraisal Process**	**Initial Injury Phase**
• Reduce swelling	Increase knowledge of injury staff and other athletes	Demonstrate support from coaching
• Reduce pain	Increase knowledge of available coping resources (particularly pain management)	
• Protect from further injury	Increase knowledge of support systems	
• Maintain existing ROM (range of motion)	Positive self-talk	
• Educate on healing, nutrition, rehabilitation, psychological factors		
Fibroblastic phase (Clinical Goals)	**Rehabilitation psychological skills and strategies**	**Sport rehabilitation strategies**
• Increase ROM	Relaxation, goal setting, Rational Emotive Therapy	Sport skill goal setting Rehabilitation social support
• Maintain cardiovascular	Knowledge of set backs	Sport skill visualizations
• Increase proprioception	Healing visualizations	Sport tactics and strategies visualizations
• Regain muscle endurance		Potential team involvement
• Promote tissue healing		
• Increase flexibility		
• Address scar tissue		
• Address other physical issues		
Maturation phase (Functional Goals)	**Psychological preparation for re-entry into competition**	**Preparation for sport re-entry**
• Increase strength	Increase confidence in body parts via functional progressions	Ensure knowledge of team tactics and strategies
• Increase power	Increase confidence in performance skills	Ensure "game fitness"
• Increase sport-specific functional activity	Knowledge of "flashbacks"	Ensure understanding of team dynamics • • •
• Increase sport-specific cardiovascular fitness	Performance visualizations	Re-entry goals
• Increase proprioception		
• Increase agility		
• Address psychological issues		

Discharge Parameters (from Athletic Therapist/Trainer)
• 90% strength (endurance and power) compared to opposite side
• Full pain-free ROM
• Full flexibility
• Pain free
• Full proprioception
• Sport-specific cardiovascular fitness
• Psychological issues addressed (or referred)

(f) gaining insight into the medical support (resources) available,

(g) gaining confidence in the sports medicine team, and

(h) becoming acquainted with a new social support group–other injured athletes.

Some of these issues can be grouped together to better provide clarity in the issues. For example, introducing the injured athlete to a group of other injured athletes provides a sense of new social support group membership and at the same time helps the athlete gain a perspective on the status of being injured. Much valuable information and many behavioral cues can be learned in an injured-athlete support group, and this one psychological strategy is a key element in a rehabilitation program (Ewing, Lewis, Magyar, & Pfaller, 2002; Flint, 1991). Certainly for a newly injured athlete, a group of currently injured athletes provides a good forum in which to express emotions about the injury. This would be a knowledgeable, empathetic, and relative peer social support group.

Education is a crucial component in the acute phase because it establishes the foundation for the athlete's behavior, decision making, and goal setting during the rest of the rehabilitation program. Not only do athletes gain valuable information, but they also form a working relationship and gain confidence in the sports medicine team through these educational discussions. Athletes want both procedural and outcome information early on in their rehabilitation primarily because they are experiencing something new. This means that they want to know what is involved in rehabilitation, how rehabilitation is going to occur, and if they are going to be as good as or better than they were before the injury. Care must be taken, however, to provide athletes with all the necessary information without overwhelming or frightening them. One National Hockey League player, who had a compound fracture of his tibia and fibula, noted that it wasn't until he received information from the surgeon on what his surgery would involve that he knew he could recover (F. A. Flint, personal communication, 1994). For some time prior to talking with the surgeon, this professional player had been looking at the bones of his leg sticking out through his sock and was imagining all the terrible things about the injury. He was devastated with the potential loss of his playing career. Knowledge about the kind of injury that has been sustained, what structures have been injured, what is involved in rehabilitation, what the athlete needs to do to recover; and most importantly, what the timing of recovery might be is critical information for the injured athlete during the acute phase. Sports medicine personnel are in a perfect position to be the primary communicators about the injury status, and once again, this helps in forming partnerships and building confidence in the recovery.

Because of partnerships and collaborations established during the acute phase, sports medicine personnel can be observant of the behavior and verbalizations of injured athletes. Often as a reaction to the injury we see negative cognitions and verbalizations become evident in athletes. Athletes may blame themselves for the injury and make statements like "You idiot!" and "How could you be so clumsy?" Also, there may be very graphic, negative comments, such as "I blew out my knee," which is often heard after a knee injury. These kinds of negative statements do not lend themselves well to a positive, encouraged outlook toward the injury or the rehabilitation. Most often, athletes are not aware that they are making these statements, or they do not realize that these kinds of negative statements can hinder gaining a positive approach or outlook toward the recovery. It is important that sports medicine personnel do not use negative, graphic statements describing injuries and that they discuss this kind of verbalization with the injured athletes. Generally, once athletes have become aware of the impact of negative verbalizations, they stop making such statements. Using positive self-talk is the key to enhancing a positive outlook toward recovery.

One important issue needing special attention during the acute phase is pain. Since pain is a multidimensional experience, there are multiple needs to be addressed in pain management. "Pain is never the sole creation of our anatomy and physiology. It emerges only at the intersection of bodies, minds, and cultures" (Morris, 1991, p. 3). To make matters worse, pain may occur in the absence of injury and injury may not result in pain (Melzack & Wall, 1988). This is particularly evident in early phases of microtrauma and situations where pain is incongruent with the extent of the tissue damage. These issues present a challenge for the whole sports medicine team and the injured athlete.

Since pain is influenced by both psychological and physiological factors (Melzack and Wall, 1988), we again need to address the whole person, not just the expression of pain. Currently, it is felt that there are three primary ways to influence the perception of pain: Gate Control Theory (Melzack and Wall, 1988, Melzack, 1997); endorphin release; and, Central Biasing Theory (Prentice, 2004):

- The Gate Control Theory proposes that the slower signals of pain from the periphery can be blocked in the spinal cord (substantia gelatinosa) by flooding the "gate" with faster signals such as touch. A Transcutaneous Cutaneous Nerve Stimulation (TENS) unit works on this principle.

- Endorphin (endogenous opiate-like neurotransmitter) release is the body's own response to tissue damage and stimulation of nociceptors (pain-related nerve endings). Electrical stimulation can also be used to aid in the release of endorphins.

- The last theory, called Central Biasing, is based on the premise that our past history in some way influences our current perceptions. The best example of this is getting a needle. Even though the needle has not yet touched the skin, most people recoil because they remember previous needle injections. Our mind has told us that it remembers feeling pain with a previous encounter with a needle.

Psychological skills and strategies can be used relative to all three pain theories with the typical approaches involving the use of imagery, distraction, and attention to the pain. Imagery can take several different directions, including a focus on the actual functioning of the modality (e.g., TENS) being used or a focus on what physiological response is occurring because of the modality (e.g., closing a gate to pain transmissions). Additionally, the athlete may be asked to use imagery to focus on reviewing the team's offenses or defenses while receiving a treatment, and this helps distract the athlete from any pain that is being experienced. This approach allows for the use of a physical modality combined with a distraction through imagery. In order to gain a sense of control over pain, some athletes benefit from focusing directly on the pain being experienced, including imagining exactly how the pain is being transmitted to the brain. This is a very advanced technique that is not as popular with athletes and has had equivocal support. Imagery scripts can be written by the therapists in conjunction with the injured athletes; sport tactics or techniques can be written by the coach and the injured athlete. This also promotes a collaborative approach to the healing process.

B. Fibroblastic Phase

During the second phase–fibroblastic or proliferative–we see a number of different situations that the recovering athlete must deal with:

(a) acceptance of the fact that rehabilitation is going to take time and effort,

(b) maintenance of a commitment to excellence even during rehabilitation,

(c) working through plateaus or setbacks in rehabilitation, and

(d) dealing with the frustration of not being a fully functioning athlete.

This phase has more to do with the work ethic of the athlete because the phase of passive rehabilitation (acute phase) when the athlete receives treatment (e.g., ice massage, cold whirlpools) is past. No longer is the athlete just quietly sitting by while the therapy staff works on the injured body part, but now must be more committed to work hard at each of the physical therapies or exercises utilized by the therapy staff. For example, the athlete will be asked to work on proprioception, increasing range of motion, and some light endurance strength exercises. Cheating on this work will not provide the desired results. The athlete must be active and engaged in this phase of healing.

One of the most important psychological strategies used during the fibroblastic phase is goal setting. Athletic therapists/trainers use goal setting every day during the designing of the rehabilitation program. For example, if the athlete is in the acute phase and there are the usual signs of inflammation, athletic therapist/trainers will identify the reduction of swelling and pain as two goals that need to be achieved. They will utilize compression and cold throughout the day in order to reach the goal of swelling and pain reduction. Thus, goal setting is part of the repertoire of knowledge of the sports medicine staff. In the same way, athletes are adept at using goal setting in their sports. Goals established by athletes and coaches would relate to learning a certain new skill in order to beat an opponent or gaining or utilizing a new tactic in order to counteract an opponent's strategy. Goals are an integral part of the athlete's life, so collaborating with the athletic therapist/trainer to use goal setting to address the athlete's need during rehabilitation would be a worthwhile psychological strategy to employ. Maintaining the athlete's highest effort and interest, as well as commitment to the rehabilitation program, especially if it a long process, are some of the benefits of using goal setting.

Because the second phase of the healing process can be long and arduous with an apparent lack of progress, there can be periods of frustration for the athlete. During this time, the body is healing, but there is often little outward manifestation of this progress. The athlete may also be dealing with setbacks, such as a return of swelling, or plateaus where no progress is achieved at all. In order to deal with the possibility of frustration, setbacks, or plateaus during this phase, we often see the recommendation that athletes learn how to use relaxation skills. This particular motor skill is valuable in dealing with increased stress and is a tool particularly pertinent to rehabilitation. The only problem with learning relaxation skills during injury rehabilitation is that the athlete is already under stress and is now attempting to learn a motor skill in order to decrease stress. This is analogous to a coach teaching an athlete a new skill in the middle of a game—something that is not done. The best case scenario involves *all* athletes learning relaxation skills *before* the season begins. In this way, all athletes learn this motor skill in low-stress situations and can then hone their relaxation skills as the season progresses and stress increases. If an injury occurs, the athlete is already prepared with relaxation training. This is not to say that learning the skills of relaxation during injury rehabilitation is not worthwhile, only that it is more beneficial to learn this type of stress-reducing skill before the season begins.

One recommendation that is constantly heard during this phase is to keep the athlete involved with the team so that the athlete remains connected to the team or sport. The typical suggestions for involving injured athletes is by having them take stats at games or helping with scouting the opposing team before games. Although this seems like a perfectly reasonable way of helping the athlete keep up with the sport and teammates, not all athletes respond positively. One athlete had a very negative experience being close to his team after a season ending medical condition:

> Once I got back to the field, it was 10 times worse because I was in a place where most of us feel most comfortable and I couldn't participate. . . . I didn't know how I was going to go on . . . watching these guys . . . running and doing drills and everything and I'm not a part of it. (F. A. Flint, personal communication, 2003)

This is only an anecdotal account, but it may highlight real, inner feelings of frustrated injured athletes. Care must be taken to ensure that involving the athlete with the team or sport is actually of benefit to the athlete. Athletes need to feel secure enough in their communication with the therapy staff and coaches to be able to state how this recommendation affects them psychologically.

As has been stated, the fibroblastic phase of rehabilitation is a long, arduous process. It is a time when the recovering athlete has a need for continued education about how the body heals, more collaborative work with the therapy staff, particularly on goal setting, and most importantly, social support. If it is possible to continue the injured athlete support group that was initiated in the acute phase, then the athlete's need for social support can be satisfied and the possibility of benefiting from a coping model in the group can be enhanced. This type of informal modelling, where the injured athlete attends to a similarly injured recovering athlete, provides valuable cues on rehabilitation behavior and commitment (Flint, 1998)

During the acute phase, there are occasions when we see negative self talk or poor verbalizations concerning the injury. In the fibroblastic phase, this trend can continue unless it was checked in the acute phase, but we can also see negative cognitions re-emerge as a result of frustration over experiencing a setback or plateau in the recovery. Here is a perfect time for a psychological strategy called Rational Emotive Therapy or ABCDE technique. This approach to negative self-talk and poor cognitions was adapted from Albert Ellis, who used this technique to deal with anxiety (Greenberg, 1987). In this approach, there is an attempt to *alter* the cognitions of the injured athlete away from negative thoughts to realistic and positive ones. In a sport injury example this is what the ABCDE approach would look like:

A. Activating stressor—injury (in this case, a knee injury)

B. Belief system—identify rational and irrational beliefs: "I blew out my knee," or "My career is over."

C. Consequences —mental, physical, or behavioral consequences: anger, depression, frustration, changes in relationships

D. Dispute irrational beliefs—"I have seen others recover from this injury and return to play," or "Hard work will get my knee stronger again."

E. Effect of changed beliefs and behavior: "I can beat this injury and get back to playing."

Rational Emotive Therapy sounds like an imposing psychological technique reserved for psychologists, but actually it is a relatively easy approach to helping athletes identify their negative beliefs about the injury and recovery and provide alternatives to achieve a positive approach. The key to dealing with a poor belief system by injured athletes is identifying it. Sports medicine personnel need to be observant of athletes' behavior and verbalizations as they progress through rehabilitation. If there is concern over dealing with a situation where an athlete has a negative approach to the rehabilitation and recovery, then this would be an example of where referral to a sport psychology consultant would be appropriate. If these negative beliefs and behavior are not identified and adjusted, then the athlete's progress into the maturation phase or return to play may be compromised.

C. Maturation Phase

The last phase of rehabilitation, the maturation or functional phase, is a time when the goals are changing from purely clinical to functional. In the case of an injured athlete, the primary functional goals relate to sport rather than just activities of daily living. So in this phase, most exercises are designed around the athlete's specific sport, skills, and position. In this way, the athlete is practicing sport skills, preparing for re-entering competition, and physically addressing sport specific needs (i.e., cardiovascular conditioning, sport actions). Some of the psychological concerns at this time involve

(a) being patient with rehabilitation,

(b) gaining confidence in the rehabilitated body part,

(c) understanding re-entry factors such as game fitness and team dynamics,

(d) recognizing flashbacks, and

(e) setting realistic re-entry performance goals.

Within the maturation phase, the main physical goals include maintaining ROM and flexibility while increasing strength (especially power), proprioception, agility, and sport-specific cardiovascular fitness. All of these physical goals become more fun, however, because they can be designed to be sport-specific. For example, a basketball player can dribble the ball while standing on a balance implement. Adjusting the maturation phase to be sport-specific is a creativity challenge for athletic therapists/trainers, but this adjustment definitely encourages more fun, interest, and enthusiasm in the athlete. It also assists with maintaining a commitment to hard work and aids in combating boredom and declining patience in doing rehabilitation.

One of the most important aspects of this phase of rehabilitation is the athlete's confidence in the previously injured body part. Confidence cannot be "given" to the athlete; it must be earned. What is the best way to build confidence in a particular body part? First, ROM and strength tests can be conducted to demonstrate to the athlete that the body part is close to or equal to the opposite body part. This is only the beginning, however, since the athlete actually needs to gain confidence by successfully completing gradually more difficult functional skills. An example of gradually more difficult functional skills for a soccer player with a previous ankle injury might involve the following:

- light jog straight ahead,
- light jog in a large figure 8,
- light jog in a smaller figure 8,
- running straight ahead,
- running in a large figure 8,
- running in a smaller figure 8,
- light jog in a zigzag pattern,
- running in a zigzag pattern,
- dribbling the ball ahead in a light jog,
- dribbling the ball in a large figure 8,
- and so on.

With successful completion of each phase, the athlete gains more confidence in the ankle. Any pain or swelling means that the athlete takes a few steps back and delays more aggressive work. Confidence is a critical factor in a successful re-entry into the sport, so it is a primary focus for athletic therapists/trainers.

During this phase also, daily goal setting helps athletes understand that the body's healing process is ongoing. There is a danger in this phase that athletes will think they are ready to participate in sport again because the body part feels strong and all the signs of inflammation are gone. This is a case where the mind does not have a clear perception of the actual strength of collagen fibers or scar tissue. If athletes have been educated about the healing process throughout the rehabilitation process, then there is more understanding that the body may not be ready even though the mind may be prepared to return.

Education and the establishing of realistic expectations of game fitness and re-entry performance is an essential ingredient in the maturation phase. This is also a time when coaches can play an important role in helping the athlete understand and prepare for re-entry. Coaches can make sure the athlete is up to date with current tactics of the team and aware of the current status of the team or sport and situation in which the athlete will be returning. Coaches can help the re-entry process by reducing the stress athletes may feel related to performance. Some athletes feel that they must show the coaches and other athletes that they are as good as they were before the injury, creating a situation in which they may try too hard and setting themselves up for re-injury. One of the most effective psychological tools to assist with performance-related issues in the re-entry process is visualizations. Coaches can provide some scripts or scenarios for performance, team offenses and defenses, and performance visualizations.

During this phase of recovery, athletes sometimes experience "flashbacks" or recreations of their injury in their minds. These flashbacks can be most disturbing for the athlete and may totally disrupt the recovery and re-entry process. One basketball player who was attempting to return to competition experienced severe flashbacks after her second major surgery. "When I would go to practice my basketball skills after the second surgery. . . . I would be doing my skill and see my knee blow out again. . . . Not only did I see it blow out, but it was really graphic" (Flint, 1998b, p. 47). In this case, the athlete was very adept at using visualizations, so her flashback was very graphic and upsetting. Her skill and experience in using visualizations also helped her recover from her flashbacks, as she used her imagery in slow motion to re-program her mind into seeing a correct biomechanical movement of her knee.

Education about the possibility of flashbacks is critical for athletes so they understand that this phenomenon may occur. Athletes have been known to keep quiet about flashbacks, thinking that there is something wrong with them. Using clear, concise visualizations may help deal with this problem as the correct movements are recreated in the visualization. In addition, keeping the lines of communication open and anticipating the need for help through potential cases of flashbacks is important for sports medicine personnel.

Discharge Parameters

Discharge parameters are key physical indicators that healing has reached a particular phase and that the athlete is ready to transition from rehabilitation exercise to sport re-entry. It is not a special "exam" that athletes must pass, but rather a gradual clearing of these criteria during the late maturation phase. In effect, discharge parameters become long-term goals for the injured athlete since these must be achieved before re-entry into sport can be completed. These criteria for return to sport should not be a surprise to the athletes. When injured athletes are educated at the outset of rehabilitation, they can see what their final targets are and can collaboratively set plans for the achievement of those goals.

Prehabilitation

Prehabilitation is a period of time between an injury and the subsequent surgery. Often surgeons wait until the effects of the initial injury have been dealt with before contemplating operating. The primary reason behind this delay is to allow the body to decrease any effects of inflammation and allow time to build up range of motion and strength. Naturally, there will be a decrease in strength, range of motion, flexibility, proprioception, and fitness after surgery, but this decrease is somewhat lessened by prehabilitation.

The period of time between injury and surgery is difficult for athletes. To them it feels like they are going nowhere because they cannot return to play until rehabilitation is complete after surgery, but they have to wait for the surgery. Many athletes question the value of doing strength training, range of motion exercise and the rest of the rehabilitation routine if they will have to do the same again after surgery. Rather than viewing this prehabilitation as being in limbo, it is important that athletes consider this as valuable preparation for surgery. Once again, sports medicine professionals are in a good position to educate the athlete about the healing process and preparation for surgery. This is also a time when the skills of relaxation and goal setting are integral in helping the athlete gain a sense of balance and stability prior to surgery. If the athlete has not previously learned these techniques, then this is good time to begin an educational process that will help to deal with stress prior to surgery and with the challenges of rehabilitation and re-entry.

Summary

Rehabilitation from major injury is a challenge for athletes, particularly those who have never faced it before. It is also a trial for sports medicine professionals in terms of identifying psychological reactions to injury and rehabilitation and integrating psychological techniques and strategies into the process of recovery. Anchoring psychological strategies and interventions to the physical healing process creates a framework for therapists. This framework helps by identifying stages where athletes are more prone to display certain psychological reactions or behaviors that can be roadblocks to recovery. Athletic therapists/trainers can then anticipate and utilize basic interventions or seek referrals from sport psychology consultants. Marrying psychological and sport aspects of injury rehabilitation to the healing process seems to provide the perfect solution to the provision of integrated injury recovery.

References

Bianco, T., Malo, S., and Orlick, T. (1999). Sport injury and illness: Elite skiers describe their experiences. *Research Quarterly for Exercise and Sport, 70*, 157-169.

Brewer, B. W., Andersen, M. B., and Van Raalte, J. L. (2005). A biopsychosocial model of sport injury rehabilitation: toward a biopsychosocial approach. In D. I. Mostofsky and L. D. Zaichkowski (Eds.), *Medical aspects of sport and exercise*. Morgantown, WV: Fitness Information Technology.

Cameron, M. H. (2003). *Physical agents in rehabilitation: From research to practice* (2ⁿᵈ ed.). Philadelphia, PA: Harcourt Brace.

Crossman, J. (2001). Managing thoughts, stress, and pain. In J. Crossman (Ed.), *Coping with sports injuries: Psychological strategies for rehabilitation* (pp. 128-144). New York: Oxford University Press.

Evans, L. and Hardy, L. (2002). Injury rehabilitation: A goal-setting intervention study. *Research Quarterly for Exercise and Sport, 73*, 310-319.

Flint, F. A. (1991). The psychological effects of modeling in athletic injury rehabilitation. (Doctoral dissertation, University of Oregon, 1991). *Microform Publications No. BF 357.*

Flint, F. A. (1998a). *Sport psychology and rehabilitation.* Paper presented at the annual conference of the Eastern Athletic Trainers' Association, Buffalo, NY.

Flint, F. A. (1998b). *Psychology of sport injury.* Champaign, IL: Human Kinetics.

Flint, F. A. (1998c). Integrating sport psychology and sports medicine in research: The dilemmas. *Journal of Applied Sport Psychology, 10*(1), 70-82.

Gordon, S., Potter, M., and Hamer, P. (2001). The role of physiotherapist and sport therapist. In J. Crossman (Ed.), *Coping with sports injuries: Psychological strategies for rehabilitation* (pp. 66-82). New York: Oxford University Press.

Greenberg, J. S. (1987). *Stress management.* Dubuque, IA: Wm. C. Brown

Iveleva, L., & Orlick, T. (1991). Mental links to enhanced healing: an exploratory analysis. *The Sport Psychologist, 4*, 25-40.

Leadbetter, W.B. (1992). Cell-matrix response to tendon injury. *Clinics in Sports Medicine, 11*, 561-562.

Ewing, M. E., Lewis, D.K., Magyar, T. M., & Pfaller, J. (2002). Support groups for injured athletes: Design, implementation, and evaluation. Symposium presented at the Association for the Advancement of Applied Sport Psychology Conference, Tuscon, AZ.

Melzack, R., and Wall, P. (1988). *The challenge of pain.* London: Penguin.

Melzack, R. (1997). *Current concepts of pain.* Paper presented at Canadian Athletic Therapists Conference, Winnipeg, Manitoba.

Morris, D. B. (1991). *The culture of pain.* Berkeley: University of California.

Podlog, L., & Eklund, R.C. (2006). A longitudinal investigation of competitive athletes' return to sport following serious injury. *Journal of applied sport psychology, 18*(1), 44-68.

Prentice, W. E. (2004). *Rehabilitation techniques in sports medicine* (4th ed.). St. Louis, MO: Mosby.

Starkey, C. & Johnson, G. (2006). *Athletic training and sports medicine.* Sudbury, MA: Jones and Bartlett.

Udry, E. (2001). The role of significant others: Social support during injuries. In J. Crossman (Ed.), *Coping with sport injuries: Psychological strategies for rehabilitation* (pp. 148-161). New York: Oxford University Press.

Vergeer, I. (2006). Exploring the mental representation of athletic injury: A longitudinal case study. *Psychology of Sport and Exercise, 7,* 99-114.

Weiss, M. R., and Troxel, R. K. (1986). Psychology of the injured athlete. *Athletic Training, 21,* 104-109, 154

Chapter Nineteen

Shades of Grey: A Sport Psychology Consultation with an Athlete with Injury

R. Renee Newcomer Appaneal
Megan D. Granquist
University of North Carolina at Greensboro

Introduction

Before introducing this case, it is important to provide the reader with information regarding my (first author) background and training, which reflects the approach I take to sport psychology consulting. I have completed graduate degree programs and postdoctoral training in both general and sport psychology. I view my work with clients as fostering their ability to achieve performance excellence, both in and outside of the sport domain. Consultation based upon this philosophy has been referred to as performance psychology (Wikipedia, 2002; Hays and Brown, 2004). During the past year, I have received professional coaching from a colleague in sport psychology, Dr. Charles Brown. One outcome of my work with Dr. Brown has been the development of a framework referred to as the Performance Continuum. In brief, the Performance Continuum illustrates that at any given time one's performance may fall along a continuum ranging from a high level (i.e., excellence) to low level (i.e., impaired), where the area in between endpoints is referred to as the vast array of grey.

Many professionals and particularly students entering the field of sport psychology are drawn to working with the high-performance athlete, where the focus of consultation is usually limited to mental skills training (MST). However, it is not uncommon (and rather frequent) that athletes encounter significant challenges due to sport participation (e.g., athletic injury) or life stress outside of sport (e.g., academic, personal and family relationships, etc.), a phenomenon that has been well documented in the literature (Brewer, Petitpas, and Van Raalte, 1999). In my clinical experience, when athletes appear to be in the grey area, athletic department staff (i.e., coaches, athletic trainers, administrators) have the most trouble in determining what to do. In the presence and/or absence of any obvious significant impairment in performance or functioning, there does not seem to be a clear protocol within the sport culture for identifying and determining how to help student-athletes in the grey.

I have introduced the Performance Continuum to athlete-clients, athletic department personnel, and graduate students for a variety of reasons, including increasing awareness of the broad range of work that is done in this field, conceptualizing a performer's presenting concern and level of impairment, and determining the most appropriate focus of intervention (e.g., MST or mental health referral). I have found it very helpful in conceptualizing where an athlete may be along the continuum at any given point in time, and depending upon that location, determining the most salient issue(s) to address. This, in turn, enables me to establish what might be the most appropriate course of intervention, where the closer an athlete lies to the "excellence" end-point, the more likely he or she will benefit from MST. On the other hand, the closer an athlete is toward the "impairment" endpoint, the more likely it is that a mental health referral or evaluation is most needed. This framework is not meant to replace or expand upon existing assessment tools (or clinical training) in determining an athlete's need or level of impairment. Instead, it is merely introduced here to illustrate in a concrete and straightforward manner what is occurring when athletes are performing below their potential.

Athletes are highly likely to become injured at some point during their career, as illustrated by injury rates around or above 30% (Petrie and Perna, 2004), and many of these injuries will result in at least some degree of performance impairment or limitation. Therefore, an athlete whose location on the Performance Continuum is toward its "excellence" end almost always moves towards the grey area after sustaining an injury. At this point, an athlete's cognitive-appraisal of the situation and subsequent response determines whether he or she will capably return to excellence, remain stuck in the grey, or perhaps continue to deteriorate, moving further along the continuum toward significant impairment.

Competitive athletes are often expected by others to handle the demands placed upon them in sport (e.g., intense physical training, injury risk, travel schedules, etc.) as well as any issues that emerge outside of sport (e.g., difficulty in relationships, schoolwork, death or loss of loved one, etc.). The athlete's coping ability, as well as the ability of his or her injury support network (e.g., athletic trainers, sport psychology consultant, etc.) to recognize the most salient issues and determine the most appropriate course of intervention is essential. To that end, the Performance Continuum is particularly germane to this case in that at the onset of my intervention with Scott[1] my focus was at one end, whereas later it shifted to the opposite end due to a variety of factors. Hence, the case of Scott is intended to illustrate the dynamic nature of sport psychology consultation, where the focus of intervention is likely to change as the athlete's life unfolds and attempts to cope are made. The information provided is presented in the same manner in which it evolved in the consulting relationship (i.e., chronological order of events). Within the intake, a SOAP-note format is used to organize the information obtained from

- the client's self-report: (S: subjective),
- my clinical observations (O: objective),
- and how both S & O were evaluated (A: assessment)
- to determine an intervention plan (P).

The Case of Scott

The Referral

I was initially introduced to the client through a referral from the athletic training staff at an NCAA Division 1 university. Scott, a sophomore student-athlete on the varsity men's basketball team, had been experiencing severe back pain for several months. In the initial referral, it was suggested that the athletic training staff, team physician, and head coach were all in agreement that Scott's symptoms may be in large part due to "his psyche" and his being "too intense." The Certified Athletic Trainer (ATC) who initially contacted me further noted that Scott acknowledged that his intensity was at times too high and he was willing to take whatever steps necessary to resolve the issue.

I must admit that I was quite skeptical of the staff's assessment, yet very curious as to what might really be occurring with Scott. It should be emphasized here that a referral for sport psychology services in response to an athlete's "psyche" allegedly contributing in some way to physical symptoms is worthy of serious consideration. On my university campus, I am known to be a member of the sports medicine treatment team, which enables me to gain access to athletes' protected health information. I was therefore able to obtain additional information from the sports medicine staff regarding Scott's symptom history, existing medical conditions, and current (or planned) treatment recommendations beyond sport psychology intervention.

Through a review of Scott's medical chart and brief dialogue with the sports medicine staff, I learned that his pain had been occurring since last season, at which time Scott was referred to several specialists, including the team physician and a Certified Strength and Conditioning Specialist. Considering that Scott's symptoms remained problematic and apparently did not subside at all, I suspected that a referral to sport psychology may have been seen as a last resort. Nonetheless, I decided to meet with Scott and assess the potential for my being of help. I was aware that Scott was under medical supervision and working with other specialists.

The Intake Interview—Session 1

Subjective

Scott's back pain began in his freshman year during one of his first high-pressure conference games. He recalls feeling the pain spreading from mid to lower back and eventually affecting his legs. By half-time the pain was so severe that despite trying to stretch and take pain medication, he had to leave the game. The pain did not subside with receiving treatment during half-time and rest through the second-half. Due to the extreme nature of the pain, one of the medical personnel in attendance transported

Scott to the local emergency room. There, he received an IV sedative and muscle relaxant. This emergency room experience was quite upsetting to Scott, and he admits being scared at the prospect of having a condition that warranted such a visit. He continued to have pain episodes throughout his freshman season, including one so severe that another trip to the emergency room was necessary. Scott clearly exhibited anxiety about these experiences and feared returning to the emergency room.

When playing, Scott would feel the initial twinges of pain that reminded him of what might follow. When this would occur, his anxiety level would increase. Scott reported he had not found a connection between intensity or duration of play and the pain he experienced. Interestingly, he recalled not having had any episodes during practices or during summer play while at home. In compliance with the advice of the athletic training staff and team physician, he had been receiving back rehabilitation treatment consisting of flexibility and strength training exercises.

As an incoming freshman, he was one of the most highly recruited players on the team. Further, in his freshman year he led the team in many categories. As a sophomore, he believed he was expected to do the same. Scott's present goal, as aligned with his coach's expectations, was to be among the nation's leaders for assists and scoring. He also felt that he "must be there for the team to win."

In addition to basketball, Scott maintained a 16-hour academic course load as a pre-medicine major, consistently earning higher than a B average. Scott also indicated that his relationships with teammates and other friends at school were "okay." He felt that he got along well with his roommate. His roommate was not a member of the basketball team; therefore, their interaction was minimal. Scott felt that he sustained a good relationship with family members. His family resides within a reasonable distance from campus, which permits him to visit with them occasionally during the weekend.

Objective

Scott arrived on-time to the intake session and was dressed in athletic attire. He was listening to an MP3 player, commonly used by college students. He was fairly soft-spoken and tended to respond to questions rather than volitionally providing information. Scott had a pleasant demeanor but appeared nervous and uncomfortable as indicated by incongruent verbal and nonverbal behavior. For example, he smiled frequently throughout the intake, particularly when talking about difficult or stressful experiences such as multiple injuries he had sustained in the past few years (i.e., ankle sprains, wrist injury and a nagging shoulder injury). He also fidgeted in his chair and played with his hands frequently during the intake session.

I provided Scott with a brief overview of MST that included various examples (e.g., activation management, attention control, mental rehearsal, etc.) and a basic structure for how we might proceed. Scott indicated having had prior exposure to MST at a summer basketball camp, although he could neither identify specific skills or how they were taught with any notable detail.

Assessment

Information Scott provided and my observations seemed consistent with the original referral from the ATC, in that Scott did appear to have a high level of activation. He seemed to demonstrate both physical and psychological symptoms, where an obvious focus on physical cues of arousal was present. This heightened sensitivity might have resulted in an exaggerated or anticipatory response to somatic cues. As Scott explained, often he would feel an initial "twinge" of pain and/or tightness and then feel "on edge" in anticipation of another episode of severe pain.

In view of Scott's presentation and personality, it seemed that his level of activation might be contributing to the onset and/or progression of his back pain. Scott's self-report and my intake observation demonstrated definite symptoms of somatic anxiety, such as increased muscle tension and a general feeling of tightness in his body. A few comments he made during the session suggested that his cognitions (e.g., irrational thoughts, negative self-talk, etc.) might play a significant role. Scott's high expectations clearly extended beyond sport and into other domains of his life (e.g., academic). The expectations, whether his own or internalized from his coach or parents, seemed unrealistic based on statements such as, "I must play well for the team to win."

Plan

Since there seemed to be no obvious "impairment" outside of sport (e.g., academic, social, sleep, appetite, etc.), I felt that it would be appropriate to work on a few areas in the domain of mental skills training. We agreed to meet 3–4 times during the next month, where the focus of our work would be to develop strategies to better manage his anxiety.

Based on Scott's high expectations and apparent "irrational beliefs" about self-worth and approval, and the resultant anxiety, the initial plan for intervention was to develop strategies for anxiety management. During the intake, Scott had described mainly somatic symptoms of anxiety (i.e., tightness, muscle tension, etc.). Therefore, it seemed best to begin with a few somatic relaxation techniques (i.e., diaphragmatic breathing and progressive muscle relaxation) aimed at reducing his physical tension. I decided that at some point during the next session, I would further explore his thoughts and expectations and perhaps incorporate cognitive strategies, such as thought stopping, cognitive reframing, or concentration training, into the consultation plan as part of a multimodal anxiety intervention.

MST Intervention—Session 2

The objectives during the first follow-up session were to
(a) further assess Scott's experience of being "too intense," and
(b) initiate relaxation training.
We began the session by reviewing the relevant information obtained during the intake that warranted relaxation training. This served to establish the rationale for intervention and to reinforce Scott's interest and commitment to MST.

Assessment of intensity

I asked Scott to remember a time when he felt his heightened intensity had interfered with performance. He thought for a moment and then began describing a particular game that occurred last season. When he finished I asked him to clarify certain issues and noted that he primarily referred to physical rather than psychological factors. When prompted to describe thoughts that typically occur during a game, it took a while for Scott to provide examples. Eventually he described thoughts that were unrelated to a specific basketball tasks (e.g., homework, upcoming exams, injury versus shooting a free-throw, dribbling, playing defense, etc.) or the game overall. In fact, he indicated that his pain level and associated impairment in physical activity were usually on his mind. Since pain and pain appraisal (i.e., interpretation of the pain and its consequences) may significantly affect mood and concentration, it is quite common that his response was to heighten sensitivity to somatic sensations (e.g., tightness, cramping, etc.).

The issues about which he thinks before or during a game were then elicited and recorded. Among these were upcoming academic tests and school work, muscle cramping and pain, and other physical ailments, including his recurring ankle injury. When asked how often (0%: not at all, to 100%: all the time) these distractions occur, he replied, "Approximately 80% of the time." Scott described these distractions as being overwhelming at times, especially toward the end of a game when multiple time-outs, fouls, and other disruptions to continued play often occur.

Next, I provided a brief overview of concentration skills by using a focus checklist[2]. The checklist contains important and relevant performance focus cues for a specific task (e.g., playing defense, dribbling on a fast break, running an offensive play, etc.). There are several benefits to creating a checklist. For example, it helps the athlete identify the important cues, it makes it easier to identify distractions that are allowed on the list, and it may foster communication with the coach regarding how to distinguish between relevant and irrelevant cues. I created a second column next to the distractions list, and asked Scott to generate two or three relevant cues that he felt he would help his performance. He quickly identified the following three: (a) following through on passes and shots, (b) focusing on the next play, and (c) adhering to his defensive assignment.

I asked Scott to look at both the list of distractions and his focus checklist. He was clearly surprised at how often he thinks about things unrelated to basketball during a game. When asked how the distractions affected him, he admitted that they usually result in increased anxiety, self-doubt, and muscle tension. This was a nice opportunity to increase Scott's awareness of being distracted, as well as provide him with additional insight as to how one's thoughts can influence emotional and/or physical responses (for better or for worse). Since we had also planned to begin relaxation training this session, I recommended a continuation of the focus checklist in a future session in order to enhance concentration. However, it would first be necessary to learn a few strategies to better manage his level of physical arousal.

To begin relaxation training, I provided Scott with a brief explanation of two different types of activation (i.e., cognitive and somatic) and of how they are related to performance, based upon a multimodal approach (Weinberg & Gould, 2003). Previously, I had provided Scott with only examples of somatic-based relaxation techniques. However, his intensity (activation) appeared to be driven by a combination of cognitive (i.e., distracting or irrational thoughts) and somatic (i.e., muscle tension) factors. This also served to support the expectation that cognitive and/or concentration skills acquisition would eventually be forthcoming. We began working on ways in which Scott might better manage his tension. Relaxation training was introduced, according to procedures recommended by Weinberg and Gould (2003, p. 247).

Education phase

I introduced Scott to two relaxation techniques that might be helpful in managing his physical activation. The first was diaphragmatic breathing. I asked Scott to demonstrate how he takes a deep breath. Clients typically respond with inhalation that emphasizes use of upper body, so that the chest and shoulders move up and down. I used both verbal and visual cues to describe how diaphragmatic breathing was different from his deep breathing. I explained how filling the lungs from the bottom to the top is similar to filling a balloon with water at the faucet. (Most clients have some prior experience of this, having taken part in water-balloon fights). I asked Scott whether he had ever filled a balloon with water and if so, to describe how it fills up. He told me that the water goes to the bottom and then fills to the top. I reinforced his response, and instructed him to watch my hands while I demonstrated diaphragmatic breathing. I placed my right hand on my chest, my left hand on my belly-button, and slowly inhaled. As I did, my stomach expanded pushing my left hand outward while my right hand remained unaffected until I had nearly completed a full inhalation. Then, I began to exhale slowly, whereby my right hand fell inward before my left hand. Scott acknowledged seeing the difference.

Acquisition phase

One of the advantages of beginning relaxation training with diaphragmatic breathing is that it is a very simple skill to acquire, and clients notice results after practicing only a few times. I instructed Scott to try it himself and take several deep breaths using one or both hands as cues. I recommended using a 3:6 time ratio between inhalation and exhalation. I assisted him by counting to 3 as he inhaled and to 6 as he exhaled. At first he was a bit tense, as indicated by considerable chest breathing. However, after a few inhalations and exhalations, Scott began to allow his stomach to expand, allowing his lungs to fill up fully with air. I reinforced his effort and encouraged him to keep trying until he noticed feeling a bit more relaxed. When he indicated being more relaxed, we began discussing ways he might practice this new skill.

Practice phase

I informed Scott that diaphragmatic breathing was something he could do nearly anywhere and almost anytime (e.g., in class, during practice, at bedtime), but just like any basketball skill he may have mastered, practice is necessary for its acquisition. Diaphragmatic breathing might also provide psychological as well as physiological benefits, in that when it is being practiced, he clearly wasn't thinking about any of the distractions mentioned earlier. Scott acknowledged that was likely true, and he agreed to practice his diaphragmatic breathing at least once a day while he was in class and at practice. I suggested that he might also try it at times when he felt "too intense," and I introduced the idea of keeping a log on his mental skills practice. Scott nodded in agreement, and we scheduled our next session for the following week.

Session 3

The objective for this session was to assess Scott's progress with diaphragmatic breathing. It was important to first determine whether he had practiced sufficiently to experience benefit before introducing progressive muscle relaxation, a more advanced skill. In addition, this assessment permitted reinforcement of his practice and discussion of any challenges he might have encountered during the week.

Scott reported having practiced diaphragmatic breathing both in class and at basketball practice about every other day, and claimed improvement by the third or fourth day of practice. He was most successful with relaxation when he engaged in it before he went to bed, but he also noticed being more relaxed and focused when he did it just prior to basketball practice. I reinforced his effort and explained that he should continue with his relaxation efforts and that he would become more proficient with regular practice. I also mentioned that diaphragmatic breathing would be an integral part of a more advanced relaxation technique, known as progressive muscle relaxation, as well as something that is often helpful when needing to refocus from a distraction. Since we had also spent last session identifying distractions, we turned our attention to his focus checklist from the previous week.

I briefly discussed the multidimensional nature of Scott's intensity, using his words to illustrate both cognitive and somatic reactions. The connection between cognitive and somatic anxiety was discussed in order to introduce the idea that Scott's thoughts affect his physical reactions. I referred to the list of distractions we developed the previous week, and we began reviewing times during basketball practice or games when he was distracted. Distracting thoughts seemed to occur during breaks such as after a foul had been committed, prior to shooting free-throws, or during timeouts. He admitted that during these times he should probably be thinking about cues from his focus checklist. However, when the team was behind or he hadn't been playing particularly well, other thoughts would occur. We discussed the importance of self-awareness and agreed that the next step would be to identify the time of distraction earlier (i.e., after becoming noticeably more tense, anxious and/or wrought with self-doubt). He offered to begin taking notes (i.e., self-monitoring) after practice or games, or perhaps at other times throughout the day (e.g., studying, at biology lab, etc.) when he might notice being distracted. It would be important for Scott to enhance his awareness before developing and implementing attention control and refocus strategies. Therefore, his homework was to keep a training log of situations when he was distracted, as well as the nature of his distractions, and any other pertinent observations.

Session 4

The objective of this session was to review Scott's training log from the previous week and to develop and implement a refocusing plan. Scott had taken detailed notes over the previous week, and we briefly discussed his observations about his distractions. I asked him what he considered to be the most frequently occurring distractions. His response was that during that past week most of his distracting thoughts were focused upon his back.

Scott had been experiencing severe low back pain since his freshman year in college, which was more than a year ago. I asked what was being done to manage the pain, and he described the various strategies the ATC had prescribed. Scott indicated that neither the ATC or team physician could identify the pain's cause. Scott clearly seemed frustrated, and when I shared this observation with him, he acknowledged its validity, stating that this had been going on for a long period of time. In fact, a specialist he had seen his freshman year had recommended surgery. However, the team physician discouraged such action, advocating rehabilitation strategies instead.

Scott was visibly annoyed; he stated that he had done what they asked and it had not worked. He went on to say that he would have preferred to have had the surgery as a freshman rather than now as a sophomore and in the middle of the basketball season. Again, I shared my observation that he was angry and tense. He nodded, and I asked him what he had been doing to cope with these emotions. He said he had made only occasional attempts at diaphragmatic breathing the past week, but that he was most bothered by the fact that these frustrations with the medical staff and his low back pain were now affecting his ability to study for exams. When I asked whether he had noticed any change in his sleep or appetite, he replied no and that he was only having difficulty studying, which made him nervous about his grades this term. After talking more about his concerns, we decided to add "low back" to his distractions list and move up "academic concerns" (i.e., need for high marks to get into a good medical school), so that both of those were at the top of the list. I reminded Scott that focus skills were not only useful for basketball but also might be helpful to him when trying to study. He expressed an interest in learning more and seemed desperate to try anything that might help him study. He responded enthusiastically to my suggestion that we develop a refocus plan using thought stopping based upon the focus checklist.

Education phase

The first step in refocusing training is to identify a specific time when distraction prevailed. Therefore, reference was made to Scott's self-monitoring log, which enabled selection of one such incident during practice a few days earlier when he was shooting free-throws. Scott was to complete 25 shots before finishing practice and going to see the ATC in order to schedule an appointment with the team physician. He shot 8 for 25, which is significantly below his average of 68%. When he reported his score, the assistant coach asked him what was wrong. He replied "I don't know," which prompted him to think about what had happened and make notes in his log. He had written "back hurts" and "want to skip doctor appointment, go to the library." It was immediately obvious to Scott that he wasn't focused on shooting but on thoughts about his back and studying later that night (as well as his lack of confidence in rehabilitation). This example was incorporated in the construction of a refocusing plan.

The next step in this process is to pause and disengage from irrelevant thoughts or negative self-talk. Scott was therefore instructed to clear such thoughts from his consciousness when able to identify their occurrence. An analogy was offered between achieving this and attempting to locate his focus checklist cues scattered among the same list as his distractions. It was suggested that he wipe clean an imaginary chalkboard that contained negative thoughts and self-talk, and rewrite only the one or two cues that are relevant or helpful to the task of shooting free-throws. A few examples were offered, such as saying "Stop," visualizing a stop sign, or anything that would indicate a cessation of counterproductive ideation. Scott responded favorably to the stop sign image and decided to use it. Scott was also reminded that diaphragmatic breathing might work well instead of, or in conjunction with the image of a stop sign, to help clear his mind.

The last step in refocus training is to recall the focus checklist for shooting. I removed the list from his visual field, and asked Scott to recite at least two of the three cues he had chosen. After thinking for a second, he recited all three: center, set, extend. I wrote down the three steps in his refocus plan, which included:

(a) catch himself distracted,

(b) stop and clear his mind,

(c) recall cue(s) from focus checklist (i.e., center, set, extend).

Next, we rehearsed his new plan.

Acquisition phase

Scott was instructed to take a few deep breaths, and while he complied, I asked him to imagine himself at practice, standing at the foul line and missing shots. I told him he could close his eyes if he felt it would help, and that I wanted him to recite his distracting thoughts aloud. Scott began talking about his back and the need to study, all the while expressing a feeling of being rushed and eager for practice to conclude. I then asked him to stop shooting, hold the ball and imagine seeing a stop sign on the back wall of the gym. Next he was asked to produce the image, and take one or two deep breaths. After his second breath, I asked him to recall his focus checklist and when he felt ready, take another shot. After approximately one minute, he opened his eyes and smiled timidly at me.

I asked him what that was like, and he indicated that he was in the correct fashion but that he had difficulty producing the stop sign image. He had felt a little more focused and relaxed before taking another shot, but he missed the basket. I told him that it was completely normal to have unclear or uncontrollable images, and that imagery was a skill like any other. The ability to generate clear, controlled images was contingent upon practice. I then asked him to describe a stop sign to me, to which he replied "Well, it's red and has six sides." We both laughed at his wrong answer, as I proceeded to draw an octagon on a blank sheet of paper. I asked him whether he recalled seeing the color red, and he shrugged. He was then asked what came to mind that was red. His best friend's racing bike was candy apple red with white accents. So,

I asked him to picture the stop sign again with the red color of that bike. He closed his eyes and smiled, indicating success.

Practice phase

Scott was told that he would become more proficient after regular practice, as was the case with acquisition of the diaphragmatic breathing skill. In two days he was to leave for a four-day road trip with the team. We identified a few times in which he might be able to attend to his refocus plan, and I gave him the paper on which I had written down its three steps.

Introduction to Progressive Muscle Relaxation (PMR)

The final portion of this session included an introduction to PMR. I provided an overview of the process that incorporated a script designed to guide Scott in alternating contraction and relaxation of specific muscles in the body. The script also emphasized awareness of the difference between muscular relaxation and tension. I cautioned that before we could proceed accordingly, his ATC should be informed of the strategy and allowed to determine if there were any contraindications or necessary modifications to the script in view of Scott's propensity towards back pain. I offered to talk with the ATC myself if he felt disinclined to do so himself. Scott indicated that he would be able to speak with her.

I gave Scott a sample PMR script (Porter & Foster 1990; Davis, Eshelman & McKay, 2000), and indicated that we would practice it during our next session. I instructed him to read the script and edit it as needed. He was to replace words with which he would feel more comfortable. For example, if a phrase such as "squish your eyelids together" sounded funny to him, he could rewrite it as "squeeze your eyelids together." I reminded him that PMR was also a skill as were diaphragmatic breathing and refocusing. We agreed that Scott would try using the PMR script and determine the degree to which it might be helpful.

I thanked Scott for agreeing to talk with the ATC about the PMR script and reminded him to practice his refocusing plan. We would start our next session with his refocus practice, discussing potential effects and/or challenges he may have encountered. Then, we would rehearse PMR based on his own edits and any ATC recommendations.

Session 5

The objectives for this session were to revisit Scott's diaphragmatic breathing practice, review his first attempts at refocusing using his 3-step plan, and introduce PMR. Since our last meeting, Scott's ATC had a few questions about relaxation training and eventually indicated that PMR appeared suitable. Scott had dutifully practiced all aspects of the refocusing plan. He said it seemed to be helpful during game situations but it had not been very efficient (i.e., one time he skipped over the second step). We discussed strategies for remembering the plan, such as one reminder or cue word for each of the three steps. When asked about diaphragmatic breathing, he said that he had been practicing. Although it continues to be effective for relaxation, he reported being very busy this past week and, as a result, he had not practiced every day. I reinforced his attempts, and then proceeded to discuss PMR with Scott.

Scott had talked with his ATC and had changed the wording in at least two places. We addressed issues that related to my office environment in an effort to optimize his comfort, such as use of a table lamp rather than fluorescent lighting, and the availability of a reclining chair. I explained that I would read through the revised script taking approximately 15–20 minutes, while he focused on my verbal instructions. I reminded him that when I instructed him to take deep breaths, he was to initiate the diaphragmatic breathing he had been practicing.

I gave Scott a few minutes to get comfortable, and then I informed him I would turn down the lights. I did my best to reassure him this was just a rehearsal, and that once we had completed the script, we would talk about the experience. Scott reclined in a comfortable chair, and I instructed him to take three slow deep breaths before we began. Similar to previous sessions, he began with short, shallow breathing, but eventually seemed to relax as I read through the script.

At the end of the script, Scott was taking very slow, deep breaths, as indicated by the rise and fall of his belly. Based upon his initial apprehension, I had some concerns; however, to my relief, PMR seemed to be quite effective for him. When asked how it went, he nearly yawned and said it was great. He had felt self-conscious at first but by the end was very relaxed and comfortable. He reported hearing very few distractions (i.e., internal or external), such as an occasional conversation between people walking by my office. But, for the most part, he was able to maintain his focus on my voice. He liked how the script had been edited to fit his needs, and he acknowledged it would be useful to practice regularly. We discussed a few language modifications and agreed to have a digital audio recording made of the script for him to play on his MP3 player.

To conclude the session, we talked about the benefits of the PMR script and his focus checklist. He understood PMR could be a useful tool for increasing his awareness of his tension and alleviating this stress. He felt the refocusing plan was useful during practice, and that with further practice, he could begin to incorporate it during games and thereby focus only on items that were part of the checklist. We agreed that we would meet in two week and that, in meantime, I would produce a digital file of the PMR script and he would continue to practice his diaphragmatic breathing and refocusing plan.

MST Intervention Summary

During these five sessions with Scott, we were able to make some encouraging progress with his awareness of tension and improved management of activation (i.e., diaphragmatic breathing) and attention (i.e., refocusing plan). The benefits of increased control over both cognitive and somatic arousal seemed to be reinforcing his efforts. He had used what he had learned during each session and diligently applied it to both practice and games, as well as occasionally while studying for tests. Scott was a self-disciplined and conscientious student-athlete, and he clearly approached MST with the same degree of effort and level of commitment he had for school and basketball. So far there had been nothing to be concerned about . . . at least not that I was aware of at the time.

When Things Started to Change

Scott e-mailed me a few hours before our next scheduled appointment, indicating that he needed to cancel. He indicated the reason was due to upcoming tests and labs, so I sent a brief reply that he could reschedule when he had time and wished him luck with his studying. Scott contacted me a few days later to reschedule our appointment, but then, just prior to our meeting, cancelled again. I began wondering how he was doing with the obvious travel schedule the team had that month and these difficult classes, but I concluded that he would contact me when he was ready to get back into MST.

Over the next few weeks, Scott continued to cancel and reschedule appointments. This went on for at least four or five weeks. Scott did not show up for the last appointment we had scheduled, nor did he contact me to cancel. This was disconcerting since it was uncharacteristic of him; up to this point, he had always remained in contact with me via e-mail. When an athlete misses an appointment, I typically send a brief e-mail in which I ask that he or she check in with me when available. Scott did not reply.

I would occasionally see Scott in the athletic training room, but I refrained from saying anything. Since I attend regular athletic training room staff meetings, I often see athletes with whom I am consulting. However, I talk with clients only if they initiate a conversation or interaction, which I then limit to casual conversation. Beyond the occasional hello while passing through the athletic training room, Scott and I had not spoken for over a month. Although I had received updates on his medical status during staff meetings, I decided to speak with the Athletic Training Room Director who worked with Scott's ATC.[3] To my dismay, the director indicated that Scott had been complaining of severe low back pain, and he had already been referred to another specialist by the team physician. The director seemed exasperated with the situation, suggesting that Scott was clearly needing help. The basketball coach had been talking with the director, and the entire medical staff seemed uncertain about the appropriate next step. Surgery had now become the only remaining treatment option.

At this point, I was eager to know Scott's perspective, and in particular how he was coping with his problematic situation. The director offered to tell Scott's ATC to mention that talking with someone about the situation might be helpful. We hoped that with a subtle reminder of the available support resources, Scott might open the door for a referral to the counseling center or perhaps might contact me again.

One week after my conversation with the director, I received an e-mail from Scott. He apologized for missing his last appointment and indicated recognition of the importance of relaxation training for him, particularly in view of what happened over the past weekend. He asked if we could meet sometime in the next few days to continue with the relaxation training. I replied and indicated when I would be available. I was unaware of what might have transpired recently, but based upon what the medical staff had reported, I suspected that Scott and I would be revising our consultation goals.

Mental Health Intervention—Session 6

Scott slowly entered my office, slumped in a chair and looked at me uneasily. To get things started, I asked, "So what's been going on since we last met?" To which he replied "A lot." He proceeded to talk about his worsening back pain and the fact that the doctors were now encouraging him to have surgery as soon as the season ended. During practice last weekend, he had pulled his left hamstring muscle, which made things worse. I inquired about how he was holding up, and he mentioned that his (paternal) grandmother had passed away a few weeks ago. He was clearly distraught and revealed guilt about not being there for his family, especially his father. His mother had taken care of all the details, including the arrangements with his basketball coach for Scott's flight home to attend the funeral. When I asked again how he was coping with all of this, he just stared blankly and said, "I'm not."

Referrals for mental health counseling

Although I am a Licensed Professional Counselor (LPC), I do not currently provide mental health counseling to student-athletes. However, I do believe that my hybrid training in sport and counseling psychology enables me to connect more easily with the existing yet disparate support services available to student-athletes. I find myself acting in many ways as liaison or bridge between two different cultures on campus, namely collegiate athletics and the student counseling center.

As Scott and I talked during session 6, it became obvious that he now needed a different intervention, namely a mental health referral. Based upon how he looked and sounded during the meeting, it seemed likely that he had been in need of a referral for a while.

Armed with new information about his grandmother's family, impaired sleep and appetite, frequent crying, and his falling grades (i.e., he had barely passed two of his last exams), I suggested to Scott that he would benefit from seeing someone at the Campus Counseling Center. He seemed shocked at my suggestion. My many referrals of students to the counseling center have taught me that its mere suggestion, particularly to student-athletes, often does not result in client compliance. I knew it would therefore be necessary to go beyond this initial step of offering a recommendation.

The referral process. I follow a referral process similar to the one outlined by Brewer et al. (1999). If possible, I choose an appropriate time and place for the conversation(s), which are usually more effective when I have identified in advance what influences I might have with the athlete (e.g., solid or long-term relationship, knowledge of his or her sport and/or life goals that are blocked by current dilemma, etc.) as well as anticipating potential barriers I might encounter when suggesting counseling (e.g., final exams coming up soon, conference play starts this weekend, prior negative experience with counseling, etc.).

I began the referral process by expressing concern for Scott's well-being. This was intended to convey my interest in his overall success—beyond sport. Next, I began summarizing my observations, which remained limited to what he had shared directly with me in this session. These observations included obvious impairments in mood (i.e., sadness, guilt, and frequent crying), poor daily functioning (i.e., taking 2-3 hours to fall asleep, inability to concentrate, loss of appetite), as well as his increasingly limited social activity (i.e., he had not talked with any of his teammates about recent events and admitted to "avoiding his roommate" in the evenings).

Scott seemed to acknowledge he needed help. I gave him the phone number for the counseling center and described the steps involved in making an appointment, such as completing an intake and attending follow-up sessions with a counselor. He admitted it would be hard to talk to someone he did not know, and I acknowledged that until this moment he had not talked about his issues with anyone from his existing support system (i.e., teammates, roommate, family, medical staff including myself). I reminded him that not too long ago, he did not know me either, but that clearly he seemed comfortable enough to share his difficulties and struggles with me now. He smiled, recalling for a moment what is was like when we first began MST. At last, he agreed to follow up on my recommendation to see a counselor.

Case Summary

A few days later, I ran into Scott in the hallway. As always, I refrained from contact until he said hello to me. Most of the athletes I have referred to counseling seem to disclose whether or not they followed my recommendation and the results of what transpired. Scott quickly looked around to see if anyone else was nearby and then revealed he had been seeing a counselor. He professed that he was coping better than when we last met. I admit feeling a little relieved that he had not only made it through the counseling center's intake process but had remained in counseling and seemed better for it. He expressed an interest in perhaps continuing the relaxation training, and we laughed a little in response to his tendency to take on everything at once. I offered to talk more with him in the future and suggested that presently it would be in his best interest to stick with this current plan, which seemed to be producing positive results.

The purpose of this firsthand account is to illustrate a sport psychology consultant's clinical intervention in assisting a collegiate student-athlete to better cope with pain and injury-related affective responses. Various kinds of mental skills were initially applied, eventually followed by referral for mental health intervention. The need to introduce a variety of interventions is emphasized, as is recognition that services beyond mental skills training (i.e., mental health) are sometimes necessary for consultants to react and adapt successfully as circumstances unfold as they did with Scott. As sport psychology professionals we ought to have knowledge of mental strategies that could be of use in these situations (e.g., coping and refocus plans for consultation, diaphragmatic breathing, etc.) as well as mental health resources to help navigate athletes through the grey area.

References

Brewer, B. W., Petitpas, A. J. & Van Raalte, J. L. (1999). Referral of injured athletes for counseling and psychotherapy. In R. Ray and D. M. Wiese-Bjornstal (Eds.), *Counseling in sports medicine* (pp. 127-141). Champaign, IL: Human Kinetics.

Davis, M., Eshelman, E. R., & McKay, M. (2000). *The relaxation & stress reduction workbook (5th ed.)*. Oakland, CA: New Harbinger Publications.

Hays, K. F. & Brown, C. H. (2004). *You're on! Consulting for peak performance*. Washington, DC: American Psychological Association.

Petrie, T. & Perna, F. (2004). Psychology of injury: Theory, research, and practice. In T. Morris and J. Sommers (Eds.), *Sport psychology: Theory, application, and issues* (2nd ed., pp. 547-551). Hoboken, NJ: John Wiley & Sons.

Porter, K. & Foster, J. (1990). *Visual athletics: visualizations for peak sports performance.* Dubuque, IA: W.C. Brown Publishers.

Weinberg, R. S. & Gould, D. (2003). *Foundations of sport & exercise psychology* (3rd ed.). Champaign, IL: Human Kinetics.

Wikipedia (2002). *Performance psychology.* Boston: Free Software Foundation, Inc. Retrieved March 16, 2006, from http://en.wikipedia.org/wiki/Performance_psychology.

Chapter Notes

[1] The athlete's name and specific details of the case have been altered to maintain confidentiality.

[2] The focus checklist was based on a technique used by Dr. Paul Salitsky.

[3] As a member of the sports medicine treatment team, I can obtain information on an athlete client from medical records or a staff member (i.e., athletic training students, ATCs, and approved clinical instructors). Considering the inherent challenges in maintaining confidentiality within the athletic training room environment, I discuss only relevant details of a specific case directly with the clinic director and always in a private location.

Chapter Twenty

The Role of Intra-Individual Responses to Injury Rehabilitation: A Case of a Repeat ACL Injury

Barbara B. Meyer
University of Wisconsin-Milwaukee

Kyle T. Ebersole
University of Illinois

Introduction

The literature in the area of the psychology of sport injury has grown markedly over the past two decades. Included in this profusion are theoretical models that identify not only the multitude of interdisciplinary factors that act as precursors to sport injury, but also those factors that influence successful rehabilitation, recovery, and return to sport. The trajectory of this work includes abandonment of the "one-size-fits-all" stage-based approach to sport injury (Kubler-Ross, 1969) and acceptance of a dynamic, process-based approach that acknowledges individual difference in response to sport injury (Brewer, 1994; Mainwaring, 1999; Rose & Jevne, 1993; Wiese-Bjornstal, Smith, Shaffer, Morrey, 1998). Proponents of the process-based approach, particularly Wiese-Bjornstal et al. (1998) in their Integrated Model of Response to Sport Injury, suggest that personal (i.e., injury history, individual differences, demographics, physical characteristics) and situational (i.e., sport, social, environmental) factors interact to influence an athlete's cognitive appraisal of the injury, which influences recovery outcomes through behavioral responses (e.g., adherence to rehabilitation, use of social support, effort and intensity) and emotional responses (e.g., positive attitude, emotional coping, fear of unknown).

The aforementioned process-based models and the research they inform (Bianco, 2001; Granito, 2001) speak to the importance of appreciating inter-individual differences in response to sport injury (i.e., sport hernia in two different athletes), but they do not explicitly acknowledge the need to consider intra-individual response to sport injury (e.g., sport hernia in the same athlete two years apart). While injury history has been identified as a personal factor that may influence the response to athletic injury (Wiese-Bjornstal et al., 1998), most research to date has failed to identify participant injury status as either a first injury or a subsequent injury. By failing to consider this variable, researchers and practitioners are assuming that responses to injury are minimally affected by previous injury experience. Examination of related medical literature illustrates valid reasons for distinguishing between an initial occurrence and subsequent occurrences of a similar health event. For example, research with cancer patients suggests that there may be different psychological and emotional reactions to initial versus recurrent cancer, which ultimately affect the information and care given to the individual (Burnet & Robinson, 2000). Additionally, literature on relapse prevention in alcohol and substance abuse programs suggests that previous experience with recovery may positively or negatively influence the responses to subsequent or repeated exposure to a treatment or intervention program (Marlatt & Gordon, 1985).

While it is impossible to generalize the psycho-emotional health of cancer survivors and addicts to those of injured athletes, results of that body of literature lend support to the need to look carefully at other individuals (i.e., athletes) who incur multiple health concerns. The paucity of research on multiple injuries in the same athlete and the processes that underlie and distinguish these repeated injuries demonstrates the need to further examine this topic and highlight implications for scientific and practicing professionals. As such, the overarching purpose of this chapter is to compare and contrast the biopsychosocial factors influencing the rehabilitation and return to sport of an elite freestyle aerial skiier who incurred two separate tears to the anterior cruciate ligament (ACL) in the right knee within a 51-week period. Throughout the case study presented below we demonstrate how contextual factors in the athlete's milieu contributed to the disparate responses to the two ACL injuries. These differences underscore the importance of considering intra-individual differences in the practice of sports medicine and the need to examine empirically the factors that influence individual response to repeat injury. To frame this case, we first provide an overview of freestyle skiing and ACL injuries.

Freestyle Skiing: An Overview

Freestyle skiing, consisting of the two disciplines of moguls and aerials, gained international recognition in 1988 as a demonstration sport in the Olympic Winter Games. The popularity of the sport for spectators and participants alike has been steadily increasing, with moguls becoming an official Olympic medal sport in 1992 and aerials following suit in 1994. Although injuries are common in both freestyle disciplines, the nature and frequency of injury in aerials prompts the focus of this chapter. To better understand the nature of the sport in general, and the risk of injury in particular, a brief overview of aerials and common training protocols follow.[1]

In freestyle aerials, athletes ski down a 20–25 degree in-run at speeds of 33–45 miles per hour and off 14-foot-tall snow-packed ramps or *kickers*. The kicker launches the athletes as high as 50 feet (i.e., five stories) into the air where they perform combinations of flips and twists before orienting themselves to their feet on a 37-degree landing hill of chopped snow. In competition, aerialists must perform two different jumps, varying by at least one flip or twist. Points are awarded for take-off (i.e., 20% of score), form in the air (i.e., 50% of score), and landing (i.e., 30% of score), which are multiplied by a degree of difficulty (DD) factor to arrive at a total score for each jump. The point total of both jumps is then added together for a final score. The aforementioned skill executions are required; that is, they comprise the competitive components that an athlete or a coach can control and plan for, to some degree. Less controllable factors, such as the weather (e.g., wind, snow and air temperature, falling snow or rain, sun), add to the difficulty and danger of aerial skiing.

In an effort to eliminate as much danger as possible, athletes in freestyle aerials spend the off-season months learning or *perfecting* skills in a way that is supposedly less risky than doing so on snow. Trampolines with bungee assisted spotting harnesses as well as outdoor pools are commonly used for this purpose. When water training, aerialists climb upwards of 150 stairs wearing their training attire (i.e., ski boots, wet or dry suit depending upon the air temperature, life preserver, helmet, braces or other protective equipment) and carrying their skis. Once at the top of the stairs (i.e., in-run), the aerialist skis down a plastic surface and then off of the same size kicker used on snow, landing in a swimming pool. A burst of air (i.e., bubbles) is sent up from the bottom of the pool just before landing in an effort to soften the impact. It is not uncommon for an athlete to take 20–40 jumps each day during the off-season.

Consistent with Zuckerman's theory of sensation seeking (Goma-i-Freixanet, 2004; Zuckerman, 1983), aerial skiing is classified as a medium-risk sport whereby participation involves a higher probability of injury than death. Aerialists understand that injury is an inherent part of the sport, and while all involved do whatever they can to minimize risk, the prevailing attitude among participants is not a question of *if* they will get injured but rather one of *when*. The most significant injuries occur when athletes fail to land properly on their skis, which can result in chronic back pain, concussions, shoulder separations, and ACL tears, to name just a few. The elite freestyle aerial skier in the current case study incurred two separate ruptures to the ACL in her right knee within a 51-week period. Although the second rupture to her ACL in such a short time period is obviously of clinical concern, the uniqueness of this particular case was the demonstrated role of intra-individual differences as key determinants in the response to a repeat ACL injury and the subsequent management of rehabilitation in an elite athlete.

ACL Injuries

The primary function of the ACL is to control forward movement of the tibia on the femur and is the most frequently torn knee ligament in athletes (Beynnon, Johnson, Abate, Fleming, & Nichols, 2005a). Movements such as landing in freestyle aerial skiing can place great stress on the ACL. The incidence of ACL injuries in World Cup freestyle skiing has been estimated to be 1.08 injuries per 1000 skier days (Heir, Krosshaug, & Ekeland, 2004). In addition to being devastating to athletes' careers, ACL injuries have become a major healthcare cost, with an estimated annual cost of about 1.5 billion dollars for reconstruction, not including the cost for post-surgical rehabilitation (Boden 2000). As a result, a significant amount of research has been conducted to identify the causal factors for ACL injury. However, the literature has not fully examined the factors and/or characteristics that contribute to a successful recovery from ACL injury and return to sport.

In the 1970s, the basic science studies suggested that a newly reconstructed ACL graft could take as long as 12 to18 months to fully mature (De Carlo, Klootwyk, & Shelbourne, 1997). Thus, ACL rehabilitation was extremely conservative, often involved placing the limb in a cast for several weeks, and generally resulted in a total recovery time of the approximately 12 months or longer. The significant growth in the scientific literature since the 1980s has provided key insight into the healing properties of ACL grafts and the efficacy of various rehabilitative strategies. The improved understanding has resulted in a reduction in the total recovery time for ACL injuries to approximately 6 to 8 months before returning to sport (Harner, Fu, Irrgang, & Vogrin, 2001). Although most individuals are able to return to sport or strenuous activity, the outcome of ACL reconstruction varies across individuals. It has been suggested (Beynnon, Johnson, Abate, Fleming, & Nichols, 2005a, 2005b; Cascio, Culp, & Cosgarea, 2004; Kvist, 2004; Podlog & Eklund, 2006; Poehling et al., 2005; Roi, Creta, Nanni, Marcacci, Zaffagnini, Snyder-Mackler, 2005) that ACL reconstruction recovery (i.e., return to sport or daily activities) is related to a variety of factors, including but not limited to

(a) associated injuries (e.g., meniscus, collateral ligaments);

(b) surgical factors (e.g., technique, selection of graft);

(c) physiological parameters (e.g., restoration of strength, motion, balance, and functionality);

(d) psychological factors (e.g., motivation, fear of re-injury, social support); and

(e) sociological factors (e.g., sport ethic, access to rehabilitation).

The relative contribution of these factors to the outcome of ACL reconstruction remains unclear, and it is likely that a multi-factorial relationship among these parameters exists. Even less apparent is the importance of the aforementioned factors to the ACL reconstruction recovery of individuals who have incurred multiple ACL tears.

The average failure rate of ACL grafts across a variety of populations has been reported to be only 2% (Kvist, 2004). Perhaps due to the low failure rate, there is a paucity of available literature on the rehabilitation of a repeat ACL rupture. This scarcity of information is somewhat surprising given anecdotal evidence that more and more elite athletes are incurring second and even third ACL tears. While the literature identifies factors related to successful return to sport following an ACL rupture (e.g., motivation, goal setting, pain/fear management, social support) (Bianco, 2001; Podlog & Eklund, 2006; Roi et al., 2005; Scherzer et al., 2001) as well as reported reasons for not returning to sport despite restoration of normal knee function (e.g., fear of re-injury, secondary gains) (Bjordal et al., 1997; Kvist, 2004; Kvist, Ek, Sporrestedt, & Good, 2005), it does not speak to the need to consider whether the rupture is a first time or subsequent event. By failing to consider injury history, researchers and practitioners alike are assuming that responses to second or third injury are minimally affected by previous injury experience and that similar injuries in one particular athlete can be treated alike.

As suggested above, the contribution of intra-individual differences to the success of recovery from repeat ACL injuries, especially in elite athletes, remains unclear. It is likely that such differences are key determinants of how athletes respond to a devastating injury like an ACL tear and subsequently approach their rehabilitation. The lack of available literature has slowed our understanding of the influence that the history of injury, specifically of repeat injuries, may have on developing an appropriate rehabilitation protocol as well as on the recovery outcomes. The case study presented below demonstrates that an appreciation of intra-individual differences may enable those in an athlete's support network to identify and facilitate the most effective rehabilitation strategies to meet the individual's outcome goals.

Case Study Profile

Athlete Background

At the time of the initial injury, the female athlete was a 29-year-old veteran of the World Cup ski circuit. Her list of athletic accomplishments was extraordinary (e.g., 19 World Cup podiums, world record two-jump total score, two World Cup Overall Grand Prix titles, Olympic gold medal), particularly given that most of her success had been achieved over the previous two or three seasons. These achievements did not come without a price, as the athlete had incurred numerous injuries along the way (e.g., broken collarbone, dislocated shoulder, multiple concussions, stress fractures, etc.). These injuries, most of which occurred during snow training or competition, are viewed as "standard operating procedure" in the sport, even for athletes like the one in question who was diligent about her in- and out-of-season training regimen (i.e., general as well as sport-specific strength and conditioning, nutrition, etc.). Although she had sustained numerous injuries, she had never "been in plaster," as noted by a sport organization official in her home country.

The 2004–05 aerial ski season was important relative to the Olympic cycle, as it marked the point when performance plans for the Olympic Games in Italy were formed and enacted. Athletes and coaches worked together to determine which jumps should be developed and/or improved over the next two years, for possible competition in the 2006 Games. This decision was informed by a number of factors, including but not limited to the athlete's own physical and technical capabilities, predictions of which jumps would be performed by competitors, and the point total that was thought necessary to win. Aerial skiing is an ever-evolving sport where athletes are rewarded (through degree-of-difficulty weighting in the scoring/judging procedure) for taking risk and "pushing the envelope." Accordingly, the athlete and her coach decided to begin working on new and more difficult jumps for the next Olympic Games. These jumps included two variations of a quad-twisting double somersault (i.e., four twists on two flips), one of which had never before been performed by a woman.[2]

ACL #1—October 2004

Injury background. Water ramp training of one of the new jumps (full-triple-full) began in September 2004 at a training site in the United States. The athlete's progress was consistent and hopeful until approximately the 30th attempt on October 9, 2004. On this particular attempt, when she entered the water after coming out of the fourth and final twist, the resistance of the water placed the body in a vulnerable position. It is thought that the bubbles, which were infused into the pool to soften the landing, rotated and shifted the ski underwater, placing her knee in valgus and an externally rotated position, which resulted in a full tear of her right ACL. The athlete vividly recalled feeling a distinctive "snap," which is a classic sign associated with ACL tears. Subsequent clinical evaluation in the U.S. and later in her home country indicated excessive joint laxity with the Lochman test (Magee, 2002), leaving little question that the ACL was fully torn.

Injury management. Immediately after the injury, the athlete expressed the desire to have the ACL repaired, and when possible, resume training for the 2006 Olympic Winter Games. In an effort to tie up loose ends at the summer training venue, and because time urgency was not a major concern of the medical staff, the athlete remained in the U.S. for a week before flying to her home country in the Southern Hemisphere. During this time the athlete, independently and whenever possible, engaged in commonly utilized strategies to control pain and swelling (i.e., icing, elevation of limb) and maintain range of motion. She also initiated general psychoemotional preparation for the forthcoming challenges of ACL surgery. Given her previous experience with psychological skills training for performance enhancement, she and the first author spent time discussing how some of those same skills could be transferred to injury rehabilitation and return to sport (Brown, 2005; Cupal & Brewer, 2001; Green, 1999; Heil, 1993; Ievleva & Orlick, 1999; Jam, n.d.; Wiese-Bjornstal et al., 1998).

Upon returning to her home one week post-injury, the athlete underwent reconstructive ACL surgery. The surgery confirmed a full tear of the ACL, but no damage to surrounding structures. A portion of the hamstring tendon from the athlete's right thigh was used to replace the torn ACL. The surgical procedure was unremarkable and no complications or concerns were noted. A multi-phase rehabilitation protocol began five days after surgery and was designed to have the athlete ready to return to competition in September 2005, approximately 11-months post-surgery (Table 1). The progress of the athlete's rehabilitation was consistent with clinical expectations as well as that of comparable injuries in other known athletes. The athlete did, however, report noticeable pain in the hamstring at the site where the graft was harvested and this pain resulted in minor delays in progress.

Contextual factors. Although there is never a good time for a serious injury in elite sport (Gayman & Crossman, 2003; Podlog & Eklund, 2006; Wiese-Bjornstal, 2005), the fact that the current injury came one full season (i.e., 16 months) prior to the 2006 Olympics allowed for enough time to complete a traditional 9-month ACL rehabilita-

Table 1.

General description of rehabilitation protocol

Phase	Objective	Phase Duration	
		ACL Injury #1	ACL Injury #2
Prehab	Prior to surgery; maintain strength and motion	Minimal formal pre-hab was performed in weeks preceding surgery	1 week prior to surgery
1	Post-operative; control pain and swelling	Week 1 post- surgery	Phases 1 & 2 were integrated across Week 1 post-surgery
2	Range of motion (ROM) and initiate strength exercises	Weeks 2 -4	
3	Continue ROM; progress strength; initiate balance and neuromuscular control	Weeks 5-9	Weeks 2-5
4	Advanced strength; initiate agility and plyometric exercises	Weeks 10-16	Weeks 6-9; Began water ramp training in Week 8
Return to Sport	Return to skiing and progressively perform jumps	Weeks 16-43; Returned to basic snow skiing in week 16 Returned to aerial ski training in Week 29	Weeks 10-12; Returned to snow skiing in week 10 and aerial skiing in Week 11
Competition	Full return to competition	Week 44	Olympic qualifying competitions in Week 14; Olympics in Week 19

tion and prepare for the 2006 Games in Italy. Although the athlete chose a surgeon who was not directly affiliated with her sport's usual network of medical providers, she embraced a more standard or conservative approach to post-operative rehabilitation. Having been witness to the knee reconstructions and complicated return to sport trajectories of several teammates, the athlete admitted in hindsight to being "too careful," beginning in pre-hab (i.e., exercises prior to surgery) and continuing through the rehabilitation process. Afraid of ruining the graft, the athlete limited activities of daily living (ADL), including basic walking, and avoided situations (e.g., shopping malls, crowded streets, and book stores) in which she may be jostled or otherwise lose her balance. Not surprisingly, self-reported quality of life also decreased during this time. Nonetheless, the luxury of time prompted the athlete's approach, which was reinforced by her support system.

Outcomes. Upon receiving the clearance to travel freely, the athlete joined friends and teammates in Europe for the last month of the 2004-05 World Cup season, which included a trip to an Olympic test event in Italy. This trip provided the athlete with an opportunity to evaluate her recovery progress (e.g., skiing for the first time post-surgery, riding the ski jump, etc.), familiarize herself with the surroundings of the Olympic venue (e.g., positioning of the aerial site, transportation patterns, etc.), and begin planning for the 2006 Games (e.g., jumps to attempt, lead-up events, qualification time frame, etc.). In regard to the latter, despite her position as the reigning Olympic gold medalist, the athlete still needed to meet criteria for team qualification. That said, there was an air of calm and patience within the team. The Olympics were a year away, and there appeared to be ample time to continue physical rehabilitation and return to top aerial form.

Overall, the athlete demonstrated a dedication and commitment to rehabilitating the ACL tear that was commensurate with her sport-specific and all-around work ethic. Although she remained goal-oriented and focused, there was little if any pressure (internal or external) to rush her return to the sport. There was a sense that she and the coaches had enough time to train and prepare for the upcoming World Cup season and the Olympics. Regardless, the athlete returned to ski training (i.e., water ramp) with her team in June 2005, incurring few if any complications. Her overarching goal was to earn a spot on her country's Olympic team as early as possible, thereby maximizing autonomy vis-a-vis competition schedule going into the Games, but the more immediate goal was to remain healthy while gradually working back into top jumping form. The health of the knee would clearly dictate the pace.

ACL #2—October 2005

Injury background. After placing fourth at the first World Cup event of the 2005–06 season, thereby earning an important Top 6 finish in terms of Olympic qualification, the athlete and her coaches focused on preparing jumps for the Games. It was determined to be too risky to continue training the quad twisting double (i.e., full-triple-full) on which injury occurred in 2004, so thoughts turned to training the other quad (i.e., double-full double-full). This new jump had a higher degree of difficulty than the triple twisting doubles performed in the 2002 Games, and athletes from one or two other countries were training for it in water. The athlete and her coach agreed that it would be good to have a jump of this difficulty in her repertoire, bringing it out if needed at the Olympics. The athlete continued with general strength and conditioning exercises as well as usual care (e.g., massage, icing, etc.) in an effort to maintain function and minimize pain in the surgically repaired leg. Despite these efforts, the athlete experienced, throughout rehabilitation and training, occasional pain in the hamstring where the graft was harvested. This report of pain was consistent with the outcomes of using a hamstring tendon for ACL reconstruction. Outside of this general discomfort, the athlete experienced minimal complications and expressed little concern about re-injury.

During water-ramp training the last week of September 2005, the athlete attempted and completed the aforementioned quad-twisting double. Over a period of several days she made consistent improvements on that jump while perfecting the other jumps in her repertoire. While training the quad twisting double on October 1, the athlete came into the landing pool with too much speed and rotation. Similar to the first ACL injury, she reported feeling the tell-tale snap in her right knee. Excessive laxity with the Lochman test left little doubt that the ACL had ruptured again. Five days later, the athlete returned to her home country.

Injury management. The athlete immediately kicked into pre-hab mode, using her previous experience to dictate icing, wrapping, elevating, using crutches, and mental training. Among all those in her sport network, talk immediately turned to the meaning of the injury for the 2006 Olympics. The first author was present at the time of injury, and spent a great deal of time talking to the athlete about her desire to move forward, facilitating discussion of options as well as of the advantages and disadvantages of working toward the goal of competing once again. Through all of these discussions, the athlete never wavered in her desire to move forward.

Part of this progress involved determination of the surgical approach that would be taken to reconstruct the ruptured ACL. Unlike with the first injury, where a luxury of time framed the recovery process, now little time was available to consider which surgical alternative, including graft type (i.e., allograft vs. autograft) and ultimately graft material (i.e., cadaver vs. synthetic), would provide the greatest possibility of recovering within 14 weeks and allow the athlete to compete in Olympic qualifying competitions (Table 1).

Contextual factors. Clearly, the overarching contextual factor associated with ACL #2 was the timing of the injury vis-a-vis the 2006 Olympic Winter Games. The proximity of the Olympics dictated not only the immediate medical approach to management of the injury, but also the ongoing physical as well as psychological management of rehabilitation and return to competition. The former is evident in the athlete's immediate involvement in pre-hab activities as well as the decision to pursue an allograft. The athlete perceived the harvest site (i.e., hamstring tendon) in ACL #1 as a source of discomfort and encumbrance that slowed her rehabilitation. She wished to avoid a repeat of this physical and mental drain on ACL #2.

Ongoing management of rehabilitation and return to competition was likewise informed predominantly by the proximity of the Olympic games and the athlete's desire to compete in them. Rather than relying upon usual standard-of-care guidelines and replicating the programs of previously injured teammates, as had been done following ACL #1, the athlete and her rehabilitation team (i.e., surgeon, physiotherapist, strength and conditioning specialist) developed a program dictated by the Olympic schedule. If she were to begin water-ramp training at Week 8, for example, then certain physical markers would need to be met by Week 4. As the athlete describes it:

> My mind set the goals and my body kept up. "Of course I can do this (e.g., achieve full range of motion) because next week I'll be doing this (e.g., working on strength and balance)." I truly believed I could do it.

The timing of the athlete's second ACL injury along with the fact that it was her *second* injury of this type also served to influence the other primary contextual factor that separated ACL #1 from ACL #2—her approach to ADLs. Within minutes of reporting the tell-tale snap in her knee, the athlete adopted a dedicated system of icing, elevating, and participating in activities to maintain maximum range of motion and strength. This more aggressive and regimented approach continued throughout the rehabilitation process, where the athlete welcomed clinic-based (e.g., landing drills, agility drills, etc.) and in-vivo (e.g., going to movies, wearing sandals and high-heeled shoes, etc.) opportunities to challenge herself both physically and mentally. A nothing-to-lose attitude (e.g., "If the knee can't survive my skiing this week, then it can't survive my landing next week") prevailed throughout the process and was embraced by all members of the athlete's support network. The athlete attributed this more balanced approach to rehabilitation with facilitating both her return to sport and quality of life along the way.

Outcomes. The athlete's aggressive physical rehabilitation protocol and reliance on physical and mental challenges to assess readiness to compete proved successful, as she was water-ramp training at 8 weeks post-op and snow skiing at 10 weeks post-op. As the late January deadline for naming the Olympic team approached, the relaxed and patient return-to-form time line previously adopted by the ski team network was replaced with a sense of urgency. Preferring not to rely on a discretionary appointment to the team, the athlete needed to compete in several of the January World Cup events and perform at a high level. As such, she was required to train and perform more difficult jumps than initially planned, in less than ideal weather conditions, with suboptimal rest cycles, any of which had the potential to increase the probability of injury. When questioned about the soundness of this expedited schedule, which was contrary to that taken after the first ACL injury, the athlete responded: "Like I have a choice."

In the end, the athlete qualified for the Olympics 14 weeks post-op and competed in the Games 18 weeks post-op, with only 20 days of snow jumping to her credit after the second ACL repair. Despite the abbreviated training schedule, weather delays, and an injury to a teammate during the competition (i.e., ACL tear), the athlete was able to stay physically healthy and mentally focused throughout the Olympic Games, winning a bronze medal along the way.

Summary

The elite skier profiled in the case study above exhibited distinct responses to her two separate ACL reconstruction and recovery experiences. Specifically, the previous ACL injury experience and the temporal proximity of the injury occurrence to the 2006 Olympic Winter Games were the overarching themes that contributed to the different biopsychosocial responses. While these two themes must be discussed separately, it appears that they (and related factors) operated concurrently to influence the athlete's return to sport. The identification of differential responses to two separate occurrences (Table 2) of the same injury highlights the need for researchers and practitioners in sport psychology and sports medicine to consider intra-individual difference in theory development, theory testing, and clinical practice. Key aspects of the aforementioned differences and implications for practice are discussed below.

Temporal Aspects of Recovery

The timing of the two ACL ruptures in relation to the Olympics played an important role in the athlete's approach to rehabilitation and return to sport. The luxury of time prompted a more traditional and conservative timeline for recovery after ACL #1; a

Table 2.

Comparison of unique aspects of ACL Injury #1 and #2

	ACL Injury #1	ACL Injury #2
Date of injury	October 1, 2004	October 8, 2005
Mechanism of injury	Entering the landing pool with foot attached to ski	Entering the landing pool with foot attached to ski
Diagnosis	Full tear of right ACL	Full tear of right ACL with partial tear of medial meniscus
Surgical technique	Hamstring tendon autograft	Cadaver patellar tendon graft using graft tunnels from initial ACL surgery
Total time for return to competition	44 weeks	11 weeks
Identifiable differences in rehabilitation	Cautious and protective approach. Followed traditional 9-month rehabilitation plan. Encountered considerable hamstring pain at site where graft was harvested. Significant anxiety relative to progressing too fast and compromising graft integrity. Looked to teammates and known others as models for rehabilitation.	Definitive timeline to Olympics. Expeditious rehabilitation plan. Significantly less pain in comparison to ACL #1. Modified lifestyle and environment to make rehabilitation accessible. Nothing-to-lose attitude. Quick return to ADLs. Sought opportunities to test physical and mental readiness vis-a-vis ACL repair. Used self (as opposed to others) as barometer for progress.

lack of time prompted a more expeditious and innovative rehabilitation timeline for ACL #2. This issue of time dictated in part the surgical, physiological, psychological, and sociological parameters associated with the return to sport following each injury. Specific differences, prompted by the perception of time following the second ACL tear, included

(a) the immediate adoption of and commitment to pre-hab activities;

(b) the type of surgical repair undertaken;

(c) the pace of rehabilitation and return to ADLs;

(d) the athlete's adoption of problem-focused coping strategies (e.g., distinguishing between good pain and bad pain, use of goal setting, etc.); and

(e) the athlete's temporary relocation to an apartment closer to the rehabilitation facility. While many of these factors have been identified as important to rehabilitation and return to sport (Gayman & Crossman, 2003; Kvist et al., 2005; Morrey, Stuart, Smith, & Wiese-Bjornstal, 1999; Podlog & Eklund, 2006; Scherzer et al., 2001; Wiese-Bjornstal et al., 1998), they have not been explicitly discussed in the context of injury history.

As this case study suggests, the athlete's cognitive appraisal of the two separate injuries (vis-a-vis time to prepare for the Olympics) was different, prompting a change in her behavioral response. Her goal to compete in the upcoming Olympics prompted an aggressive timeline for recovery, resulting in emotional and behavioral responses that were quite different from those exhibited following the earlier ACL tear. It appears inappropriate for researchers and practitioners to assume that a particular individual will respond similarly to each injury, even if the injuries are similar or the same. This case report also suggests that early return to elite-level sport after a second ACL reconstruction is possible and may be partly determined by attention to psychosocial parameters such as facilitating appropriate goal and motivational orientations as well as coping strategies, utilizing a systems approach to treatment, and including psychological skills training.

Injury Experience

The athlete's previous experience with ACL injury was another major factor that contributed to her unique psychological and behavioral responses. Upon reflection, the athlete acknowledged that the "aura of knee reconstruction" permeated her approach to rehabilitation and return to sport following the first ACL tear. One of the ways in which this aura manifested itself was in the athlete's approach to recovery. In an effort to promote full maturation of the graft and provide additional protection following ACL #1, the athlete relied upon assistive devices for mobility, avoided ADLs that might have challenged her knee, and assumed a "sick role" of sorts, all of which undermined the competence and autonomy necessary to facilitate return to sport (Podlog & Eklund, 2006). Concomitantly, the aura of knee reconstruction and the fact that it was uncharted territory for the athlete prompted her to rely on others for advice and feedback about goals and objectives that would lead to success. Anecdotal and empirical evidence suggests that an athlete's support network may be a valuable source of informational support, emotional support, and vicarious learning (Granito, 2001; Hagger, Chatzisarantis, Griffin, & Thatcher, 2005; Podlog & Eklund, 2006; Rock & Jones, 2002), but the literature to date does not consider the relevancy of these resources in relation to rehabilitation success or injury history. That is, listening to and/or learning from others may be of value only if the rehabilitation outcomes were positive, the context surrounding the athletes' injuries were similar, and/or an athlete had no injury experience of his or her own upon which to draw.

Learning from her own experiences with the initial ACL tear, the athlete in the current case changed her approach to the subsequent ACL tear by filtering the advice she received and focusing on individualized criterion (as opposed to normative) measures of rehabilitation success. This more autonomous approach was preceded by a demystification of ACL injury rehabilitation the second time around, as well as the athlete's realization that her own prior (positive and negative) experiences with ACL reconstruction served as the most salient source of information to guide her response to ACL #2. Literature in the areas of self-efficacy (Bandura, 1977), goal orientation (Duda, 1992), and coping style (Lazarus & Folkman, 1984) support the aerialist's expeditious and successful return to competition and can be used as a resource for practitioners working with athletes who have incurred repeat injuries.

The athlete's identification of injury experience as an important factor in response to injury is consistent with previous research involving elite athletes (Podlog & Eklund, 2006; Roi et al., 2005; Wiese-Bjornstal, 1998), yet extends that body of literature by suggesting the need to focus future work on experience with the same injury. The athlete in the current case had incurred numerous injuries over the course of her career, yet none influenced her rehabilitation and return to sport after ACL #2 more than her experience with ACL #1. Consistent with other medical literature (Burnet & Robinson, 2000; Marlatt & Gordon, 1985), researchers and practitioners in sports medicine must do more to identify the key individualized characteristics that may serve as markers of success in response to repeat injury.

This case study demonstrated that an individualized, accelerated rehabilitation protocol can be used to successfully return an elite-level athlete to competition far sooner than traditional clinical expectations. The outcome of this case study clearly identifies the importance of considering contextual factors and incorporating athletes' psychological responses into the development and management of an ACL rehabilitation protocol, especially during a repeat injury. That is, athletes may appraise the same injury differently across separate time points, thereby necessitating a different and perhaps more effective treatment paradigm. Future research that examines responses to initial and subsequent injury, such as that which has been conducted in the broader medical literature (Burnet & Robinson, 2000; Marlatt & Gordon, 1985), will help us to identify factors important in the treatment of repeat injury. Until such evidenced-based practice approach has been further examined with repeat athletic and/or ACL injury, intra-individual biopsychosocial factors such as those presented in the case above should be considered as possible contributors to the multi-factorial nature of ACL injury response and recovery.

References

Bandura, A. (1977). Self-efficacy: Toward a unifying theory of behavioral change. *Psychological Review, 84,* 191-215.

Beynnon, B. D., Johnson, R. J., Abate, J. A., Fleming, B. C., & Nichols, C. E. (2005a). Treatment of anterior cruciate ligament injuries, Part I. *American Journal of Sports Medicine, 33,* 1579-1602.

Beynnon, B. D., Johnson, R. J., Abate, J. A., Fleming, B. C., & Nichols, C. E. (2005b). Treatment of anterior cruciate ligament injuries, Part II. *American Journal of Sports Medicine, 33,* 1751-1767.

Bianco, T. (2001). Social support and recovery from sport injury: Elite skiers share their experiences. *Research Quarterly for Exercise and Sport, 72,* 376-388.

Bjordal, J. M., Arnly, F., Hannestad, B., & Strand, T. (1997). Epidemiology of anterior cruciate ligament injuries in soccer. *American Journal of Sports Medicine, 25,* 341-345.

Boden, F. W., Dean, G. S., Feagin, J. A., Garrett, W. E. (2000). Mechanisms of anterior cruciate ligament injury. *Orthopedics, 23,* 573-578.

Brewer, B. W. (1994). Review and critique of models of psychological adjustment to athletic injury. *Journal of Applied Sport Psychology, 6,* 87-100.

Brown, C. (2005). Injuries: The psychology of recovery and rehab. In S. Murphy (Ed.), *The sport psych handbook* (pp. 215-235). Champaign, IL: Human Kinetics.

Burnet, K., & Robinson, L. (2000). Psychosocial impact of recurrent cancer. *European Journal of Oncology Nursing, 4,* 29-38.

Cascio, B. M., Culp, L., & Cosgarea, A. J. (2004). Return to play after anterior cruciate ligament reconstruction. *Clinics in Sports Medicine, 23,* 395-408.

Cupal, D. D., & Brewer, B. W. (2001). Effects of relaxation and guided imagery on knee strength, reinjury anxiety, and pain following anterior cruciate ligament reconstruction. *Rehabilitation Psychology, 46,* 28-43.

De Carlo, M., Klootwyk, T. E., & Shlebourne, K. D. (1997). ACL surgery and accelerated rehabilitation revisited. *Journal of Sport Rehabilitation, 6,* 144-156.

Duda, J. L. (1992). Motivation in sport settings: A goal perspective approach. In G.C. Roberts (Ed.), *Motivation in sport and exercise* (pp. 57-91). Champaign, IL: Human Kinetics.

Gayman, A. M., & Crossman, J. (2003). A qualitative analysis of how the timing of the onset of sports injuries influences athlete reactions. *Journal of Sport Behavior, 26,* 255-271.

Goma-i-Freixanet, M. (2004). Sensation seeking and participation in physical risk sports. In R. M. Stelmack (Ed.), *On the psychobiology of personality: Essays in honor of Marvin Zuckerman* (pp. 185-201). New York: Elsevier Science.

Granito, V. J. (2001). Athletic injury experience: A qualitative focus group approach. *Journal of Sport Behavior, 24,* 63-82.

Green, L. B. (1999). The use of imagery in the rehabilitation of injured athletes. In D. Pargman (Ed.), *Psychological bases of sport injuries* (2nd ed., pp. 235-251). Morgantown, WV: Fitness Information Technology, Inc.

Hagger, M. S., Chatzisarantis, N. L .D., Griffin, M., & Thatcher, J. (2005). Injury representations, coping, emotions, and functional outcomes in athletes with sports-related injuries: A test of self-regulation theory. *Journal of Applied Social Psychology, 35,* 2345-2374.

Harner, C. D., Fu, F. H., Irrgang, J. J., & Vogrin, T. M. (2001). Anterior and posterior cruciate ligament reconstruction in the new millennium: A global perspective. *Knee Surgery, Sports Traumatology, Arthroscopy, 6,* 330-336.

Heil, J. (1993). *Psychology of sport injury.* Champaign, IL: Human Kinetics.

Heir, S., Krosshaug T., & Ekeland, A. (2004). The incidence and trends of ACL injuries in world cup freestyle skiing during a 10-year period [abstract]. *Knee Surgery, Sports Traumatology, Arthroscopy, 12,* 169-177.

Ievleva, L., & Orlick, T. (1999). Mental paths to enhanced recovery from a sports injury. In D. Pargman (Ed.), *Psychological bases of sport injuries* (2nd ed., pp. 199-220). Morgantown, WV: Fitness Information Technology, Inc.

Irrgang, J. J., & Harner, C. D. (1997). Recent advances in ACL rehabilitation: clinical factors that influence the program. *Journal of Sport Rehabilitation, 6,* 111-124.

Jam, B. (n.d.). New paradigms in rotator cuff retraining. Retrieved March 8, 2006, from http://www.aptei.com/articles/pdf/Rotator_Cuff.pdf

Kubler-Ross, E. (1969). *On death and dying.* London: Macmillan.

Kvist, J. (2004). Rehabilitation following anterior cruciate ligament injury. *Sports Medicine, 34,* 269-280.

Kvist, J., Ek, A., Sporrstedt, K., Good, L. (2005). Fear of re-injury: A hindrance for returning to sports after anterior cruciate ligament reconstruction. *Knee Surgery, Sports Traumatology, Arthroscopy, 13,* 393-397.

Lazarus, R. S., & Folkman, S. (1984). *Stress, appraisal, and coping.* New York: Springer.

Mainwaring, L. M. (1999). Restoration of self: A model for the psychological response of athletes to sever knee injuries. *Canadian Journal of Rehabilitation, 3,* 145-156.

Magee, D. J. (2002). *Orthopedic physical assessment* (4th ed.). Philadelphia: Elsevier Sciences.

Marlatt, G. A., & Gordon, J. R. (1985). *Relapse prevention: Maintenance strategies in addictive behavior change.* New York: Guilford.

Morrey, M. A., Stuart, M. J., Smith, A. M., & Wiese-Bjornstal, D. M. (1999). A longitudinal examination of athletes' emotional and cognitive response to anterior cruciate ligament injury. *Clinical Journal of Sports Medicine, 9,* 63-69.

Podlog, L., & Eklund, R. C. (2006). A longitudinal investigation of competitive athletes' return to sport following serious injury. *Journal of Applied Sport Psychology, 18,* 44-68.

Poehling, G. G., Walton, W. C., Lee, C. A., Ginn, T. A., Rushing, J. T., Naughton, M. J., et al. (2005). Analysis of outcomes of anterior cruciate ligament repair with a 5-year follow-up: Allograft versus autograft. *The Journal of Arthroscopic and Related Surgery, 21,* 774-785.

Rock, J. A., & Jones, M. V. (2002). A preliminary investigation into the use of counseling skills in support of rehabilitation from sport injury. *Journal of Sport Rehabilitation, 11,* 284-304.

Roi, G. S., Creta, D., Nanni, G., Marcacci, M., Zaffagnini, S., & Snyder-Mackler, L. (2005). Return to official Italian first division soccer games within 90 days after anterior cruciate ligament reconstruction: A case report. *Journal of Orthopaedic & Sports Physical Therapy, 35,* 52-66.

Rose, J., & Jevne, R. F. J. (1993). Psychosocial processes associated with athletic injuries. *The Sport Psychologist, 7,* 309-328.

Scherzer C. B, Brewer, B. W., Cornelius, A. E., Van Raalte, J. L., Petitpas, A. J., Sklar, J. H., et al. (2001). Psychological skills and adherence to rehabilitation after reconstruction of the anterior cruciate ligament. *Journal of Sport Rehabilitation, 10,* 165-172.

Sport description. (n.d.). Retrieved February 27, 2006, from http://www.airbergy.com/Sport%20Description.asp What is freestyle? (n.d.). Retrieved February 27, 2006, from http://www.freestyleski.com/eng/freestyle/index.htm

Wiese-Bjornstal, D. M. (2005). From skinned knees and pee wees to menisci and masters: Developmental sport injury psychology. In M. Weiss (Ed.), *Developmental sport and exercise psychology: A lifespan perspective* (pp. 525-561). Morgantown, WV: Fitness Information Technology.

Wiese-Bjornstal, D. M., Smith, A. M., Shaffer, S. M., & Morrey, M. A. (1998). An integrated model of response to sport injury: Psychological and sociological dynamics. *Journal of Applied Sport Psychology, 10,* 46-69.

Zuckerman, M. (1983). Sensation seeking and sports. *Personality and Individual Differences, 4,* 285-293. *Inside freestyle skiing.* (n.d.). Retrieved February 27, 2006 from http://www.nbcolympics.com/freestyle/inside.html?qs=;ch=0

Chapter Notes

We thank Alisa Camplin for taking the time to answer questions about her two ACL injuries and for granting permission to utilize her case in this chapter. For those who would like to learn more about aerial skiing and Alisa Camplin's experiences as a two-time Olympic medalist, her book *High Flyer* is available on the web from Dymocks Booksellers (www.dymocks.com.au/), or Angus & Robertson (www.angusrobertson.com.au/).

[1] See the following sources for additional historical and technical information on freestyle skiing: http://www.nbcolympics.com/freestyle/inside.html?qs=;ch=0; http://www.airbergy.com; http://www.freestyleski.com/eng/freestyle/index.htm.

[2] Prior to the 2004-05 season, the athlete had been competing with two variations of a triple-twisting double somersault (i.e., three twists on two flips).

About the Authors

Mark B. Andersen is a registered psychologist in Australia and the United States. He is an associate professor at Victoria University in Melbourne, Australia, in the School of Human Movement, Recreation, and Performance. He serves on the Board of the Centre for Ageing, Rehabilitation, Exercise, and Sport and coordinates the master's and doctor of applied psychology degrees (sport and exercise psychology emphasis) in the School of Psychology. He received his doctorate from the University of Arizona in 1988 and emigrated to Australia in 1994. He is a recipient of the Dorothy Harris Memorial Award from the Association for the Advancement of Applied Sport Psychology for excellence as a young scholar/practitioner. He is the former editor of the Professional Practice section of the international journal *The Sport Psychologist* and has published widely in refereed journal articles. His three edited books, *Doing Sport Psychology, Sport Psychology in Practice,* and *Psychology in the Physical and Manual Therapies,* are used around the world.

R. Renee Newcomer Appaneal is an assistant professor at the University of North Carolina at Greensboro. She completed a B.A. at the University of Kansas and an M.A. at the University of North Carolina at Chapel Hill. Dr. Appaneal completed both an Ed.D. in sport and exercise psychology and a second M.A. in counseling at West Virginia University. She was a postdoctoral research associate at Boston University and a psychology fellow at Spaulding Rehabilitation in Boston, Massachusetts. Dr. Appaneal is a Certified Consultant (CC, AAASP) and a Licensed Professional Counselor (LPC) in North Carolina. At UNCG, she teaches a graduate course in psychological aspects of sport injury and rehabilitation.

Theresa M. Bianco is an assistant professor in the Department of Psychology at Concordia University in Montreal, where she teaches undergraduate courses in sport psychology and health psychology. Theresa received her Ph.D. in sport psychology from the University of Western Australia, her M.A. in sport psychology from the University of Ottawa, and her B.A. in psychology from Concordia University. Her research focuses on the role of social support in recovery from sport injury, with a particular emphasis on coach support. In addition to her teaching and research endeavors, Theresa also runs a private consulting practice and provides sport psychology services to national team athletes through the National Multisport Training Centre in Montreal.

Kimberlee Bethany Bonura is a doctoral candidate in sport and exercise psychology at Florida State University and an instructor in the Department of Physical Education at the United States Military Academy, West Point. She earned her M.S. in sport and exercise psychology from Florida State University. Her thesis research investigated the impact of different exercise modalities on stress, anxiety, and depression responses in older adults, and her dissertation research investigates the impact of yoga on psychological health. Kimberlee is a triple-certified yoga instructor (Ashtanga, Power, and Hatha), registered with Yoga Alliance. Additionally, she is certified as a Tai Chi/Qi Gong instructor, personal trainer, group fitness instructor, kickboxing instructor, senior citizen fitness specialist, and Reiki master. She has been teaching yoga, wellness, and fitness classes for over a decade and has practiced yoga for more than 17 years. She has produced several yoga practice DVDs and CDs and has written about yoga for national and international publications.

Britton W. Brewer, Ph.D., is professor of psychology at Springfield College. He is a Certified Consultant, Association for the Advancement of Applied Sport Psychology, and is listed in the United States Olympic Committee Sport Psychology Registry, 2004–2008. He has received a series of grants from the National Institute of Arthritis and Musculoskeletal and Skin Diseases in support of his research on psychological aspects of sport injury.

Scott L. Cresswell holds a research position in the School of Human Movement and Exercise Science at the University of Western Australia. He is an accredited consultant with Sport Science New Zealand and a contracted sport psychology provider to the New Zealand Academy of Sport. Dr.Cresswell's recent research has focused on player burnout in professional rugby union. The primary aims of this program of research include developing and assessing practical strategies to help prevent and manage player burnout.

Kyle T. Ebersole is an assistant professor and director of the Graduate Athletic Training Program in the Department of Kinesiology and Community Health at the University of Illinois. He received his Ph.D. in exercise physiology from the University of Nebraska and is a Licensed Athletic Trainer and Certified Athletic Trainer. Dr. Ebersole's research has focused on the simultaneous recording of electromyography (EMG) and mechanomyography (MMG) to non-invasively examine the electrical and mechanical components, respectively, of force production during various types of muscle actions. Recent projects have integrated EMG and MMG into examining various parameters of muscle function that may serve as underlying mechanisms and/or risk factors for the etiology and progression of acute and chronic injuries of the lower extremities, as well as markers for improvement in muscle strength in response to rehabilitation protocols.

Robert C. (Bob) Eklund, is a professor in the Department of Educational Psychology and Learning Systems at Florida State University in Tallahassee. Professor Eklund received his Ph.D. in exercise and sport science from the University of North Carolina at Greensboro in 1991. His interest in sport psychology stems from his experiences as a freestyle wrestler while participating in collegiate and international competition, and as a coach of athletes participating in youth sport, intercollegiate competition, and major international sporting events. He has authored or co-authored numerous sport and exercise psychology refereed research publications, book chapters, and professional/applied practice articles and has presented papers at a range of regional, national, and international conferences. His reports have addressed issues on psychological experience associated with sport performance, as well as self-presentational and self-relevant cognition associated with exercise participation. He is the coeditor, with

Professor Gershon Tenenbaum, of the third edition of the prestigious *Handbook of Sport Psychology*. He has secured extramural funding to support his sport and exercise psychology research as well as corporate funding to support multidisciplinary research on heat stress, dehydration, and fatigue among underground and surface miners in remote locations in Western Australia. Finally, Bob has been professionally active in providing peer review service to over a dozen research journals. Bob is the current editor of the *Journal of Sport and Exercise Psychology* and has served as an associate editor for the *Journal of Applied Sport Psychology* and a section editor for the *Research Quarterly for Exercise and Sport.*

Edward F. Etzel is licensed psychologist for the West Virginia University Department of Intercollegiate Athletics. He is also an associate professor in sport and exercise psychology at WVU. He teaches graduate courses in counseling athletes, ethics and professional issues, performance enhancement, and an undergraduate course in the psychology of injury. Ed is a 1984 Olympic Gold Medalist in shooting.

A.P. "Budd" Ferrante, Ed.D., ABPP, is a psychologist in private practice in Hilliard, Ohio. Before entering the private sector, he served as psychologist for Athletics and Sport Psychology Services at The Ohio State University. A Diplomate in counseling psychology with the American Board of Professional Psychology, Dr. Ferrante served as sport psychologist with the 1988 U.S. Olympic Team in Seoul, Korea.

Frances A. Flint, Ph.D., as been a faculty member in the School of Kinesiology and Health Science at York University since 1977. She attended the University of Oregon for her M.S. (1973) and Ph.D. (1991) degrees in sport psychology and sports medicine. Her research was an integration of both areas and focused on the psychology of the injured athlete. She is a Certified Athletic Therapist (CATA) and a Certified Athletic Trainer (NATABOC). Frances was the head coach of the varsity women's basketball team at York University for 9 years and was involved with the Canadian Women's National Basketball team from 1983 to 1988. Her background with international sport includes work with the Canadian Olympic Association at three Pan American Games and at the Barcelona Summer Olympics as well as various World Student Games and World Championships. Currently, Frances is the Coordinator of the Athletic Therapy Certificate Program at York University. The focus of her research and teaching is in psychology of injury and sports medicine, and she presents nationally and internationally in these areas.

Megan D. Granquist is a Certified Athletic Trainer and doctoral student in the Sport and Exercise Psychology Program at the University of North Carolina at Greensboro. Her research is focused on the psychology of sport injury. Ms. Granquist received her master's degree in exercise and movement science with an emphasis in sports medicine from the University of Oregon. Her undergraduate degree is from Pacific Lutheran University.

Lance B. Green, Ed.D., is an associate clinical professor in the Department of Exercise and Sport Sciences at Tulane University in New Orleans, Louisiana. He has been consulting in the area of educational sport psychology since 1980 when he earned his doctorate's degree from the University of Northern Colorado. His area of teaching specialization includes courses in the psychology, philosophy, sociology, and history of sport as well as in stress management. His consulting work spans all age levels of sport participation. He has also had experience as a baseball coach at the collegiate level, as well as with the first-ever U.S.A. Women's National Baseball team.

J. Robert Grove is a professor within the School of Human Movement and Exercise Science at the University of Western Australia. He was section editor of the Sport Psychologist's Digest for the *Journal of Sport and Exercise Psychology* for 11 years, and he is currently a member of the editorial board for the *International Journal of Sport and Exercise Psychology* as well as the *Australian Psychologist*. Bob's general area of research interest is the social psychology of exercise, health, and sport. Specific areas of current interest include personality factors, coping processes, training distress, and physical self-concept. He received his Ph.D. in movement science education from Florida State University.

Jane C. Henderson teaches in the Department of Physical Education at John Abbott College in the province of Quebec, Canada. She received her Ph.D. in sport psychology from Florida State University. She is an Association for the Advancement of Applied Sport Psychology (AAASP) Certified Consultant. Her current research interests include physiological manifestations of psychological stress, as well as depression and suicide in athletes. She is a consultant to numerous athletes seeking peak performance. Her passion involves competing in distance and marathon running

Keith P. Henschen is a professor in the Department of Exercise and Sport Science at the University of Utah with an area of expertise in the psychosocial aspects of sports. Dr. Henschen received his P.E.D. from Indiana University in 1971 and has been a member of the University of Utah Faculty for the past 35 years. Dr. Henschen's research interests include the psychology of performance, use of psychological interventions in sports, and sport psychology for special populations. Dr. Henschen served as president (1997–98) of the American Alliance of Health, Physical Education, Recreation and Dance (AAHPERD). He also served as president of the International Society of Sport Psychology (ISSP) from 2001–2005.

Urban Johnson, Ph.D., is an associate professor in applied psychology at the Centre for Sport and Health Research, Halmstad University, Sweden. He is a certified elite trainer (team handball) and has been a sport psychology consultant for team and individual athletes since 1985. Dr. Johnson is currently a member of FEPSAC managing council.

Ralph Maddison is a research fellow at the Clinical Trials Research Unit, School of Population Health, University of Auckland, New Zealand. He received his M.Sc. and Ph.D. at the University of Auckland. His Ph.D. thesis focused on the role that psychological factors play in the prediction, prevention, and rehabilitation of athletic injury. His research work continues in injury rehabilitation and prevention; however, his other research focuses on physical activity promotion in clinical and non-clinical populations. He is a member of the New Zealand Sport Psychology Association and works with elite athletes through the New Zealand Academy of Sport. He is also a digest contributor to the *Journal of Sport and Exercise Psychology*.

Lou M. Makarowski is a licensed psychologist, author, and hypnotherapist who has been in full-time private practice since 1976 in Pensacola, Florida. He frequently consults on stress-related issues with elite and professional athletes, families, physicians, and other healthcare professionals. Recognized on three occasions by the American Academy of Family Physicians, he pioneered medical trauma psychology. The Makarowski Assessment of Personal Stress was used in the largest study of paramedics stress. Dr. Makarowski received his Ph.D. specializing in pediatric, school, and clinical psychology from the University of Iowa. He has been a member of the United States Olympic Committee Sport Psychology Registry, AAASP, and the Council for the National Register of Health Service Providers in Psychology. He is a Registered Traumatologist and certified by the America Society of Clinical Hypnosis. He has written approximately 400 sport psychology columns for the popular media and his book, *How to Keep Your COOL with Your Kids* (Perigee, 1996), is in print in China, Taiwan, and Mexico.

Barbara B. Meyer is an associate professor in the Department of Human Movement Sciences at the University of Wisconsin-Milwaukee. She received her Ph.D. in health education, counseling psychology, and human performance (sport psychology emphasis, counseling cognate) from Michigan State University. Dr. Meyer's interest in applied sport psychology is informed by social psychology theory, intelligence theory, and cognitive behavioral therapy. Current research is focused on (a) the assessment of emotional intelligence in athletic populations, (b) the description of emotional intelligence in athletes and coaches, and (c) the relationship between emotional intelligence, sport participation, sport performance, and satisfaction with the sport experience. Dr. Meyer's research and knowledge of theory serve as a foundation for her ongoing work as a performance enhancement consultant to world-class athletes, performing artists, and corporate groups.

Tony Morris is professor of sport, exercise, and health psychology in the School of Human Movement, Recreation, and Performance at Victoria University, where he has also been closely involved with the University Research Centre for Ageing, Rehabilitation, Exercise and Sport (CARES) for 14 years, since he led its establishment. He also conducts research in the new Victoria University Institute for Health and Diversity. Tony has been involved in more than 200 research projects on aspects of physical activity and well-being, covering areas including stress and anxiety, motivation, imagery, confidence, flow, transitions, and injury. He has published 8 books and more than 150 refereed papers in journals and international conference proceedings. He has presented more than 200 papers at international conferences. Tony was a member of the Managing Council of the International Society of Sport Psychology (ISSP) for eight years and is president of the Asian South Pacific Association of Sport Psychology (ASPASP), a position he has held for the last nine years.

Young-Eun Noh teaches in the Department of Physical Education at Chonnam National University in Kwangju, South Korea. She received her bachelor's degree from the Department of Dance in the Chosun University and completed a master's of sport psychology in the Department of Physical Education at the Chonnam National University. She received her Ph.D. in sport and exercise psychology from the School of Human Movement, Recreation, and Performance at Victoria University in Melbourne, Australia. She has published and presented internationally in the areas of sport and dance psychology, principally on the relationship between psychosocial factors and dance injury and intervention for the prevention of injury.

Frank M. Perna, Ed.D., Ph.D., is a licensed psychologist specializing in clinical health and sport psychology. He is jointly appointed in the Section of General Internal Medicine and in the Division of Psychiatry at Boston University School of Medicine (BUSM), and he is a core faculty member in the Mental Health and Behavioral Medicine Graduate Training Program at BUSM. Dr. Perna completed his doctoral work in counseling psychology and in health psychology at Boston University and the University of Pittsburgh, respectively, and post-doctoral training in clinical sport psychology at the U.S. Olympic Training Center and a NIMH post-doctoral fellowship in behavioral medicine at the University of Miami. Dr. Perna has authored numerous professional papers, has served on a number of editorial and professional association boards, and was the recipient of an early-career contribution award from the Association for the Advancement of Applied Sport Psychology.

Albert J. Petitpas, Ed.D., is professor of psychology at Springfield College, where he directs the National Football Foundation Center for Youth Development through Sport. He is a licensed psychologist in Massachusetts and a Certified Consultant, Association for the Advancement of Applied Sport Psychology. He has provided consulting services to a wide range of sport organizations including The First Tee, the NCAA, the NBA, the NFL, and the United States Olympic Committee.

Trent A. Petrie is a professor in the Department of Psychology and Director of the Center for Sport Psychology and Performance Excellence (CSPPE) at the University of North Texas. He received his Ph.D. from The Ohio State University in 1991. He is a licensed psychologist in Texas, a Certified Consultant, AAASP, and a member of the 2004–2008 USOC Sport Psychology Registry. Through the CSPPE, he consults with athletes and sport teams from all competitive levels. He also is on the Editorial Board of *Journal of Sport and Exercise Psychology* and serves as a reviewer for numerous journals. In 2000, he was named a fellow in the Association for the Advancement of Applied Sport Psychology. His current research interests include eating disorders, sport psychology, academic adjustment and performance, and athletic injury. He is the proud father of two wonderful children who are now entering the world of select sports and putting to the test all that he has learned about working successfully in the youth sport environment.

Les Podlog is currently a lecturer in the School of Human Movement Studies at Charles Sturt University, where he teaches classes in sport and exercise psychology and the socio-cultural foundations of human movement. He recently received his Ph.D. in sport and exercise psychology from the University of Western Australia and completed a master's degree in sociology at Simon Fraser University. His research interests focus on the return to sport transition following injury recovery, and he has co-authored several research publications on the topic. His interest in this area stemmed from his unfortunate injury experiences as a varsity freestyle wrestler while at Simon Fraser University.

Harry Prapavessis is associate professor in the School of Kinesiology, Faculty of Health Sciences, The University of Western Ontario, London, Ontario, Canada. He received his Ph.D. from the University of Western Australia. Dr Prapavessis works in the area of exercise and health psychology. His research program has three main foci.

First he investigates determinants of physical activity and interventions grounded in self-regulation theory in changing physical activity in diseased and non-diseased populations. Second, he studies exercise as a therapy to improve health. Specifically, he studies the role exercise plays in smoking cessation. Third and finally, he examines the role that psychological factors play in the prediction, prevention, and recovery of injury.

Michael L. Sachs is a professor in the Department of Kinesiology, College of Health Professions, specializing in exercise and sport psychology. He has been at Temple University since 1989. He received his Ph.D. in sport psychology from Florida State University in 1980 and was an assistant professor at the University of Quebec at Trois-Rivieres from 1980 to 1983. From 1983 to 1989 he served as research project coordinator in the Applied Research and Evaluation Unit in the Department of Pediatrics, University of Maryland School of Medicine. He has an extensive list of publications and presentations, including authorship as associate editor of *Psychology of Running* (Michael Sacks & Michael Sachs, Human Kinetics Publishers, 1981) and co-editor of *Running as Therapy: An Integrated Approach* (Michael Sachs & Gary Buffone, University of Nebraska Press, 1984). He is a licensed psychologist in Maryland, as well as a Certified Consultant, Association for the Advancement of Applied Sport Psychology. Dr. Sachs served as the president of the Association for the Advancement of Applied Sport Psychology (1991–92).

Gerry Schwille is the director of athletics and assistant athletic trainer at Northern York High School. He is the former head athletic trainer at Temple University. He was the founder and director of the Valley Hospital Sports Institute, Ridgewood, New Jersey, and head athletic trainer for the New Jersey Generals of the United States Football League. He received his master's degree in physical education/sports medicine from Oklahoma State University and is pursuing a doctoral degree from Temple University. He is a member of the American College of Sports Medicine, a Certified Athletic Trainer of the National Athletic Trainers Association and a Licensed Athletic Trainer in Pennsylvania and New Jersey. He is a Certified Master Athletic Administrator from the National Interscholastic Athletic Administrators Association and a member of the Pennsylvania State Athletic Directors Association Executive Council.

Gregory A. Shelley, Ph.D., is a professor and performance consultant at Ithaca College, New York. He has conducted hundreds of regional, national, and international presentations and workshops for performers across all levels of sport, academia, and business. Dr. Shelley has spent the last 13 years educating and training individuals and groups in the areas of leadership, motivation, group development, communication, stress management, conflict resolution, and peak performance. He has worked with youth, high school, collegiate, and professional level performers and is currently the applied sport psychology and performance consultant for several collegiate athletic departments and professional organizations. In addition, Greg is co-author of a performance psychology book, *Moving Toward Your Potential: The Athlete's Guide to Peak Performance,* and has authored or co-authored several book chapters, articles, and educational brochures detailing numerous performance enhancement strategies for teams, coaches, leaders, and managers.

Michael R. Sitler is a professor in the Department of Kinesiology, Temple University, specializing in athletic training/sports medicine. He received his Ed.D. in sports medicine from New York University. Prior to his arrival at Temple University, he was an assistant professor at the United States Military Academy, West Point, New York, for six years. He is a certified member of the National Athletic Trainers' Association (NATA) and is currently the chairperson of the Department of Kinesiology at Temple University. His research interests are primarily in evidence-based practice in athletic training and sports medicine, with particular focus on interventions to reduce injuries and on post-surgical outcomes. He currently serves as president of the NATA Research and Education Foundation.

Wendy F. Sternberg is an associate professor of psychology (and current chair of the Psychology Department) at Haverford College, in Haverford, Pennsylvania. She received her Ph.D. in behavioral neuroscience at UCLA in 1994, and has been on the Haverford faculty since 1995. Her research centers around understanding inter-individual variability in the experience of pain.

Judy L. Van Raalte, Ph.D. is professor of psychology and director of the Athletic Counseling master's program at Springfield College, where she served as coach of the women's tennis team for five years. She is co-editor of the text, "Exploring Sport and Exercise Psychology," and is executive producer of 13 sport psychology videos. She is listed in the United States Olympic Committee Sport Psychology Registry, 2004–2008, is a Certified Consultant, Association for the Advancement of Applied Sport Psychology, and is a past-president of Division 47 (Exercise and Sport Psychology) of the American Psychological Association.

Sam Zizzi, Ed.D., is associate professor in sport and exercise psychology at West Virginia University, where he teaches graduate and undergraduate courses in the psychology of injury, exercise psychology, sport psychology, and statistics and is program coordinator for the Sport and Exercise Psychology Program. His primary research interests include lifetime physical activity and applied sport psychology. He serves as a statistical consultant to several graduate programs at WVU, including athletic training and counseling psychology. His areas of expertise in research include survey development, univariate statistics, and psychometric testing. Dr. Zizzi supervises graduate students in their sport psychology work, works with WVU athletes on performance enhancement, and is a Certified Consultant (AAASP) and member of the U.S. Olympic Committee's Sport Psychology Registry.

Index